Atlas of Neuroradiology

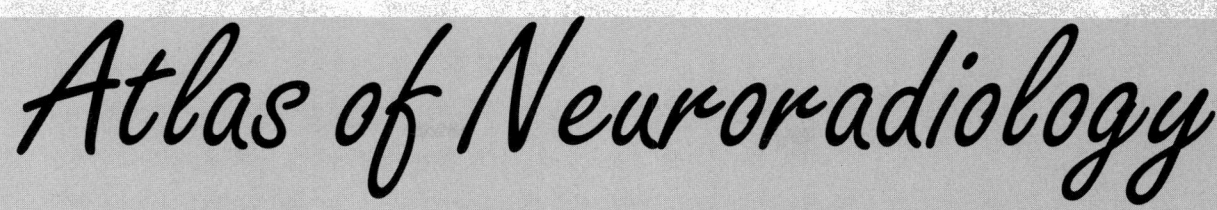

Atlas of Neuroradiology

Matthew J. Kuhn, M.D.

Chief, Division of Neuroradiology

Associate Professor of Radiology, Neurology and Neurosurgery

Southern Illinois University School of Medicine

Springfield, Illinois

Foreword by

Juan M. Taveras, M.D.

Professor of Radiology, Emeritus

Harvard Medical School

Radiologist, formerly Radiologist-in-Chief

Massachusetts General Hospital

Boston, Massachusetts

Gower Medical Publishing   New York   London

Distributed in the USA and Canada by:
Raven Press
1185 Avenue of the Americas
New York, NY 10036
USA

Distributed in Japan by:
Nankodo Company Ltd.
42-6, Hongo 3-Chome
Bunkyo-Ku
Tokyo 113
Japan

Distributed in the rest of the world by:
Gower Medical Publishing
Middlesex House
34-42 Cleveland Street
London W1P 5FB
UK

Library of Congress Cataloging-in-Publication Data
Kuhn, Matthew J.
    Atlas of neuroradiology / Matthew J. Kuhn.
      p.   cm.
    Includes bibliographical references and index.
    ISBN 1-56375-008-2
    1. Central nervous system—Radiography—Atlases.   I. Title.
    [DNLM: 1. Central Nervous System Diseases—radiography—atlases.
    2. Central Nervous System Neoplasms—radiography—atlases.
    3. Neuroradiography—atlases.   WL 17 K96a]
    RC349.R3K84   1992
    616.8'047'570222—dc20
    DNLM/DLC
    for Library of Congress   92-1421
                          CIP

British Library Cataloging-in-Publication Data
A catalogue record for this book is available from the British Library.

Editor: **Tim Condon**

Designer: **Surachara Wirojratana**

Illustrator: **Patricia Gast**

Illustration Supervisor: **Laura Pardi Duprey**

Typesetting Supervisor: **Erick Rizzotto**

Printed in Singapore by Imago Productions (FE) Pte Ltd.

10 9 8 7 6 5 4 3 2

Dedication

To my dearly loved wife, Alyssa, and our precious children, Alexis and Andrew

Foreword

It is with pride that I respond to the request of Matt Kuhn to write a foreword to this book. Following completion of his training at Massachusetts General Hospital, Matt went to Southern Illinois University to help establish a neuroradiology service in that medical center. He has accomplished this in a highly successful way. In addition, within a very short period of time, he has obviously been able to collect enough didactic material to produce a book of the quality of this *Atlas of Neuroradiology*.

As I look at the page proofs, I am rather impressed by the quality of the illustrations and the variety of the material. Practically every aspect of the subspecialty of neuroradiology is covered in this comprehensive atlas. In addition to original images of computed tomography and magnetic resonance, cerebral angiography, and myelography, this atlas contains outstanding line drawings of the pertinent anatomy and pathology, which the author has used where he felt they would be helpful, particularly for beginners in the field.

The material is so clearly presented and the illustrations are of such good quality that it will make for easy reading and reviewing for residents preparing for their boards, medical students interested in gaining more in-depth knowledge in this area, as well as general radiologists and our neurological colleagues exposed to neuroradiological imaging problems. I feel that practitioners at all levels of expertise will find this work extremely valuable.

The publishers have done a superb job in putting this together in a very pleasing manner.

Juan M. Taveras, M.D.

Preface

The objective of this atlas is to display the vast majority of the neuropathological disorders which can be imaged using contemporary techniques. These are primarily two-dimensional cross-sectional representations of the brain and spine. MRI has become the premier imaging modality for evaluation of the central nervous system; CT maintains a solid position in aiding with the evaluation of subarachnoid hemorrhage, calcified lesions, and bony abnormalities. Cerebral angiography remains the gold standard for evaluation of aneurysms, vascular malformations, and carotid disease. Even myelography is still useful in the evaluation of certain spinal disorders.

Virtually the entire spectrum of disorders studied by neuroradiologists are illustrated on the following pages. Detailed line drawings of many of the images have been created for clarification purposes. The accompanying text provides background information including key identifying features and specific findings which may help to distinguish one lesion from another.

Acknowledgments

Many individuals affiliated with the Southern Illinois University School of Medicine helped me with this text and I remain very grateful. In particular, Drs. Timothy Swan, Cynthia Hart, Stewart Couch, Bruce Hedgepeth, Scott Long, Michael Baker, and Linda Swenson, assisted with review of the galley proofs. Drs. David Binstadt and David Morris supplied several of the radiographs. John W. O'Shaughnessy helped to organize the MR images. Scott Kilbourne, RBP, provided superb photographic reproductions of the scans and radiographs. Millard Adams and Alan Bea produced the magnificent angiograms.

My family was willing to sacrifice my presence on innumerable occasions in order to give me time to create this book. Thank you. Special thanks and thoughts go to Kay Mack, whose personal battle with spinal disease has long been an inspiration.

I also thank Abe Krieger, president of Gower Medical Publishing, for originating the idea and seeing the need for this text. I am grateful to him for having chosen me to help see his plans come to fruition. Abe encouraged me to use some of the illustrations and text from E. George Kassner's *Atlas of Radiologic Imaging* chapter on the brain by George Lantos. Patricia Gast is responsible for the beautiful line drawings associated with the black and white images. Surachara Wirojratana has made the book visually exciting and unique; she has done a first-class job. Finally, I am most indebted of all to Tim Condon, the project manager/editor at Gower, who truly was my partner in preparing this text. He shared with me the enthusiasm, excitement, and pride in this project.

Contents

Part One BRAIN

Part Two SPINE

part one

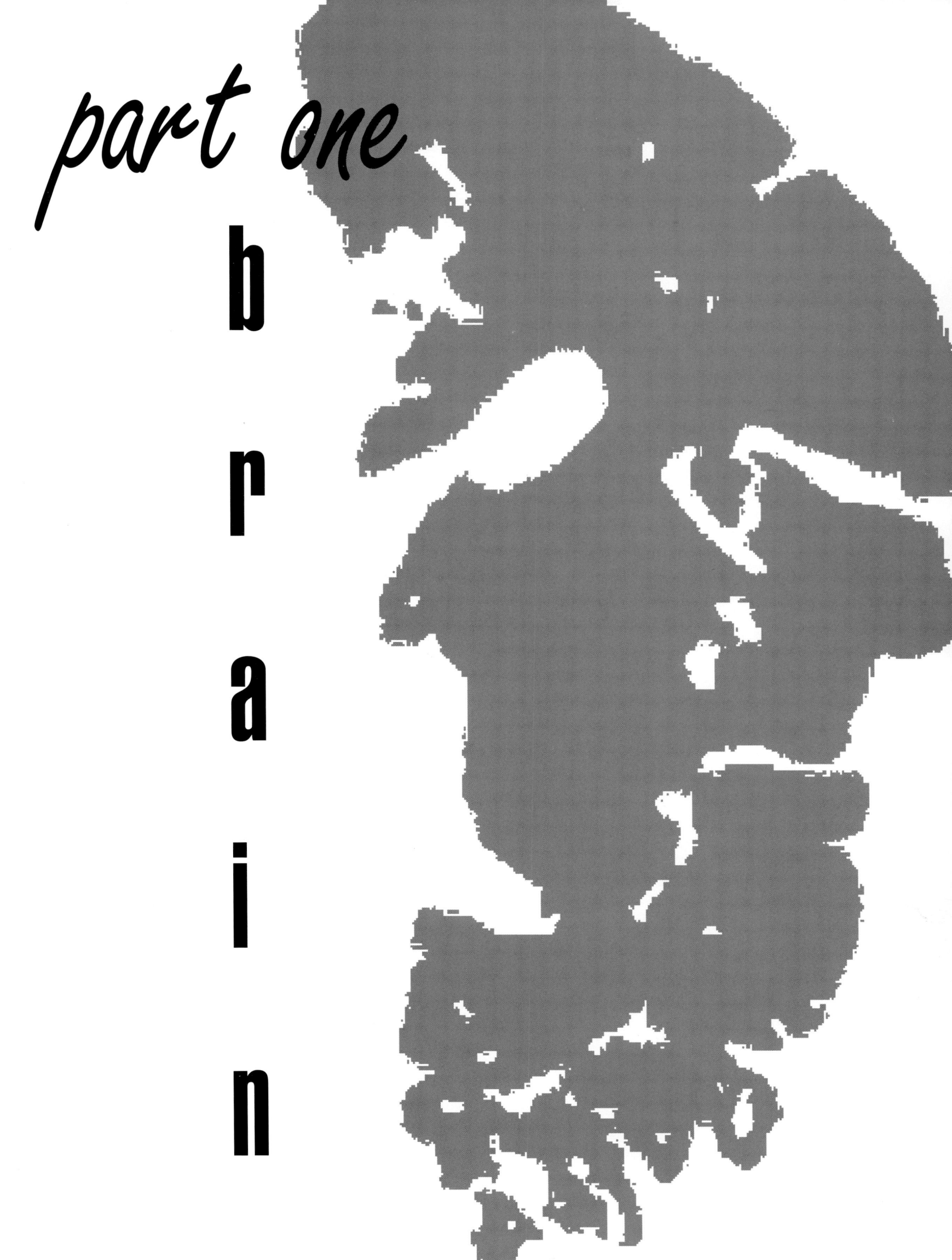

**b
r
a
i
n**

Neuroradiology today bears little resemblance to the primitive pneumoencephalographic images of just twenty years ago. Truly remarkable advances since the inception of cranial computed tomography have irrevocably changed neurological and neurosurgical practice, much akin to the revolution in the treatment of infectious diseases which followed the introduction of antibiotics. The ability to directly visualize the brain is a technological marvel which has served mankind in a dramatic and unprecedented fashion. Little wonder why neuroradiology is so exciting!

Regardless of the particular imaging technique employed, we must resist the temptation to interpret an "MR image" or a "CT scan." These two-dimensional representations of complex three-dimensional anatomy are merely our tools. Our focus should be on the **brain**, not the **scan**. Anatomy and pathophysiology will remain constant long after individual imaging techniques become obsolete.

The brain remains an elusive organ. It cannot be casually explored or reached by endoscope to confirm our diagnostic impressions. Neurophysiologists still only have a rudimentary understanding as to how it really works. The brain holds our thoughts, controls what we say and feel, and what we do. Perhaps in the decades to come we will be able to image and understand its emotions, aesthetics, logic, and its capability to process and retain information. Future authors will then be able to present more than these mere, presumptuous images of structural and signal abnormalities.

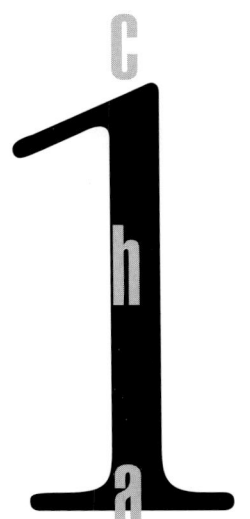

Chapter

1

Congenital Malformations
of the Brain

Congenital anomalies of the brain and its coverings result from abnormal intrauterine development of the nervous system. In some instances craniocerebral anomalies are due to a combination of genetic and intrauterine environmental factors; however, in the majority of cases, no single causative factor can be implicated. Some congenital disorders of the brain are part of the spectrum of anomalies associated with multisystem disorders and syndromes. These may be idiopathic, metabolic, or infectious in nature. Most major congenital malformations result from defective formation of the neural tube during the third and fourth weeks following conception. Others are related to events later in gestation. While some malformations are clearly related to a specific defect in organogenesis, the pathogenesis of many others is poorly understood.

A modification of the De Meyer classification of congenital brain malformations is shown in Fig. 1.1.

DISORDERS OF ORGANOGENESIS

Disorders of Closure

Meningoceles and encephaloceles result from a congenital defect of the skull that allows intracranial contents to herniate: meninges and cerebrospinal fluid (CSF) in the case of a meningocele; brain tissue in the case of an encephalocele. A meningoencephalocele is a more complex malformation, consisting of brain, meninges, and CSF.

Occipital defects are most common in the Western Hemisphere, whereas meningoencephaloceles related to the floor of the anterior cranial fossa predominate in the Orient (Fig. 1.2). The clinical

---

Congenital Malformations of the Brain

I. Disorders of Organogenesis

A. Disorders of closure
1. Cranioschisis
   - Meningocele
   - Encephalocele
2. Agenesis of the corpus callosum
3. Lipoma of the corpus callosum
4. Chiari malformation
5. Dandy–Walker malformation
6. Arachnoid cyst

B. Disorders of diverticulation
1. Holoprosencephaly
2. Septo-optic dysplasia

C. Disorders of sulcation and migration
1. Lissencephaly and pachygyria
2. Polymicrogyria
3. Grey matter heterotopia
4. Schizencephaly

D. Destructive lesions
1. Hydranencephaly
2. Porencephaly
3. Hypoxia
4. Toxicoses
5. Inflammatory disease
   - Rubella
   - Cytomegalovirus
   - Toxoplasmosis
   - Herpes simplex

II. Disorders of Histogenesis

A. Tuberous sclerosis
B. Neurofibromatosis
C. Sturge–Weber syndrome (encephalotrigeminal angiomatosis)
D. Neoplasia
E. Vascular lesions

III. Miscellaneous Congenital Disorders

A. Basal cell nevus syndrome
B. Achondroplasia
C. Hurler's syndrome
D. Craniosynostosis
E. Pseudohypoparathyroidism

Figure 1.1
Congenital malformations of the brain.

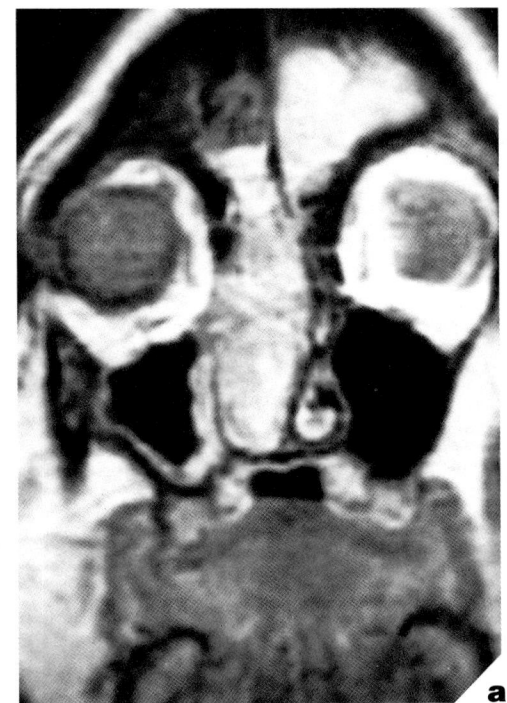

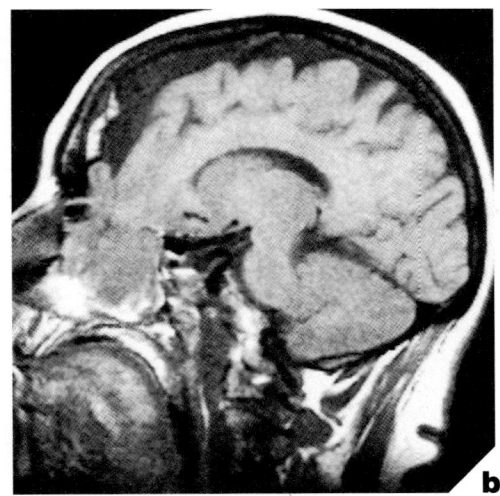

Figure 1.2

*Naso-ethmoidal encephalocele. **a** Coronal and **b** sagittal T1-weighted MR images show brain tissue of the right frontal lobe herniating through the floor of the anterior cranial fossa into the nasal cavity and ethmoid sinuses. **c** Axial proton density image might be misinterpreted as demonstrating a nasal polyp or cyst rather than an encephalocele. **d** Note the partially "empty" right side of the anterior cranial fossa on the T2-weighted axial MR images.*

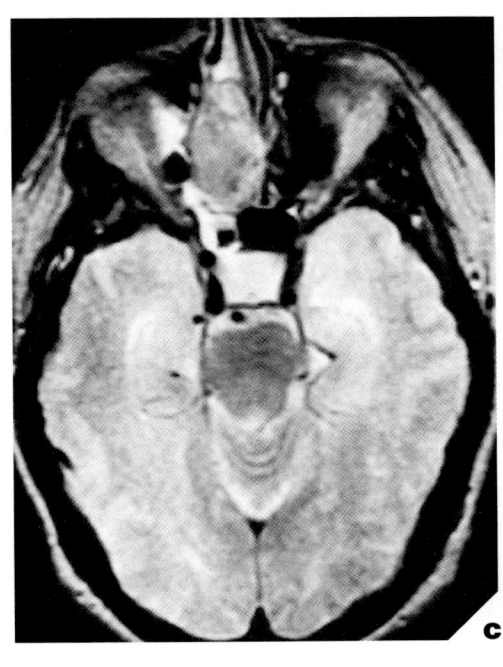

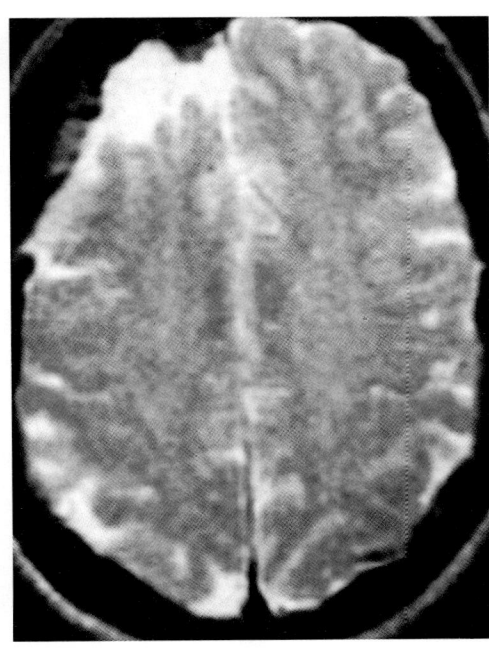

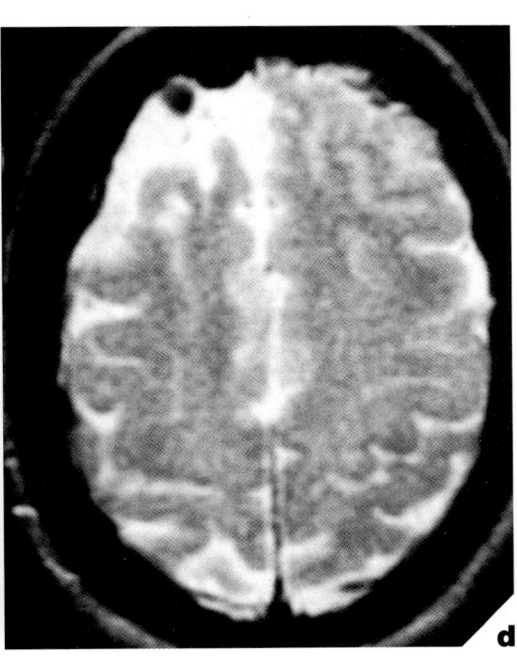

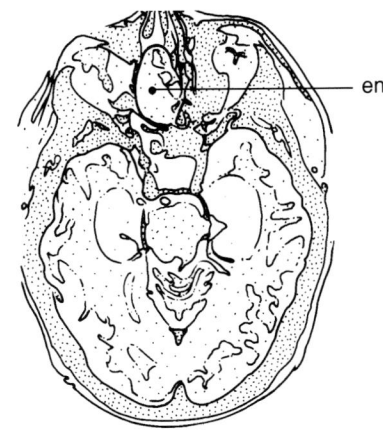

encephalocele

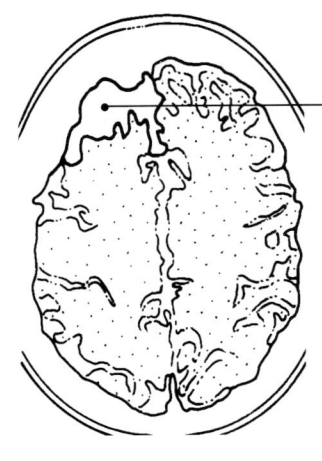

CSF-filled space resulting from herniation of anterior right frontal lobe inferiorly

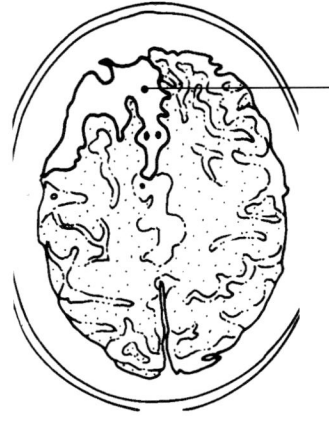

CSF-filled space resulting from herniation of anterior right frontal lobe inferiorly

1.3

spectrum ranges from a small, asymptomatic lump to a large, exophytic mass of dysplastic brain tissue. Leakage of CSF, which can lead to meningitis, is a potential complication (Fig. 1.3). This may be evaluated with positive contrast CT administered via a lumbar puncture in an attempt to identify the leakage site for surgical planning.

Absence of the brain (anencephaly) is usually diagnosed by ultrasound in utero by its characteristic head shape. Polyhydramnios and increased fetal limb motion are often seen.

Agenesis of the corpus callosum may be complete or partial (dysgenesis). It may be isolated or associated with other anomalies such as the Dandy–Walker

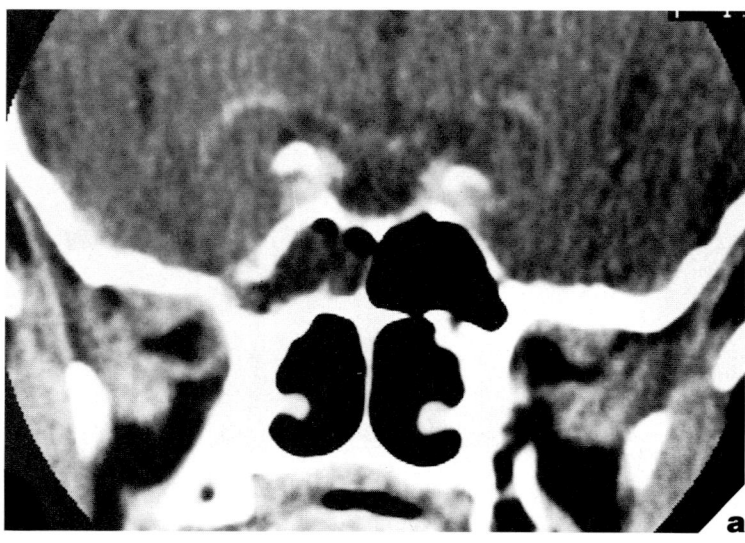

Figure 1.3

*Sphenoidal encephalocele. This 45-year-old man presented with CSF rhinorrhea. **a** Coronal CT at the level of the sella and the sphenoid sinus shows a defect in the bony margin of the right lateral wall of the sphenoid sinus, soft tissue and fluid density in the right side of the sphenoid sinus, and CSF in the*

*sella ("empty sella"). **b** After opacification of the subarachnoid space with water soluble contrast material, the source of the CSF leak is seen to be the subarachnoid space of the medial temporal region, and not the sella turcica. At operation, the contents of the sphenoid sinus proved to be an encephalocele.*

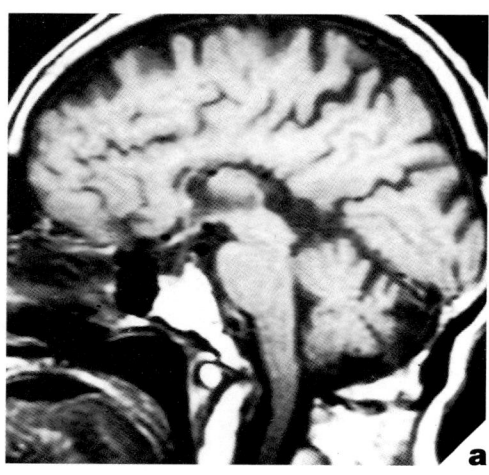
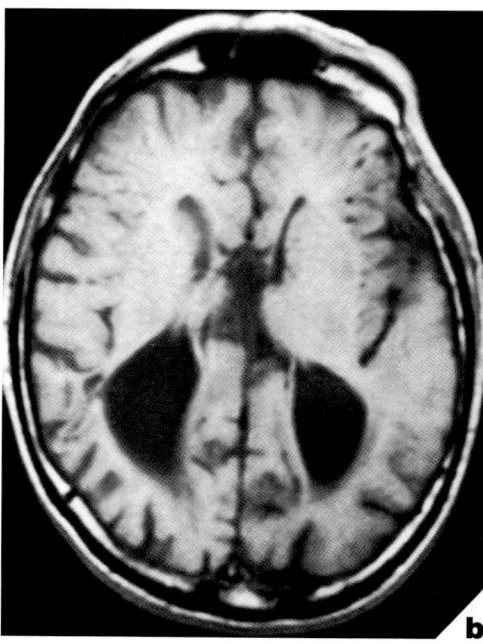
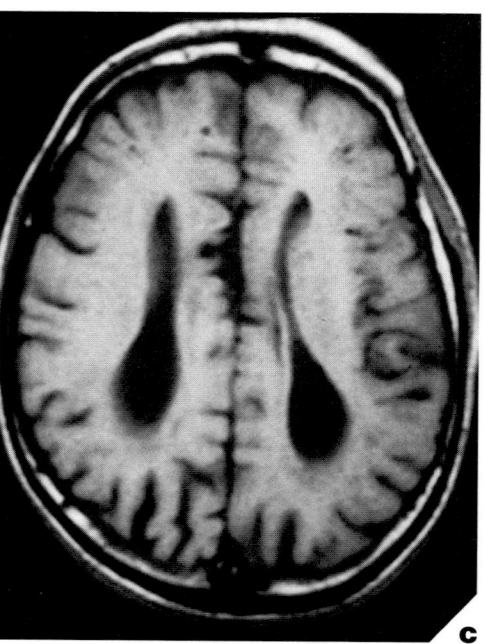

Figure 1.4

*Agenesis of the corpus callosum. **a** T1-weighted midline sagittal MR image shows absence of the corpus callosum. **b,c** T1-weighted axial images reveal a deep inter-hemispheric fissure and a parallel configuration of the lateral ventricles.*

malformation. Clinically, there is developmental delay and seizures. The computed tomography (CT) and magnetic resonance imaging (MRI) findings are characteristic: partial or total absence of the corpus callosum; lateral elongation of the foramina of Monro; wide separation of the frontal horns; a deep interhemispheric fissure and a parallel configuration of the lateral ventricles into "box-car" shapes (Fig. 1.4). Angiographic findings include tortuous or "wandering" pericallosal arteries. Lipoma of the corpus callosum, which is sometimes associated with partial agenesis, is believed to represent incorporation of mesodermal adipose tissue during the period of neural tube closure. It is easily identified on both CT and MRI by the characteristic abnormal fat density/signal. There may be adjacent calcification (Fig. 1.5).

The Chiari malformations comprise a spectrum of distinct hindbrain dysgenetic abnormalities. In the Chiari I malformation (Fig. 1.6), there is isolated downward displacement of the cerebellar tonsils often associated with syringohydromyelia. It usually presents in middle age with a variety of vague and diverse clinical symptoms including occipital headache, vertigo, and upper extremity sensorimotor abnor-

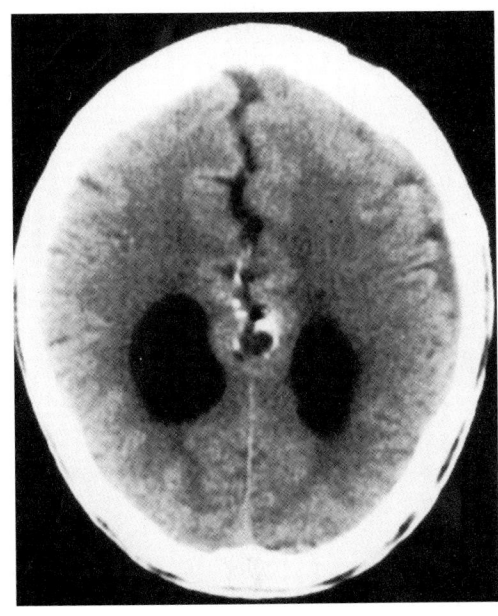

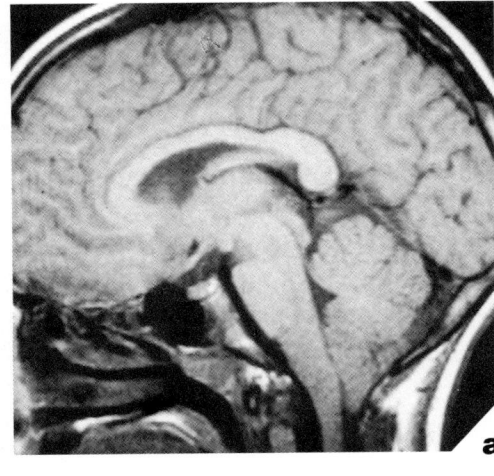

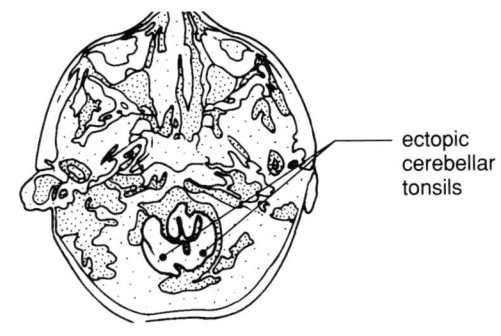

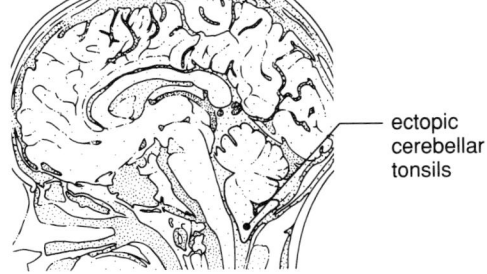

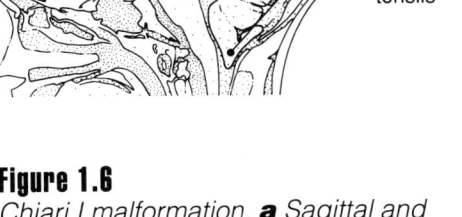

Figure 1.5
Lipoma and calcification of the corpus callosum. Calcification is seen adjacent to a small area of fat density in a patient with agenesis of the corpus callosum. Such calcification is occasionally visible on skull films. The interhemispheric tissue is deep and there is associated interdigitation of medial frontal lobe gyri. Note the dilatation of the atria of the lateral ventricles (colpocephaly). This is due to dysgenesis of the periventricular white matter, a malformation commonly associated with agenesis of the corpus callosum.

Figure 1.6
Chiari I malformation. **a** Sagittal and **b** axial T1-weighted MR images show downward herniation of the cerebellar tonsils through the foramen magnum into the cervical spinal canal. The fourth ventricle is normal in location and configuration.

Congenital Malformations of the Brain

malities. The Chiari II malformation (Fig. 1.7) occurs in nearly all patients with lumbosacral meningomyelocele and is characterized by downward displacement of the brainstem, fourth ventricle, and other portions of the cerebellar hemispheres, including the tonsils.

There are numerous radiological findings in the spine in patients with Chiari II malformation; these are discussed in Chapter 8. A variety of other intracranial anomalies are associated with the Chiari II malformation, including midbrain beaking (Fig. 1.8a), a large

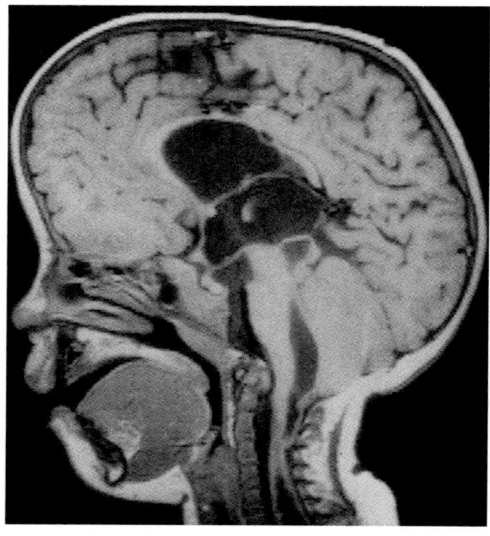

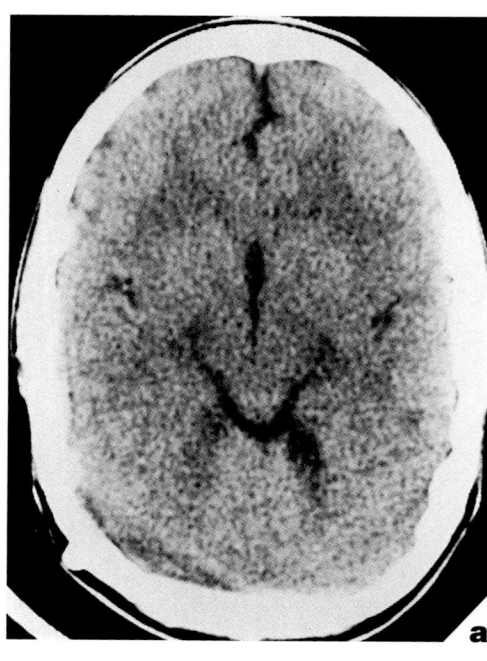

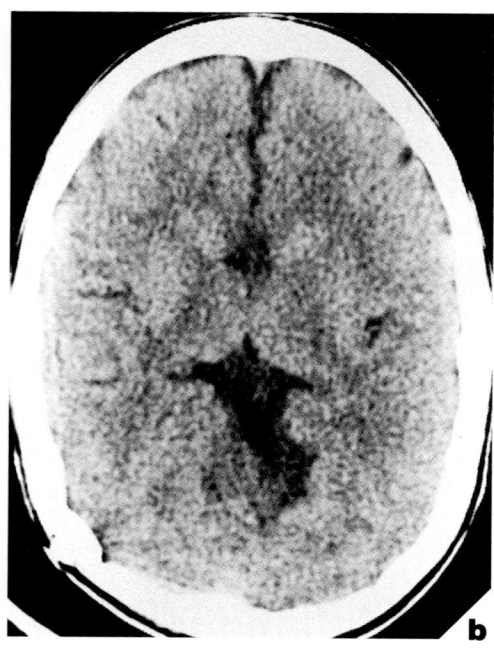

Figure 1.7
Chiari II malformation. Sagittal T1-weighted MR image shows elongation and an abnormally low position of the fourth ventricle. The cerebellar tonsils extend into the cervical spinal canal. A cervical syrinx is demonstrated and there is hydrocephalus.

Figure 1.8
*Chiari II malformation. Adjacent axial CT sections show **a** characteristic "pointing" or beaking of the tectum and **b** an enlarged massa intermedia.*

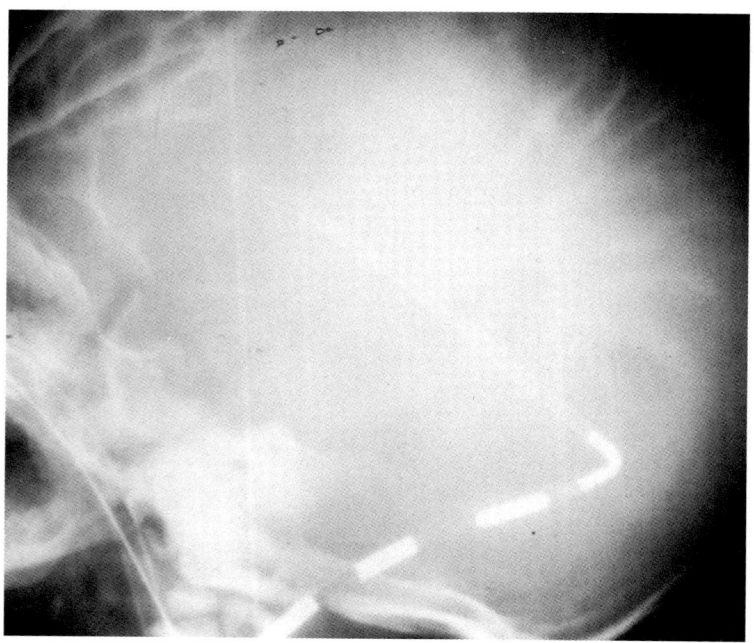

Figure 1.9
Lacunar skull. Lateral plain film of the skull in this patient who has undergone ventriculo–peritoneal shunting shows multiple areas of thinning within the frontal and parietal bones.

massa intermedia (Fig. 1.8b), varying degrees of hydrocephalus, scalloping of the clivus and petrous bones, enlargement of the foramen magnum, hypoplasia of the falx and tentorium, low insertion of the tentorium near the foramen magnum, and bulging of the cerebellum superiorly through the tentorial notch, and anteriorly around the brainstem. Infants with an associated meningomyelocele commonly exhibit a lacunar skull (lückenschädel) secondary to membranous bone dysplasia (Fig. 1.9). These bony findings disappear after six months of age.

Chiari III malformation consists of a large occipital encephalocele. In the Chiari IV malformation there is complete agenesis of the cerebellum.

The Dandy–Walker syndrome consists of a mid-line posterior fossa cyst continuous with the fourth ventricle that is usually associated with hydrocephalus (Fig 1.10). Although originally it was thought that Dandy–Walker syndrome was due to atresia of the outlet foramina of the fourth ventricle, some patients with patent outlet foramina have been reported. This suggests that hypoplasia of the cerebellar hemispheres and vermis may be the primary dis-order. The Dandy–Walker malformation must be differentiated from a giant cisterna magna (Fig. 1.11) or a posterior fossa arachnoid cyst. In both of these conditions, a clearly recognizable fourth ventricle—which is separate from the enlarged CSF space—is identified on CT or MRI. In addition, no mass effect should be associated with a giant cisterna magna.

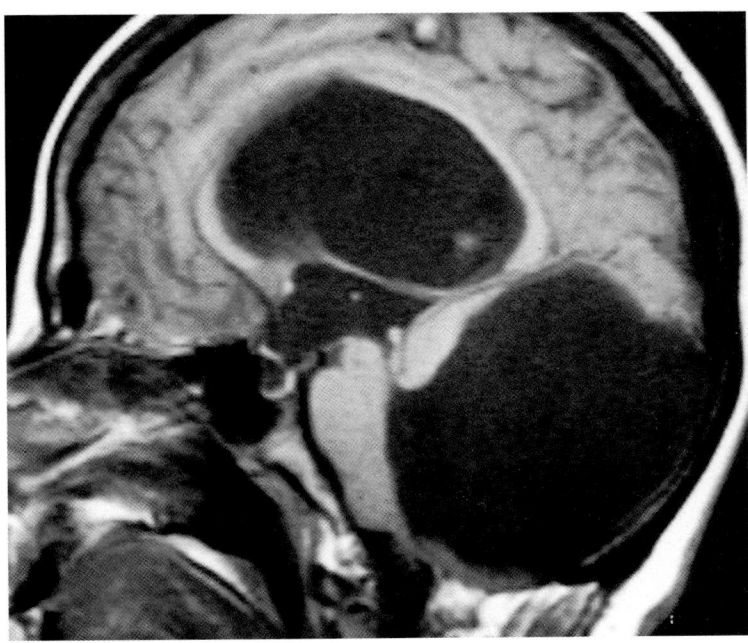

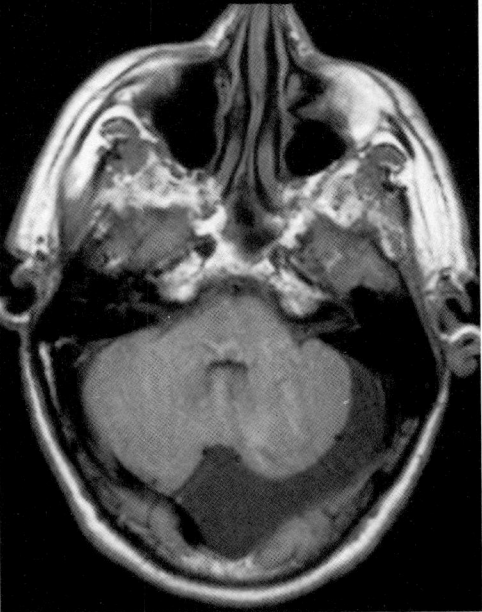

Figure 1.11
Giant cisterna magna. T1-weighted MR image shows a prominent CSF space behind the left cerebellar hemisphere which is isointense to the CSF in the fourth ventricle. Although there is some atrophy of the left cerebellar hemisphere, there is no evidence of mass effect.

Figure 1.10
Dandy–Walker cyst. Sagittal T1 MR image shows a huge posterior fossa cyst connected to the fourth ventricle. There is associated hydrocephalus.

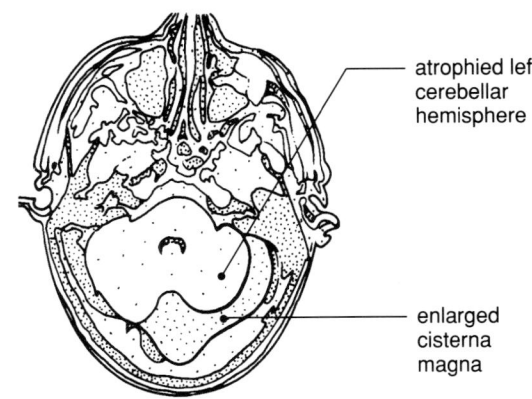

atrophied left cerebellar hemisphere

enlarged cisterna magna

Congenital Malformations of the Brain

Arachnoid cysts most commonly occur in the middle cranial fossa (Fig. 1.12), especially anterior to the temporal lobe tips. They also frequently occur in the cerebello-pontine angles (Fig. 1.13), sylvian fissures, and in the quadrigeminal plate cistern. When large, arachnoid cysts may be associated with a significant mass effect and clinical symptoms.

Disorders of Diverticulation

Holoprosencephaly is the result of failure of the first two segments of the brain (telencephalon and diencephalon) to undergo diverticulation. Depending on the severity of the malformation, holoprosencephaly may be classified as alobar, semilobar, or lobar. In the most severe (alobar) variety, there is a single

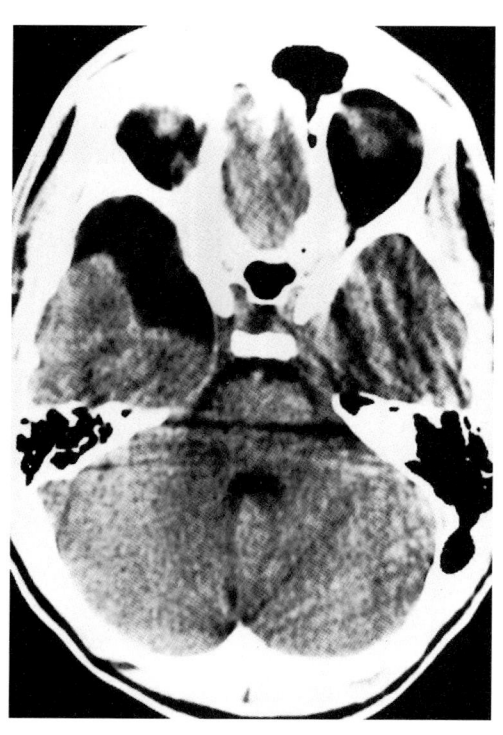

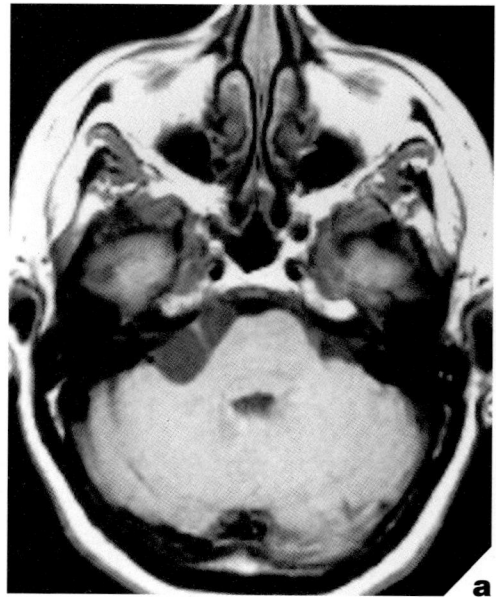

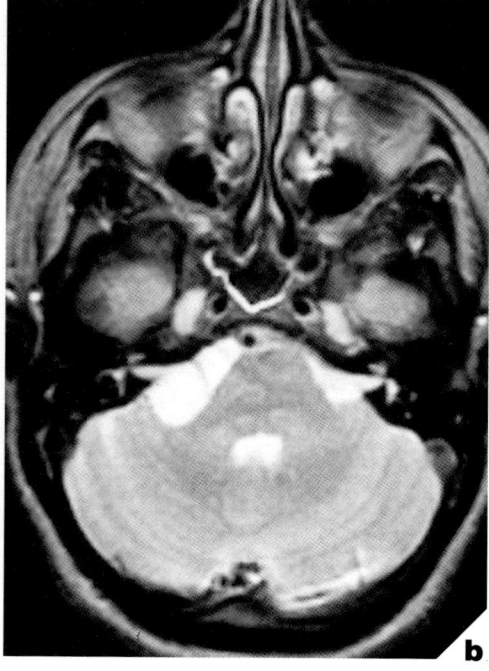

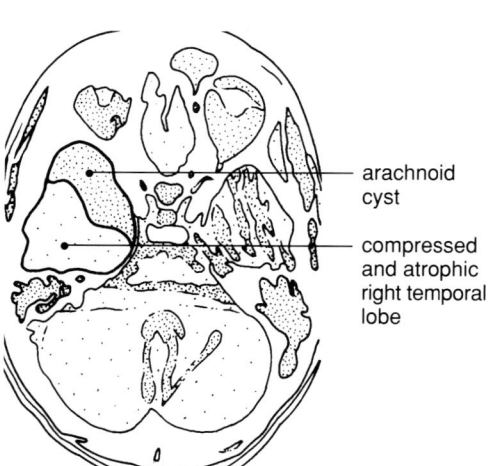

arachnoid cyst

compressed and atrophic right temporal lobe

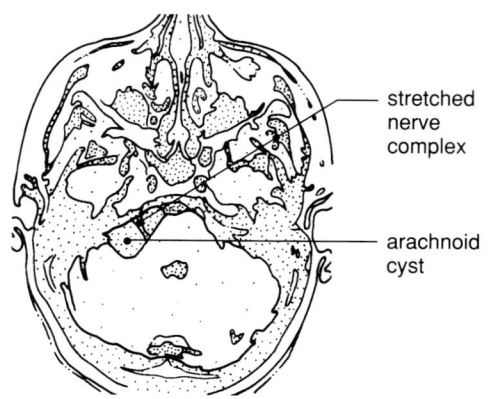

stretched nerve complex

arachnoid cyst

Figure 1.13
Cerebello-pontine angle arachnoid cyst. **a** *T1- and* **b** *T2-weighted MR images show a mass in the right cerebello-pontine angle which is isointense to CSF on both pulse sequences. This cyst may further be distinguished from a solid mass such as an acoustic schwannoma since the adjacent seventh/eighth cranial nerve complex is compressed and displaced rather than enlarged.*

Figure 1.12
Right middle cranial fossa arachnoid cyst. Axial CT scan shows a low dense mass anterior to the right temporal lobe tip which is isointense to CSF. There is some mass effect and atrophy of the right temporal lobe.

midline ventricle with absence of the interhemispheric fissure. In all cases there is absence of the falx cerebri. In the semilobar and lobar forms (Fig. 1.14) there is increasing formation and development of the cerebral hemispheres.

Septo-optic dysplasia (Fig. 1.15) is a rare anomaly characterized by absence of the septum pellucidum, a primitive optic ventricle, hypoplasia of the optic nerves and chiasm (Fig. 1.16), and hypoplasia of the pituitary stalk. Clinically, there is visual disturbance with hypoplasia of the optic discs and hypopituitarism of varying degree. There may be delayed sexual development. CT and MRI show midline defects. The septum pellucidum is absent and there is a "squared-off" appearance of the frontal horns.

Cavum septum pellucidum and cavum vergae

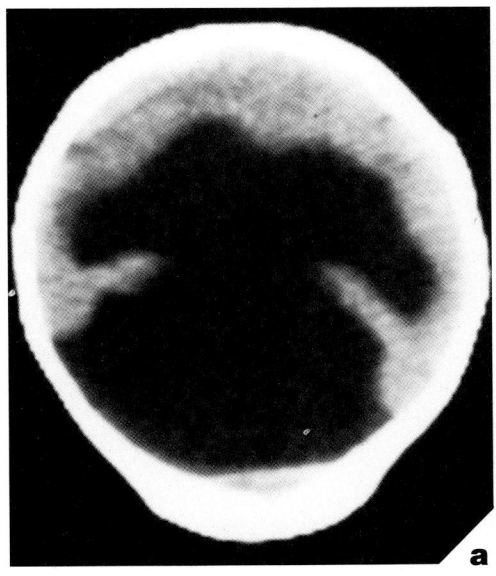 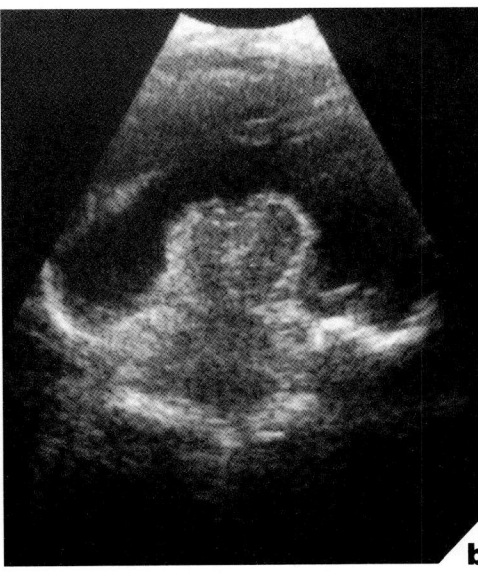 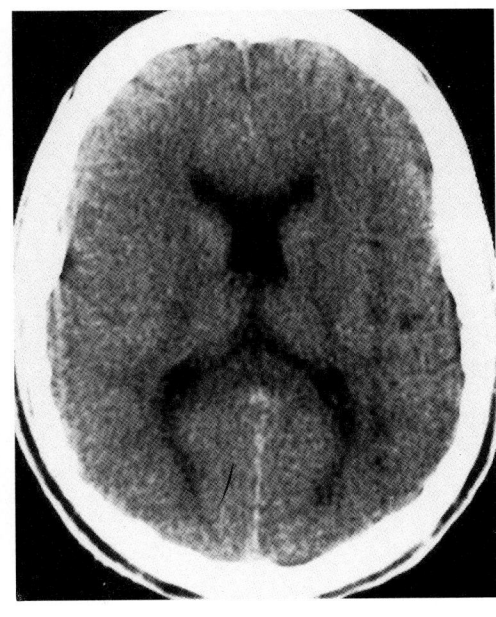

Figure 1.14
*Lobar holoprosencephaly. **a** Axial CT and **b** coronal ultrasound images of a child with severe midline abnormalities including cleft lip and palate, absence of nose and cyclopia. These demonstrate a single midline ventricle with a moderate amount of adjacent cerebral cortex. There is no falx cerebri or interhemispheric fissure.*

Figure 1.15
Septo-optic dysplasia. Axial CT scan shows a "squared off" appearance of the frontal horns and absence of the septum pellucidum.

Figure 1.16
Septo-optic dysplasia. Coronal T1-weighted image shows marked hypoplasia of the optic chiasm. The septum pellucidum is absent.

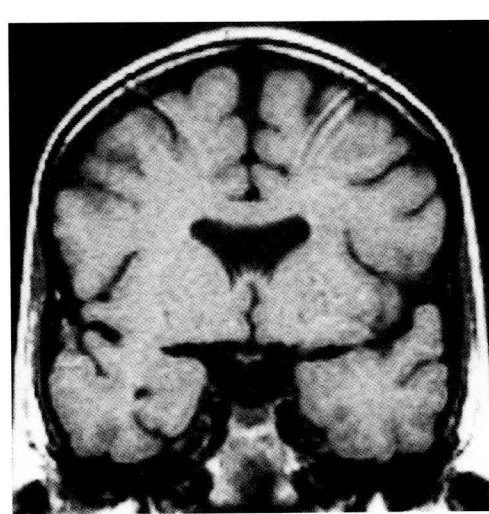 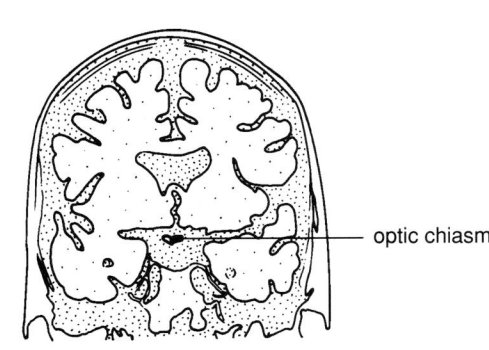

optic chiasm

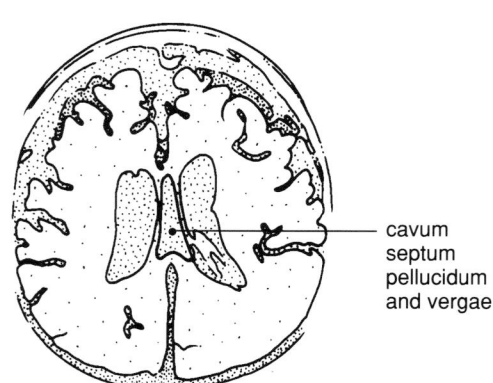

Figure 1.17
Cavum septum pellucidum and cavum vergae. Note the midline collection of CSF between the two lateral ventricles.

cavum
septum
pellucidum
and vergae

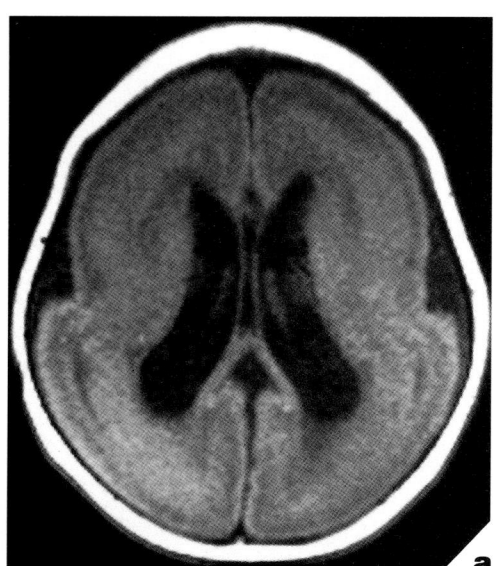
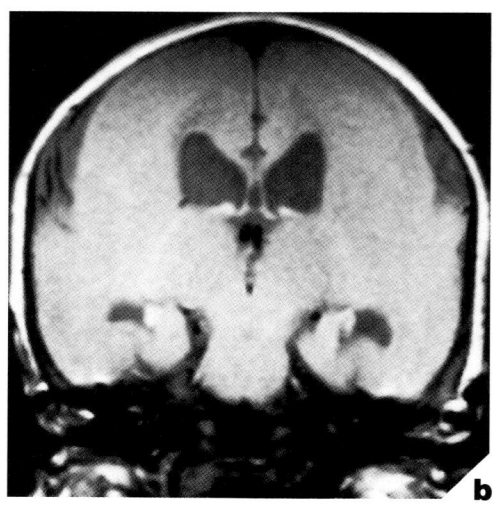

Figure 1.18
Lissencephaly. **a** Axial and **b** coronal T1-weighted images demonstrate faulty neuronal migration and lack of formation of the opercula. The cerebral surface is smooth.

b

a

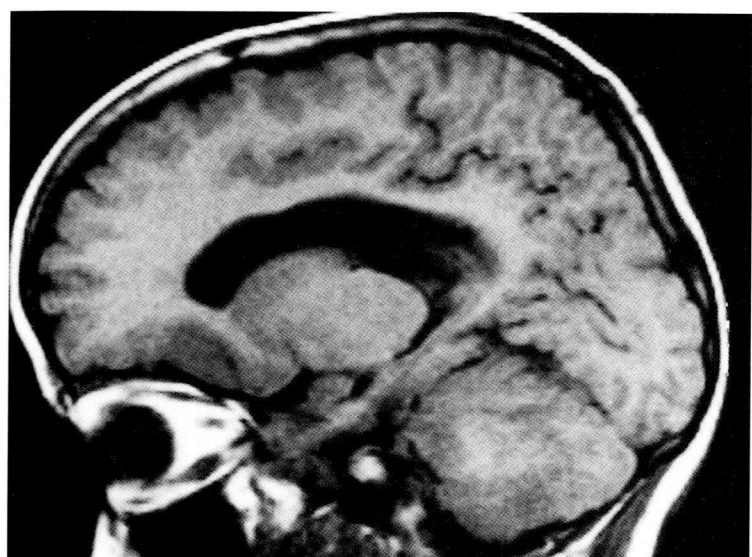

Figure 1.19
Polymicrogyria. Although more often there is an appearance of pachygyria since the gyri fuse, MRI of polymicrogyria may also demonstrate numerous, small cerebral cortical convolutions as in this T1-weighted sagittal image.

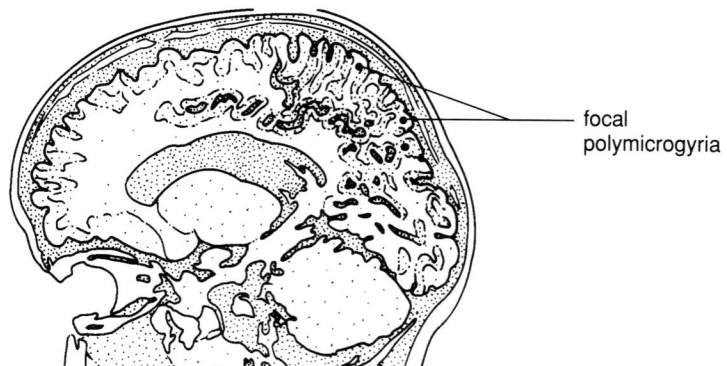

focal
polymicrogyria

(Fig. 1.17) result from persistence of the fetal separation of the two leaves of the septum pellucidum. These leaves usually fuse early in the neonatal period. The foramen of Monro is an arbitrary landmark dividing this single CSF space into the cavum septum pellucidum anteriorly and cavum vergae posteriorly. This is a developmental variant with no clinical significance.

Disorders of Sulcation and Migration

The germinal matrix, a region of the developing brain that lies adjacent to the ependymal surface of the lateral ventricles, gives rise to the neurons and glia of the grey matter structures of the cerebral cortex and basal ganglia. This process occurs during the neuronal proliferation stage (second to fourth fetal months), after which the neurons migrate to their ultimate destination (third to sixth fetal months). Lissencephaly results from failure of neuronal migration; as a result, the cortex consists of four layers rather than the normal six. Because the gyri develop from the two missing layers, there is an absence of convolutions, and the surface of the brain is thus smooth (Fig. 1.18). When this disorder is localized to one or a few specific areas of the brain, it is termed *pachygyria*.

MRI of patients with polymicrogyria (Fig. 1.19) may demonstrate excess gyri in the cerebral cortex or thickened gyri with shallow sulci. This may be generalized, focal, or multifocal. More commonly, the excess gyri are fused, resulting in a false appearance of pachygyria.

When the neurons fail to migrate normally, there may also be nodules of grey matter extending from the ventricles to the surface of the brain (grey matter heterotopias) (Fig. 1.20).

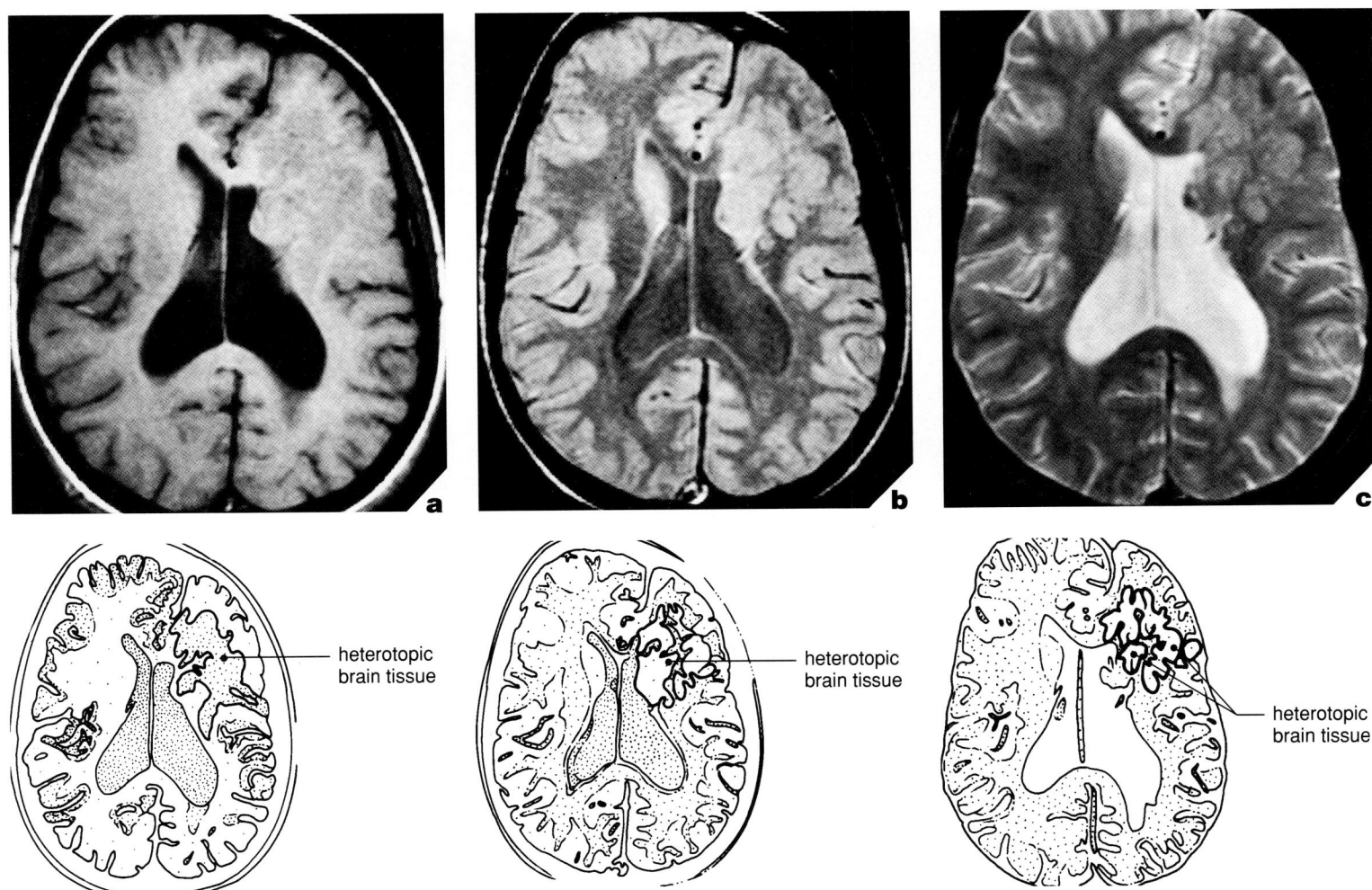

Figure 1.20
*Grey matter heterotopia. **a** Axial T1, **b** proton density, and **c** T2-weighted MR images reveal islands of grey matter in the mid-left frontal lobe which are isointense to cerebral cortical grey matter on all pulse sequences.*

Congenital Malformations of the Brain

Schizencephaly is a neuronal migration disorder which results in grey matter lined clefts extending from the ventricles towards the surface of the brain. It may be open- (Fig. 1.21) or closed-lipped (Fig. 1.22), depending upon whether the cleft reaches the brain's surface.

Destructive Lesions

Hydranencephaly results in absence of most or all portions of the cerebral hemispheres. A large fluid-filled sac replaces the rostral portion of the brain with preservation of the basal ganglia and posterior fossa structures (Fig. 1.23). It needs to be distinguished from severe hydrocephalus. Unlike hydranencephaly, in severe hydrocephalus there is a thin rind of compressed cerebrum and formation of cerebral arteries and veins.

Porencephaly is a cavity within the brain; it may be congenital or acquired. Congenital porencephaly may be due to antenatal vascular occlusion (encephaloclastic variety) or developmental factors (schizencephalic variety). CT and MRI show an area of CSF density or intensity (Fig. 1.24) that may or may not communicate with the ventricular system. The encephaloclastic and schizencephalic forms frequently cannot be differentiated radiologically.

Fetal hypoxia often results in extensive loss of brain tissue when evaluated postnatally. However, small and discrete areas of injury may also be seen. For example, Möbius syndrome (Fig. 1.25) is a congenital disorder characterized by inability to abduct the eyes and facial paralysis. Characteristic punctate calcifications are demonstrated on CT and MRI in the infarcted abducens nuclei bilaterally.

DISORDERS OF HISTOGENESIS

Tuberous sclerosis (Bourneville's disease) is a hereditary disorder manifested clinically by the triad of mental retardation, seizures, and adenoma sebaceum. The brain lesions are hamartomas (calcified or noncalcified) that are often located in a subependymal location (Fig. 1.26). Nodules located in certain critical places in the CSF pathways such as the foramina of Monro may cause obstructive hydrocephalus. Malignant degeneration may occur, typically resulting in giant cell astroblastomas at the foramina of Monro. MRI shows small bright foci of T2 signal abnormality that may represent hamartomas or low grade gliomas.

Neurofibromatosis is a widespread mesodermal dysplasia with protean clinical and radiographic manifestations. Neurofibromatosis has been categorized into two types: NF-1 (von Recklinghausen's disease)

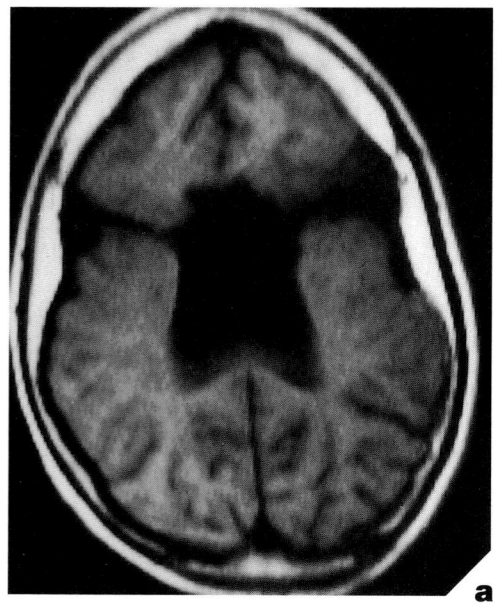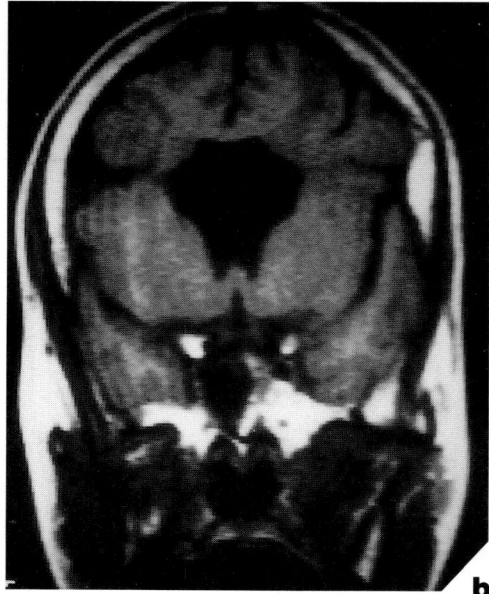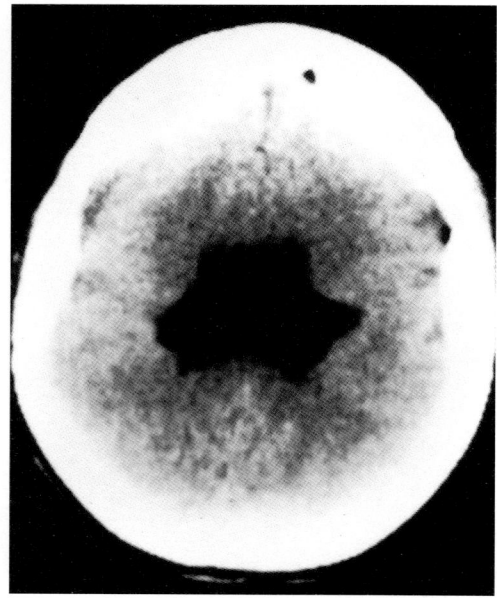

a   b

Figure 1.21
Open-lipped schizencephaly. **a** *Axial and* **b** *coronal MR sections show bilateral clefts extending from the ventricular system to the convexity subarachnoid space. The crevices are lined with grey matter.*

Figure 1.22
Closed-lipped schizencephaly. Bilateral clefts are demonstrated along the lateral margins of the lateral ventricles. The clefts do not extend to the cortical surface.

and NF-2 (bilateral acoustic neurofibromatosis). NF-1 is associated with neoplasms of astrocytes and neurons (gliomas and hamartomas) while NF-2 is associated with tumors of Schwann cells (Schwannomas) and tumors of the meninges (meningiomas). In NF-1 there may be congenital absence of the greater wing of the sphenoid (Fig. 1.27). Intracranial gliomas and hamartomas (Fig. 1.28) may be difficult to differentiate. The various types of spinal disorders associated with neurofibromatosis are discussed in Chapter 10.

Sturge–Weber syndrome (Encephalotrigeminal angiomatosis) is characterized by a port-wine nevus of the face in the ophthalmic division of the trigeminal nerve, leptomeningeal angiomatosis, and seizures;

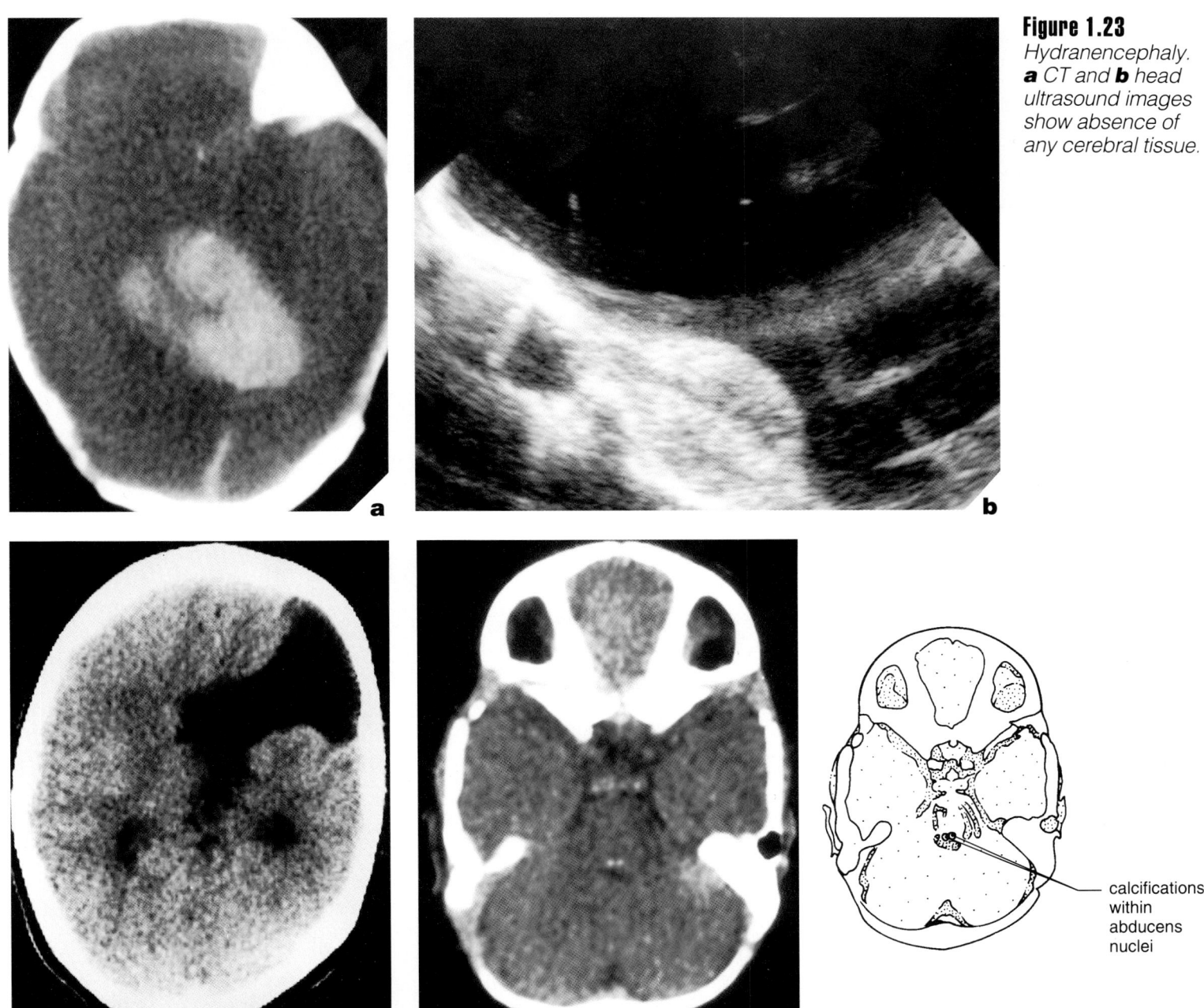

Figure 1.23
Hydranencephaly.
a *CT and* ***b*** *head ultrasound images show absence of any cerebral tissue.*

calcifications within abducens nuclei

Figure 1.24
Porencephaly. There is a large area of low attenuation in the left frontal lobe watershed zone, which is continuous with the frontal horn of the left lateral ventricle.

Figure 1.25
Möbius syndrome. Axial CT scan shows bilateral punctate calcifications in the abducens nuclei.

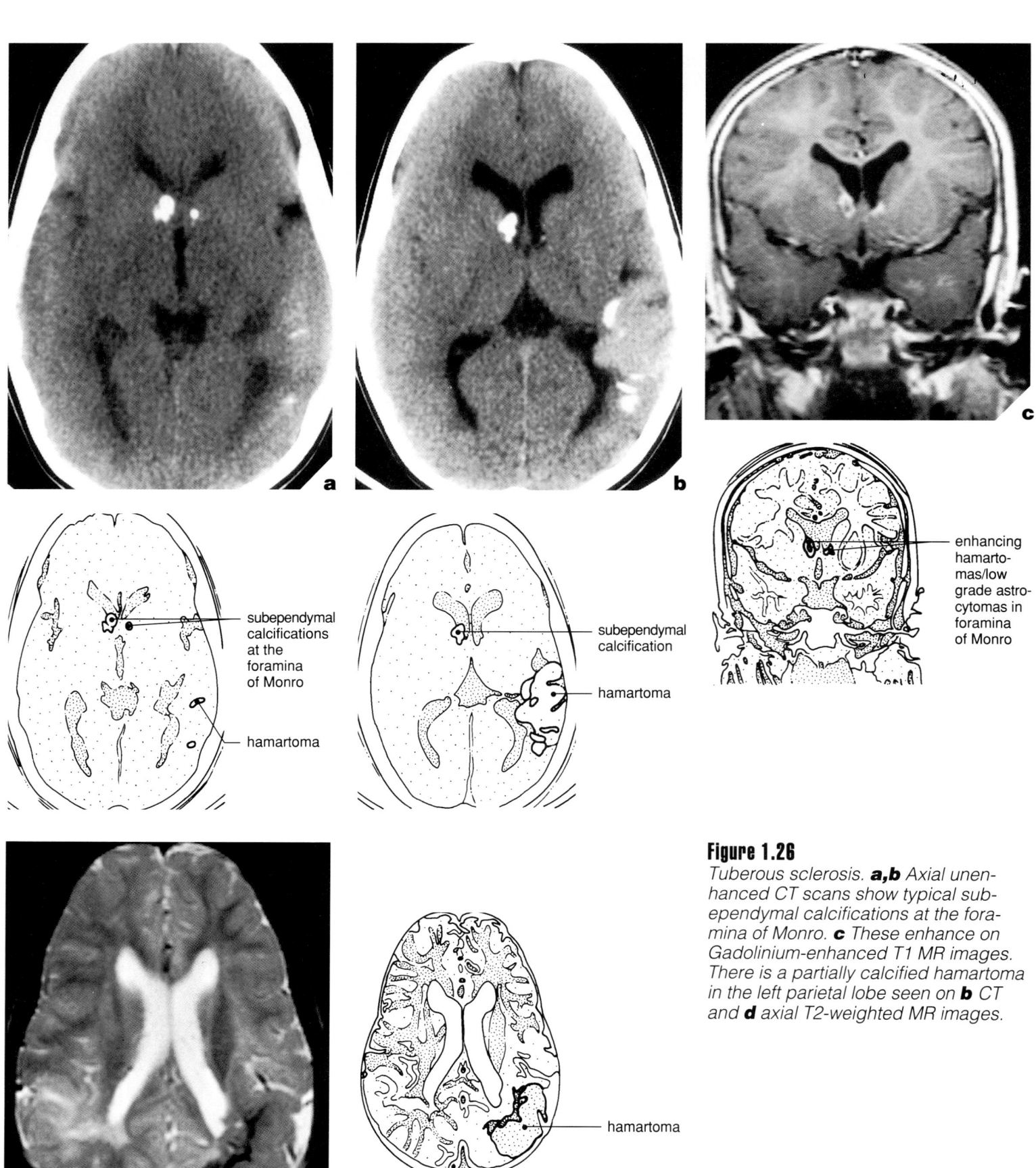

subependymal calcifications at the foramina of Monro

hamartoma

subependymal calcification

hamartoma

enhancing hamarto-mas/low grade astro-cytomas in foramina of Monro

hamartoma

Figure 1.26

Tuberous sclerosis. ***a,b*** *Axial unen-hanced CT scans show typical sub-ependymal calcifications at the fora-mina of Monro.* ***c*** *These enhance on Gadolinium-enhanced T1 MR images. There is a partially calcified hamartoma in the left parietal lobe seen on* ***b*** *CT and* ***d*** *axial T2-weighted MR images.*

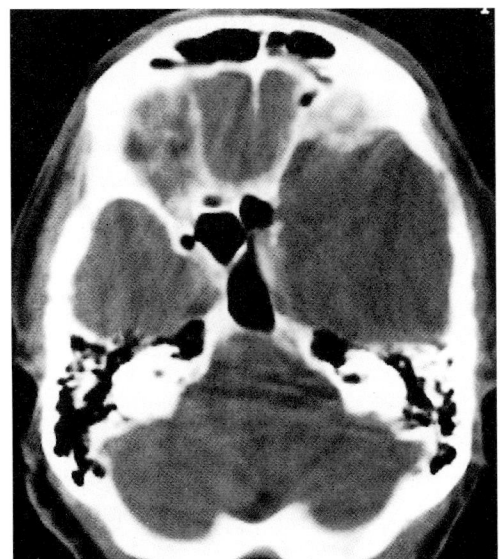

Figure 1.27
Neurofibromatosis. Axial CT scan shows congenital absence of the greater wing of the sphenoid on the left. Herniation of the temporal lobe into the orbit, resulting in pulsatile exophthalmos, may occur in patients with this congenital bone defect.

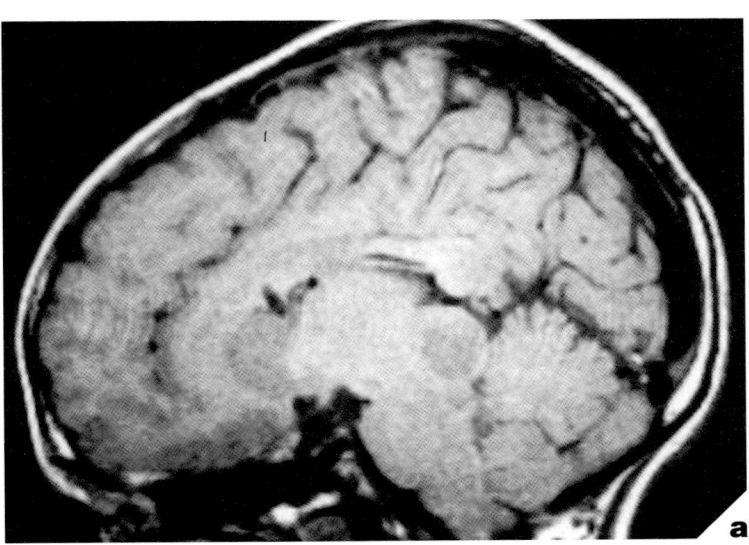

a

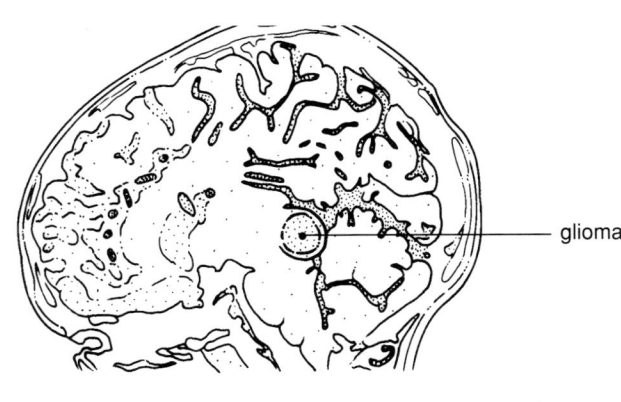

glioma

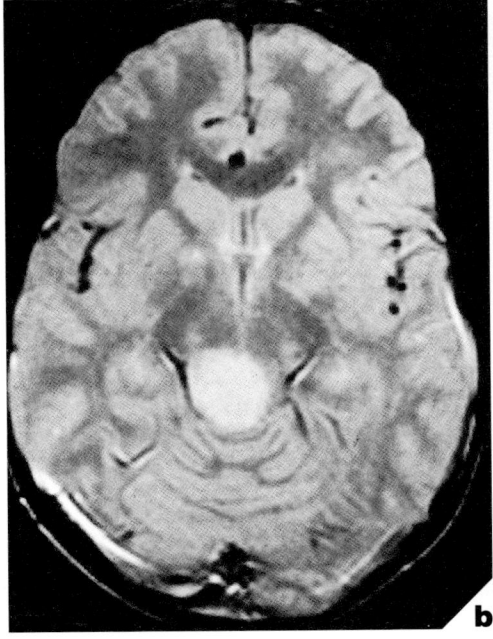

b

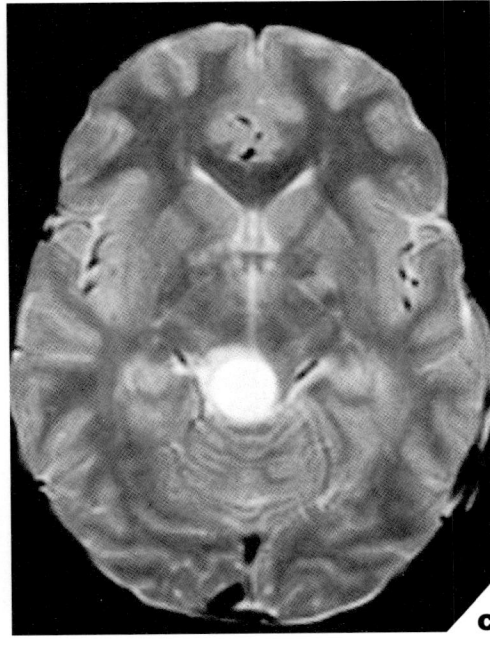

c

Figure 1.28
*Brainstem glioma in a patient with neurofibromatosis. **a** Sagittal T1 and **b,c** axial T2 images demonstrate a nodular mass in the colliculi of the brainstem which was found to represent a glioma. Intracranial gliomas and hamartomas are common in patients with neurofibromatosis.*

Congenital Malformations of the Brain

mental retardation is frequently present. Hemiparesis or hemiplegia with hemiatrophy is seen in severe cases. CT or plain skull films demonstrate the characteristic "tram-track" gyral calcifications of this disorder (Fig. 1.29). The calcifications occur in the cerebral cortex rather than within the angiomatous vessels and are believed to be a result of chronic ischemia. MR shows these gyral calcifications as areas of absent signal (Fig. 1.30). There is often ipsilateral hemiatrophy of the cerebral hemispheres (Dyke–Davidoff–Masson syndrome).

Many congenital disorders are not easily categorized into a particular etiologic grouping. Among these are multisystem congenital, metabolic, toxic, and infectious disorders. Some disorders do not present until much later in life. In others, the intracranial findings may be characteristic and interesting but of little or no clinical relevance.

Leigh's disease is an autosomal recessive disorder in which infants present with seizures and loss of head control. MRI (Fig. 1.31) typically shows bright-T2

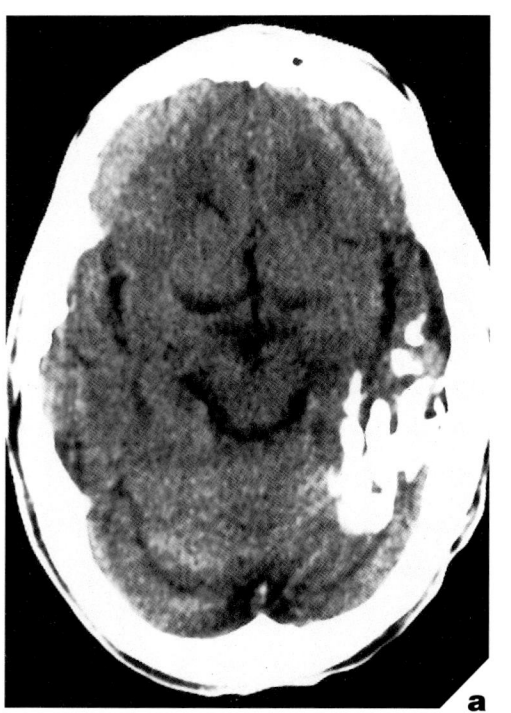
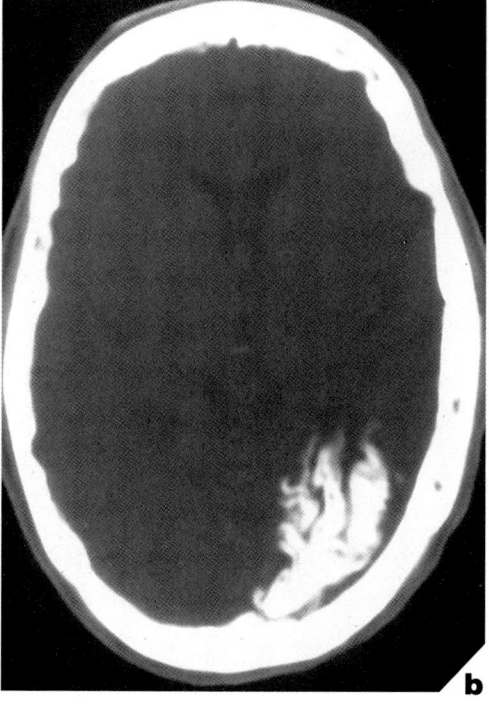

Figure 1.29
*Sturge–Weber syndrome. **a,b** CT images demonstrate "tram-track" calcifications in the left temporal and occipital lobes of this mentally retarded patient with skin discoloration on the left side of her face.*

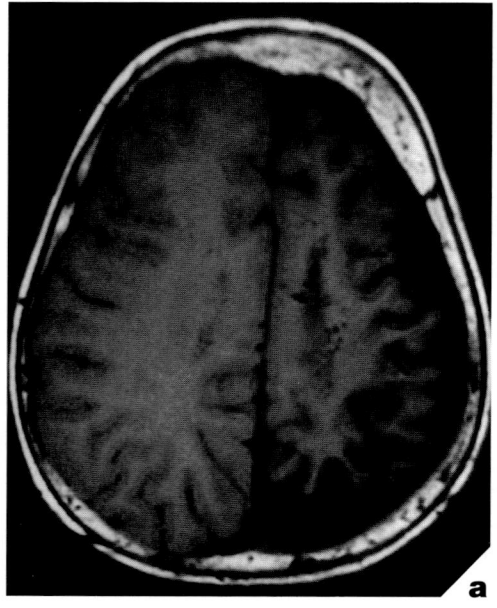
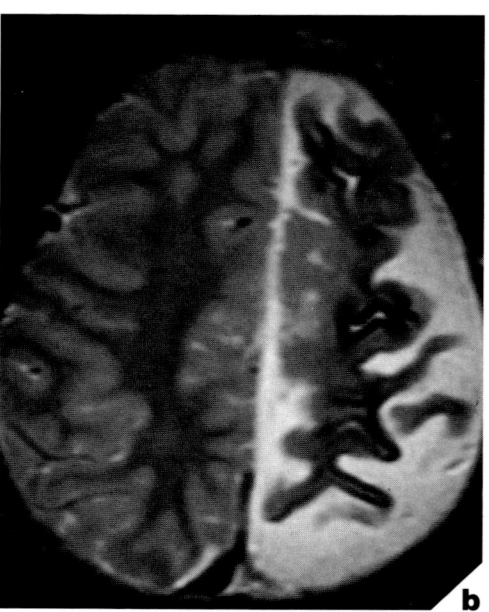

Figure 1.30
*Sturge–Weber syndrome with Dyke–Davidoff–Masson syndrome. **a** T1-weighted MR image shows atrophy involving the left cerebral hemisphere with compensatory dilatation of the left lateral ventricle and left convexity subarachnoid space. The left side of the skull is thick compared to the right—an example of the Dyke–Davidoff–Masson syndrome (cranial asymmetry associated with unequal development of the cerebral hemispheres). **b** T2-weighted MR image at a slightly higher level shows gyral calcifications as curvilinear bands of decreased signal intensity.*

signal abnormalities in the caudate nuclei, putamina, and midbrain.

Basal cell nevus syndrome (Fig. 1.32) is not usually catagorized as a disorder of histogenesis but it is an inheritable disorder that results in abnormal calci-fications which occur in specific intracranial locations: the falx cerebri and tentorium. These patients usually have multiple basal cell carcinomas in the skin, ovarian fibromas, and rib deformities.

Achondroplasia is a congenital disorder resulting in

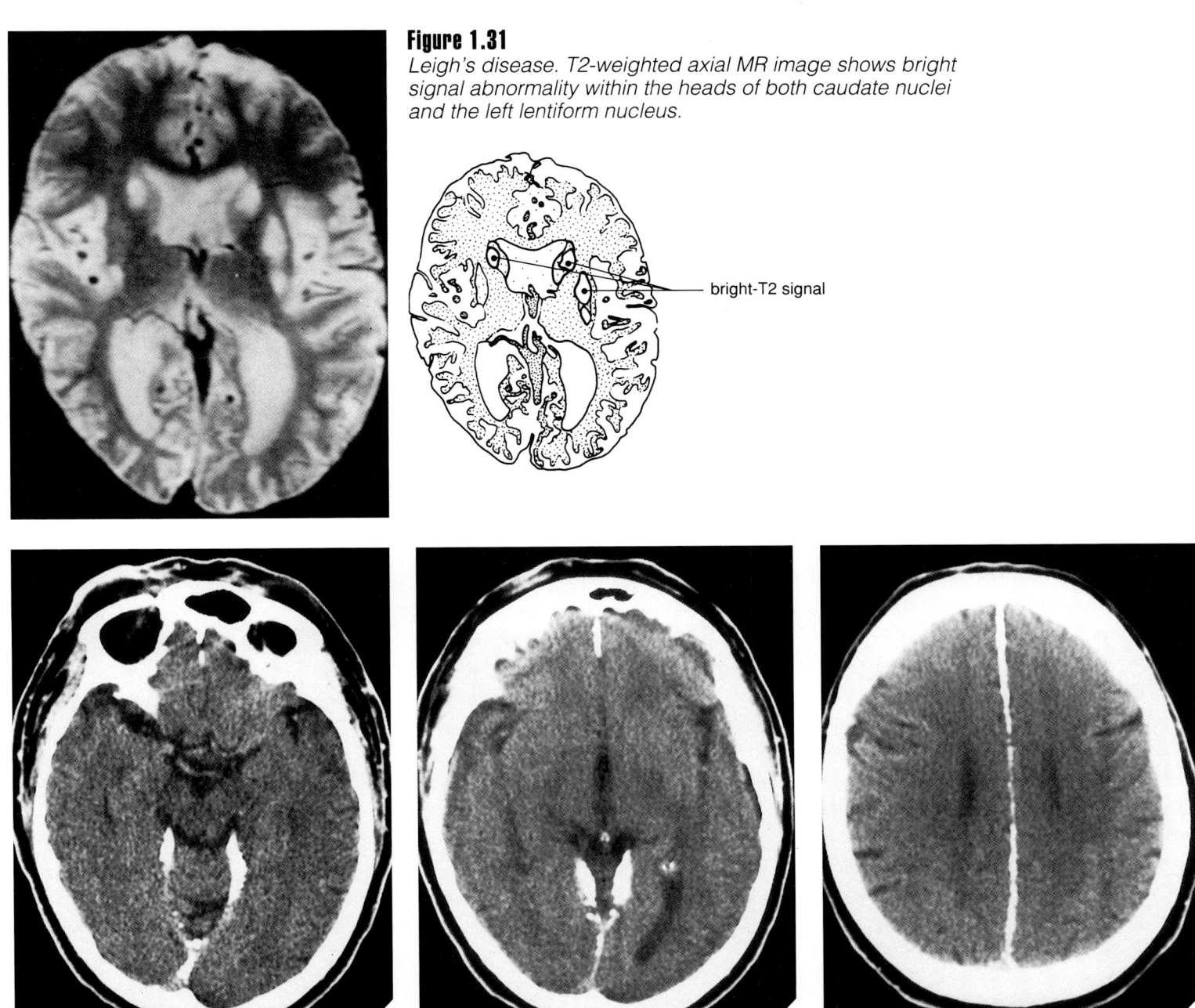

Figure 1.31
Leigh's disease. T2-weighted axial MR image shows bright signal abnormality within the heads of both caudate nuclei and the left lentiform nucleus.

bright-T2 signal

Figure 1.32
*Basal cell nevus syndrome. **a,b,c** Characteristic calcifications in the falx cerebri and tentorium are demonstrated on these unenhanced CT images.*

severe shortening of endochondral bones. Among the many radiologial findings is marked narrowing of the foramen magnum (Fig. 1.33).

Hurler's syndrome (Fig. 1.34) is a mucopolysaccharidosis caused by a deficiency of α-L-iduronidase, and as a result, heparan and dermatan sulfates are excreted in the urine. The skull is scaphocephalic and thickened. Suprasellar arachnoid cysts commonly occur and there is a deep chiasmatic recess of the sphenoid bone which results in a "J-shaped" sella turcica. Communicating hydrocephalus occurs in many patients with Hurler's syndrome.

Premature fusion of the cranial sutures is called *craniosynostosis.* When the sagittal suture fuses prematurely, the skull is elongated in its antero-posterior diameter; this is termed *scaphocephaly* or *dolichocephaly.* Asymmetric, premature sutural closure is called *plagiocephaly* (Fig. 1.35). Premature fusion of the coronal or lambdoid sutures results in *brachycephaly* (Fig. 1.36).

Basal ganglia mineralization is very common in the elderly population. Rarely, basal ganglia calcification may be secondary to a pathologic entity such as pseudohypoparathyroidism (Fig. 1.37). The dentate nuclei of the cerebellum are also often affected, and irregular areas of additional brain parenchymal calcification may be present. Other causes of basal ganglia mineralization include other disorders of calcium metabolism including hyperparathyroidism, Fahr's disease, and Cockayne's syndrome.

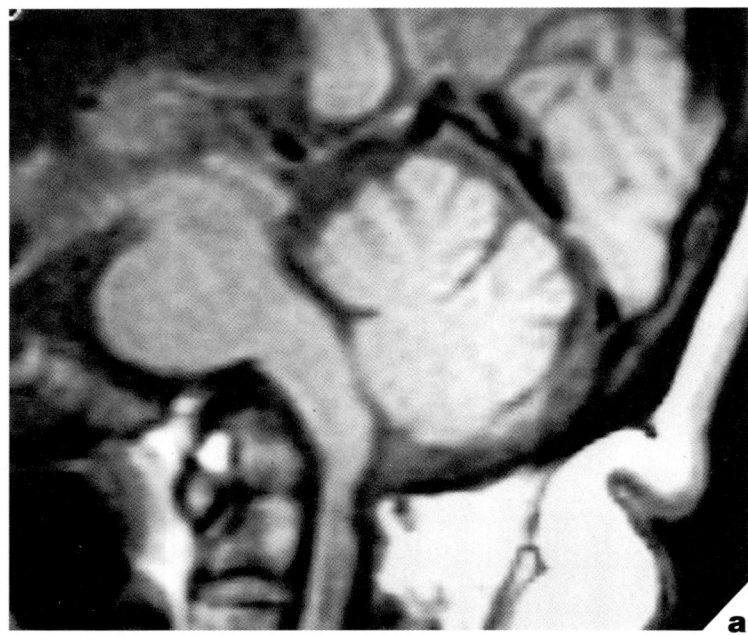

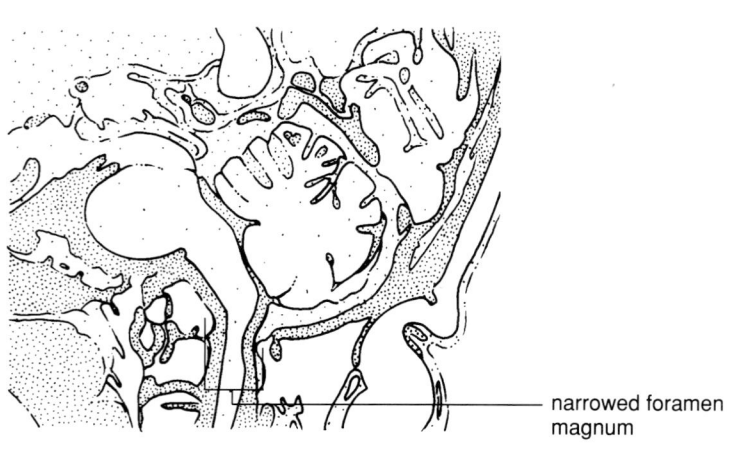

narrowed foramen magnum

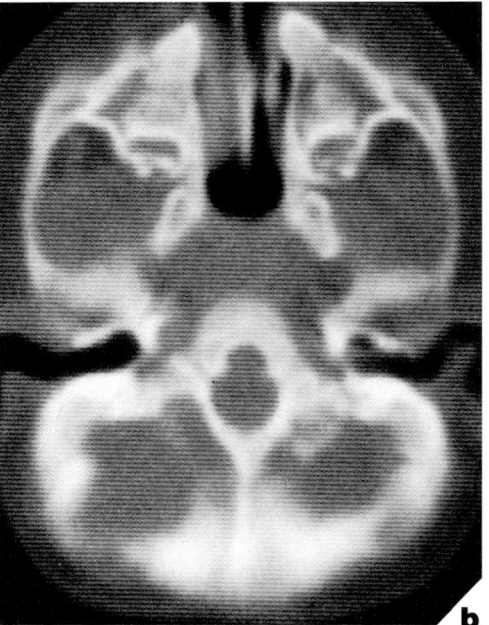

Figure 1.33
*Achondroplasia. Severe narrowing of the foramen magnum with associated compression of the cervico–medullary junction are demonstrated on **a** MR and **b** CT images.*

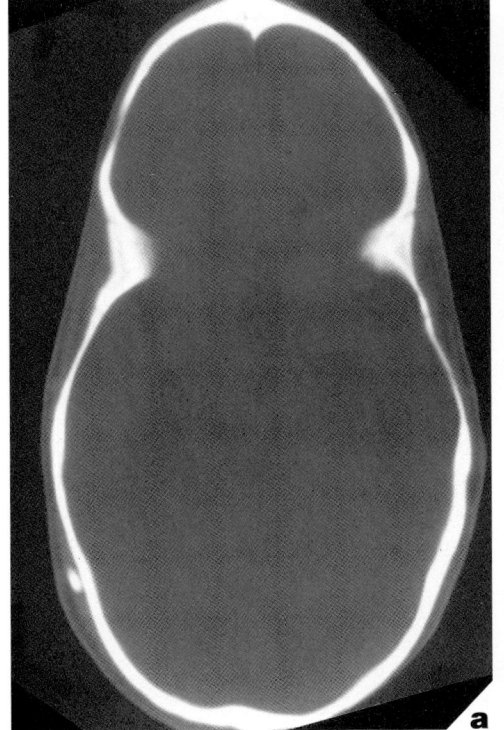

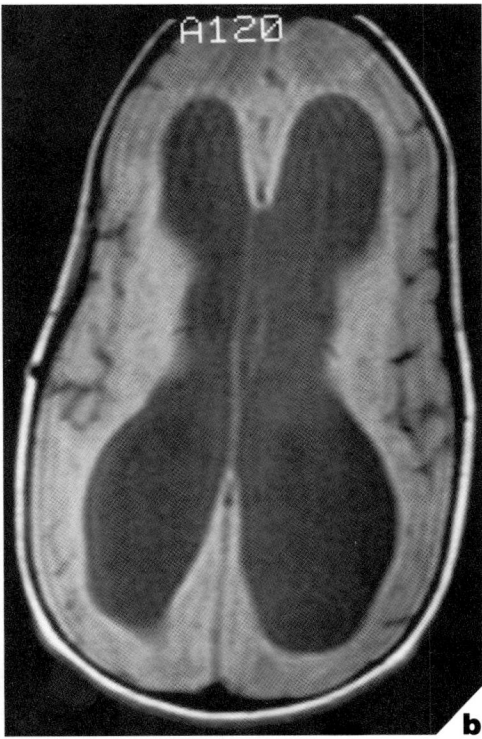

Figure 1.34

Hurler's syndrome. **a** *A scaphocephalic skull with* **b** *communicating hydrocephalus and* **c** *frontal bossing and a small posterior fossa are demonstrated. There is a deep, "J-shaped" sella turcica.*

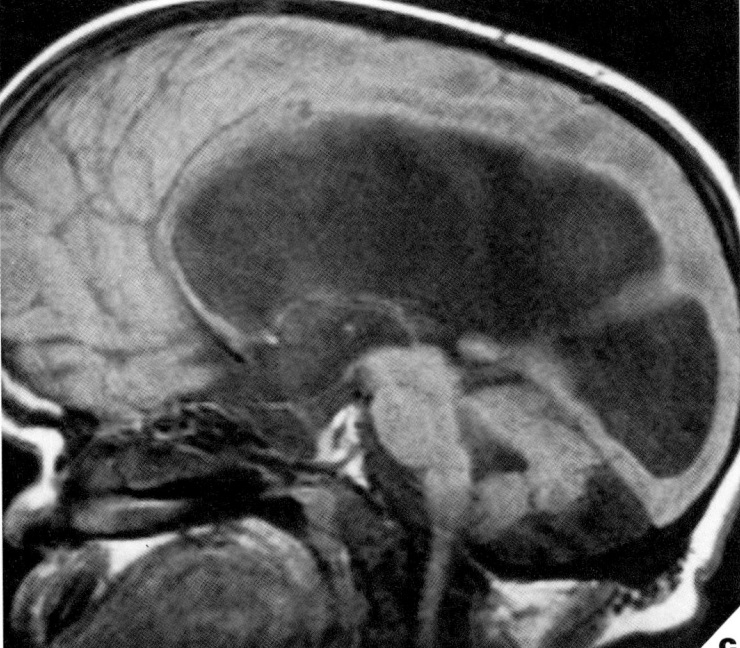

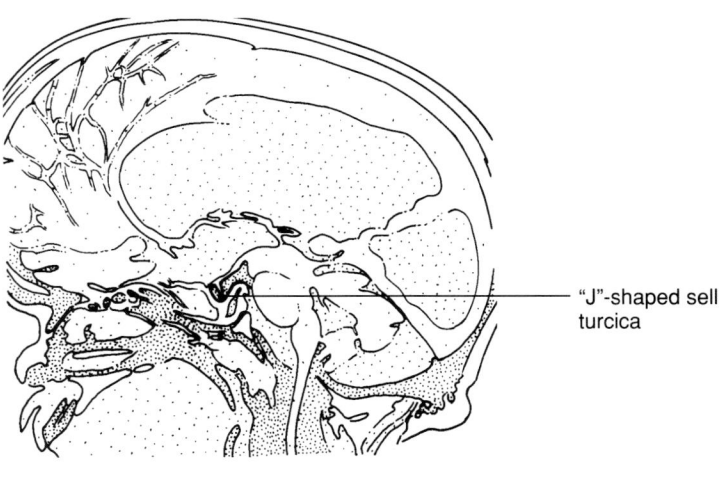

"J"-shaped sella turcica

Congenital Malformations of the Brain

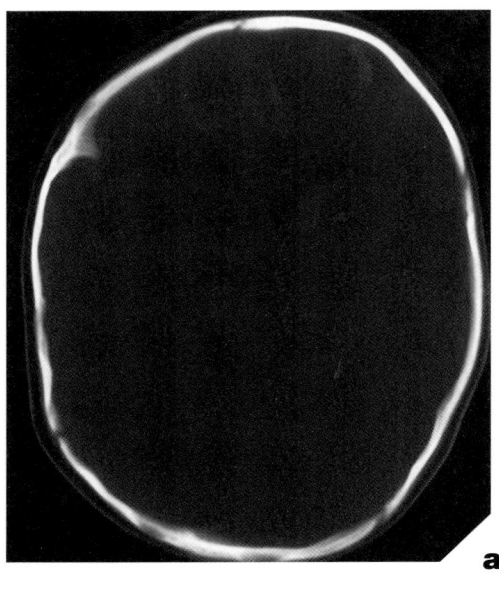

Figure 1.35
*Premature closure of the right coronal suture. **a** CT section (bone window) shows premature fusion of the right coronal suture resulting in marked cranial and facial asymmetry with **b** elevation of the right orbit. Incidentally seen is a persistent metopic suture.*

a

b

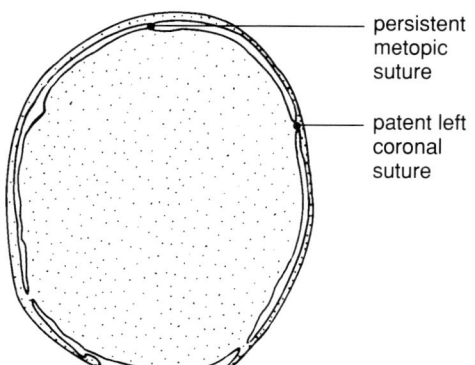

persistent
metopic
suture

patent left
coronal
suture

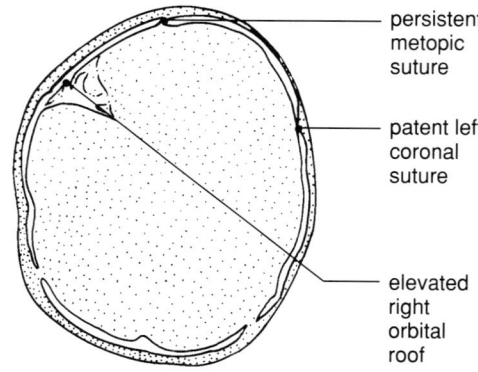

persistent
metopic
suture

patent left
coronal
suture

elevated
right
orbital
roof

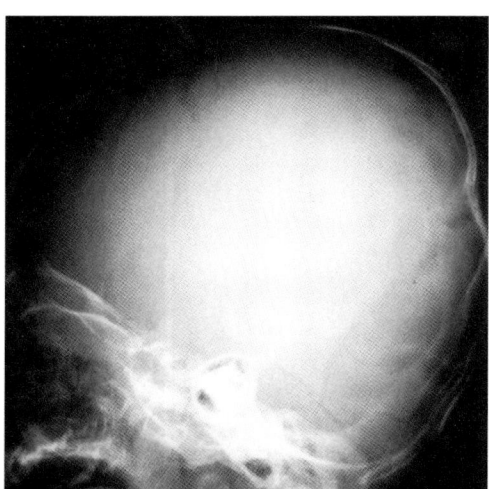

Figure 1.36
*Brachycephaly.
The antero-posterior diameter of the
skull is diminished.*

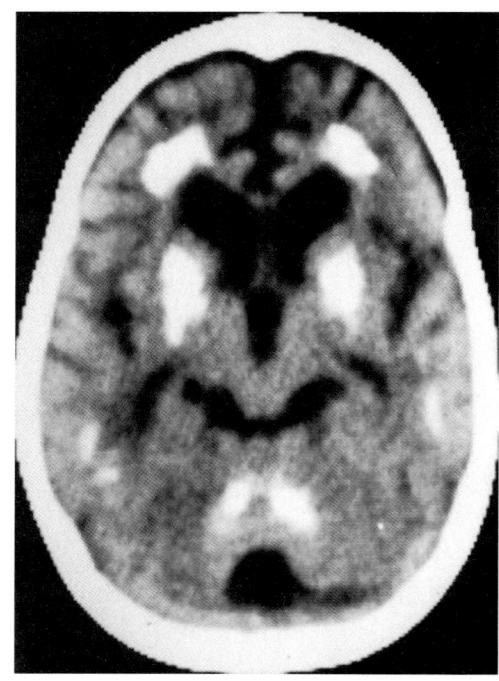

Figure 1.37
*Pseudo-hypoparathyroidism.
Axial CT image
shows heavy calcifications within the
basal ganglia and
dentate nuclei.
Other parenchymal calcifications
are also present.*

2

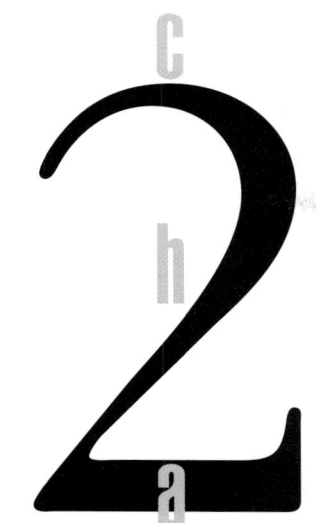

White Matter Disease

White matter diseases include a group of primary and secondary disorders that usually involve myelinated nerves. The lesions may be primarily infectious, vascular, iatrogenic, or idiopathic. Many white matter disorders demonstrate what on first inspection appear to be similar MRI findings. Detailed evaluation of the size, shape, symmetry, and locations of the lesions plus correlation with the clinical history often helps to make a specific diagnosis possible.

Cerebral white matter is composed of bundles of axons and their respective phospholipid, cholesterol-containing coverings. Overall, white matter contains approximately 12% less water than grey matter; it has a shorter T1 than grey matter and is therefore relatively bright on T1-weighted images

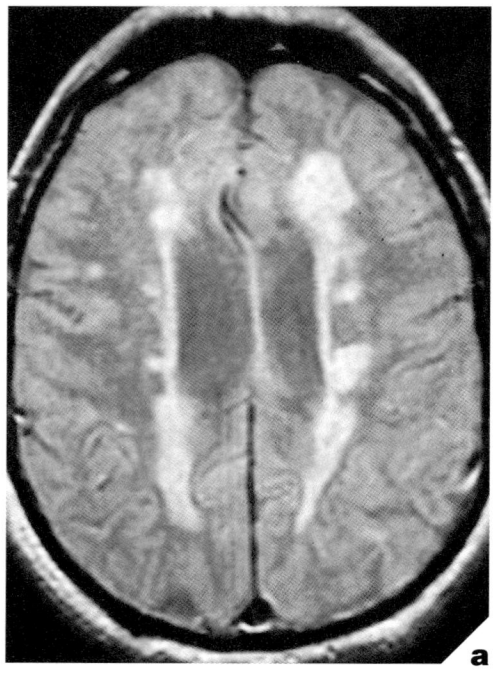

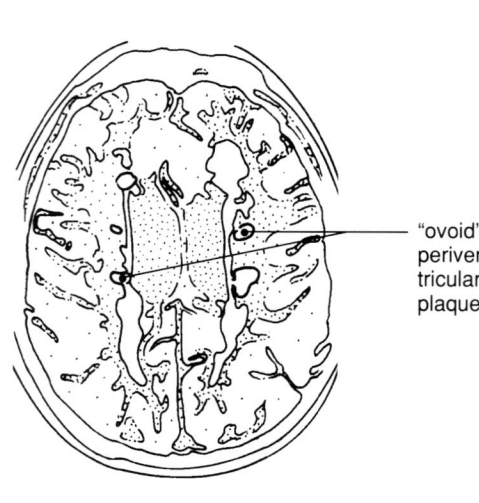

"ovoid" periventricular plaques

Figure 2.1

*Multiple sclerosis. **a,b** Proton density and **c,d** more heavily T2-weighted MR images at and just above the level of the lateral ventricles show the classic size, configuration, location and signal characteristics of plaques. These small and confluent bright-T2 lesions are predominantly periventricular. In addition, many are "ovoid" in shape and are oriented perpendicular to the lateral and superior margins of the lateral ventricles.*

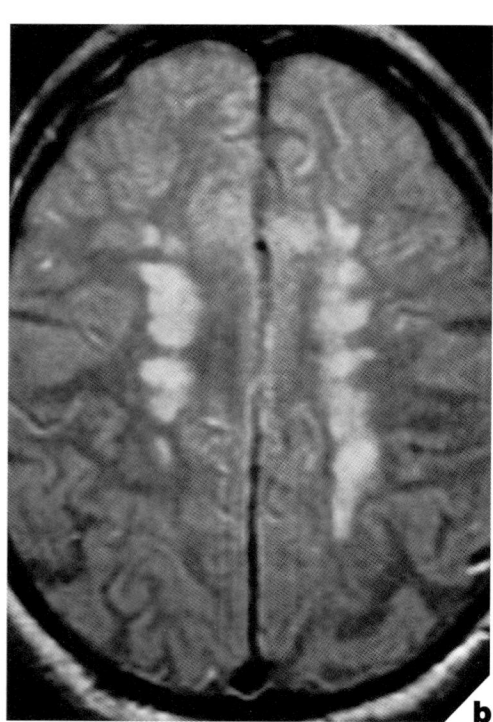

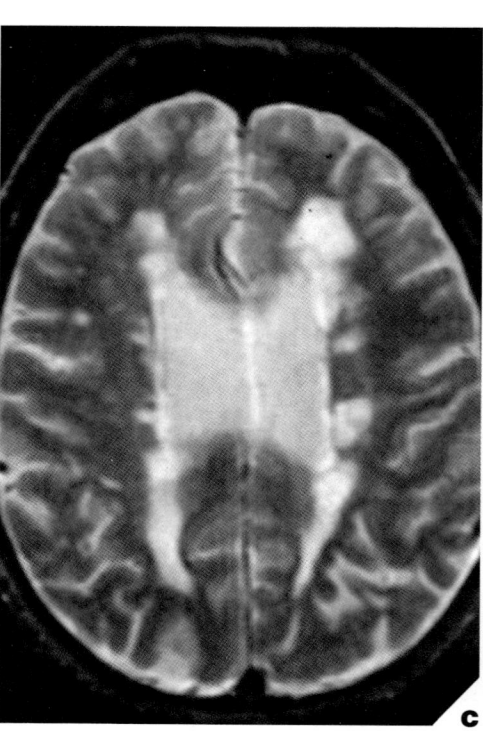

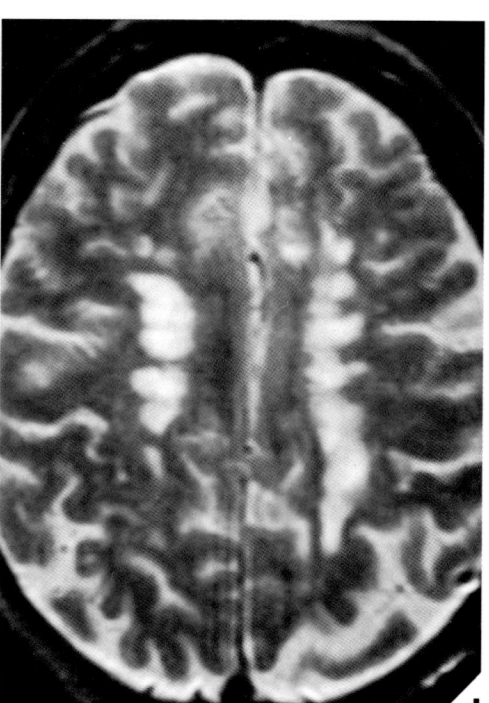

and has a shorter T2 and is thus relatively dark on T2-weighted images.

Traditionally, this group of diseases which have the common feature of myelin destruction have been categorized together. They are divided into two groups: (l) the *demyelinating* group, in which the myelin is initially normal but is subsequently destroyed by a pathologic process; and (2) the *dysmyelinating* group, in which an enzymatic disturbance, usually due to an inborn error of metabolism, causes the formation of abnormal myelin or interferes with myelin maintenance. White matter diseases are further categorized by their etiology; thus, multiple sclerosis, progressive multifocal leukoencephalopathy, degenerative microangiopathy, and adrenoleukodystrophy would be classified as idiopathic, infectious, vascular, and metabolic disorders, respectively.

The concept of white matter disease has the advantage of emphasizing prominent pathological and radiologic features shared by a diverse group of disorders. Many white matter disorders demonstrate small bright foci of T2 signal abnormality on MRI and/or broad areas of low attenuation on CT. The challenge then, is to identify, categorize, and differentiate these disorders from one another.

DEMYELINATING DISEASES

Multiple Sclerosis and its Variants

Multiple sclerosis (MS) is an idiopathic disorder, usually of young adults, which presents with a wide variety of sensorimotor neurological signs and symptoms that vary in time and space. Optic neuritis is a common early symptom. Transient motor weaknesses, altered sensorium, visual symptoms including internuclear ophthalmoplegia and altered affect are other common clinical manifestations. Laboratory findings upon CSF examination and electrodiagnostic studies are often very helpful in confirming the clinical diagnosis but the demonstration of plaques on MRI is particularly critical in making the diagnosis of MS.

MRI shows multifocal small bright foci of T2 signal abnormality which are typically periventricular (Fig. 2.1). Characteristic lesions are "ovoid" in shape, and their long diameters lie adjacent and perpendicular to the lateral margins of the lateral ventricles. MS plaques often occur in specific white matter tracts of the brain that are rarely affected by other lesions, particularly the corpus callosum and the middle cerebellar peduncles (Fig. 2.2). Although plaques do tend to predominate in the areas just described, they fre-

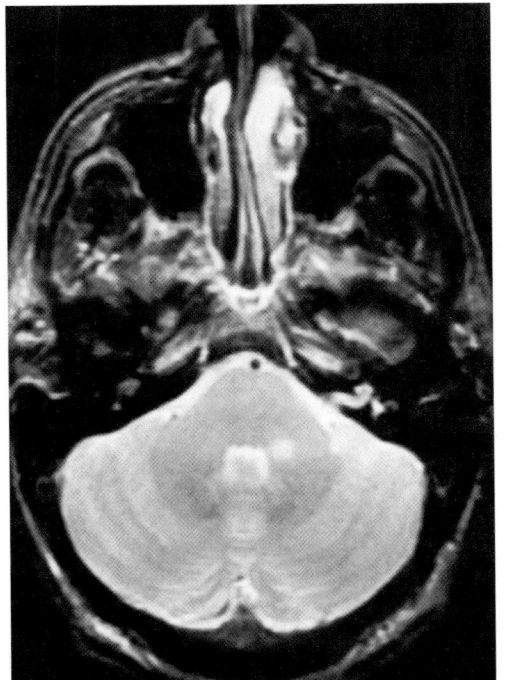

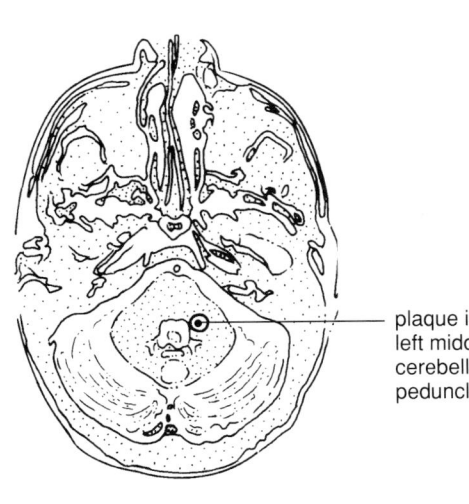

plaque in left middle cerebellar peduncle

Figure 2.2

Multiple sclerosis. Axial T2-weighted MR image in a patient with multiple sclerosis demonstrates a plaque in the left middle cerebellar peduncle (brachium pontis). This white matter tract is a common and characteristic location for multiple sclerosis. Other types of lesions rarely occur in this location.

White Matter Disease

quently occur throughout the brain (Fig. 2.3), including grey matter structures such as the basal ganglia or cerebral cortex. When these lesions occur in noncharacteristic locations, the diagnosis may still be consistent with, although not totally specific for, multiple sclerosis since vascular or other processes may have overlapping MR findings.

Old plaques may shrink and rarely, become invisible on MRI. Cerebral atrophy is a common finding with chronic multiple sclerosis.

MS plaques may enhance when Gadolinium or iodinated contrast material is administered intravenously; this typically occurs in active plaques and is due to breakdown of the blood–brain barrier. In some instances, there are multiple small enhancing white matter lesions that may be difficult to distinguish from metastases (Fig. 2.4). However, metastatic deposits tend to favor the grey matter/white matter junction, a helpful differentiating factor. Occasionally, an active plaque may become quite large and exert significant mass effect. It may then be difficult to dis-tinguish from a glioblastoma multiforme or other solitary neoplasm.

Acute disseminated encephalomyelitis (ADEM) (Fig. 2.5) represents a solitary episode of cerebral demyelination. It is due to an immune complex reaction and may follow measles, rubella or chicken pox infection. Postvaccination demyelination may follow immunization for rabies, influenza, or tetanus.

Infectious Disorders

Progressive multifocal leukoencephalopathy (PML) is a distinctively white matter lesion due to infection by the papova virus. Most of these infections are caused by the JC strain (a minority are caused by the simian virus 40 [SV 40] strain). Since the advent of the AIDS epidemic, PML has been seen with increasing frequency. Previously, it occurred almost exclusively as an opportunistic infection in patients with systemic malignancies or patients receiving immunosuppressive drugs for renal transplantation. MRI and CT

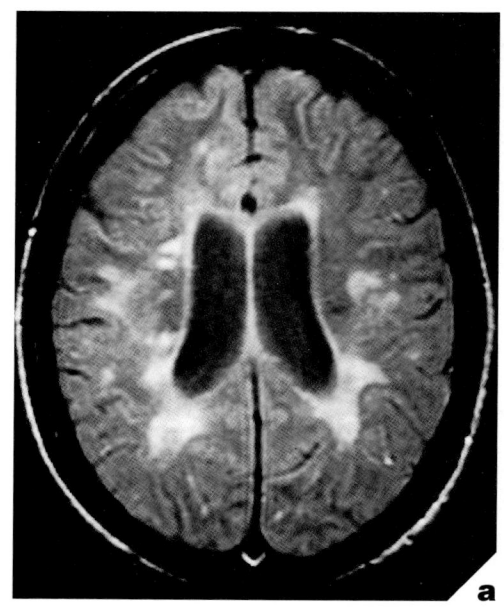 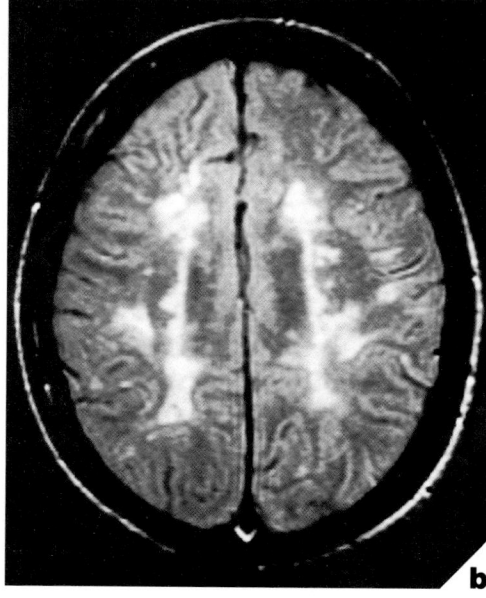 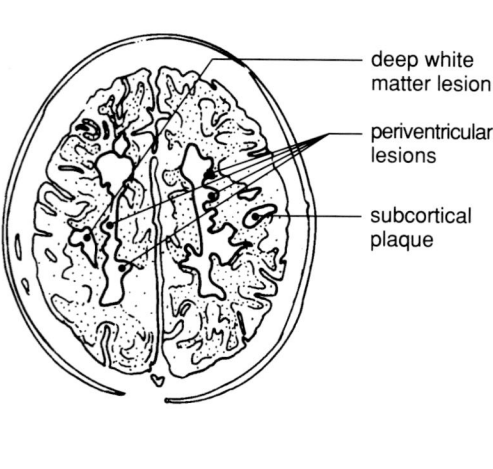

deep white matter lesion

periventricular lesions

subcortical plaque

Figure 2.3

*Multiple sclerosis. **a** Proton density and **b** more heavily T2-weighted MR images demonstrate characteristic "ovoid" periventricular lesions. However, there also are numerous plaques in the deep and subcortical white matter of both cerebral hemispheres. Such multiplicity of location is common and may hamper the differential diagnosis.*

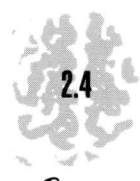

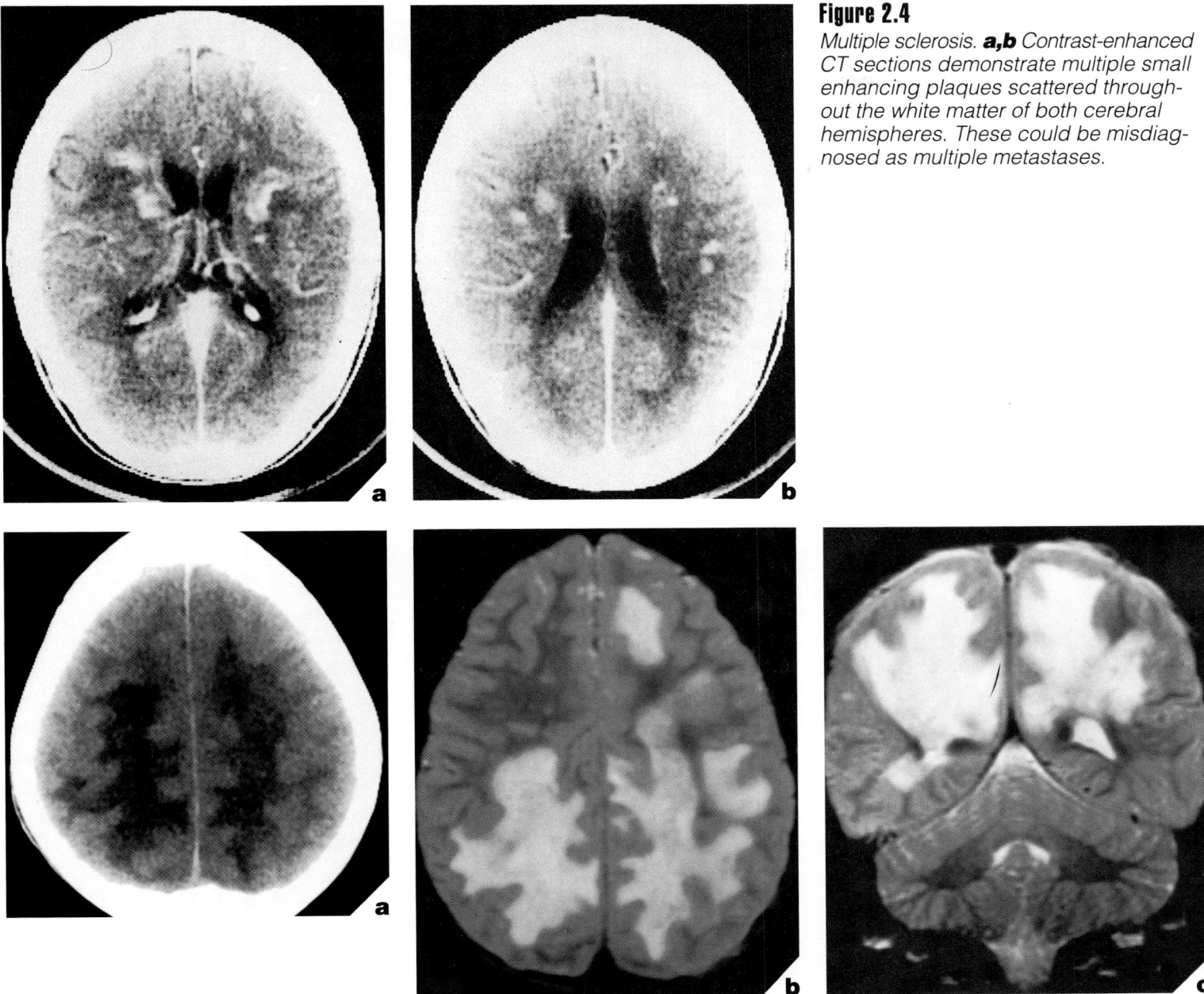

Figure 2.4

*Multiple sclerosis. **a,b** Contrast-enhanced
CT sections demonstrate multiple small
enhancing plaques scattered throughout the white matter of both cerebral
hemispheres. These could be misdiag-
nosed as multiple metastases.*

Figure 2.5

*Acute disseminated encephalomyelitis (ADEM). **a** CT and
b,c T2-weighted MR images show diffuse, homogeneous ab-*
*normality within the cerebral white matter in this patient with
postinfectious demyelination.*

show discrete or confluent areas of abnormality in the deep white matter. The lesions do not enhance and usually exert no mass effect (Fig. 2.6).

Numerous other infectious disorders may result in signal abnormality which exclusively or predominantly involves the cerebral white matter. Vasculitis associated with Lyme disease may cause small bright foci of T2 signal abnormality in the cerebral white matter (Fig. 2.7). Cysticercosis, bacterial abscesses and parasitic infestations may rarely predominate in the white matter. These infectious processes will be discussed in greater detail in Chapter 3.

Central pontine myelinolysis (CPM) is a disorder of unknown etiology characterized pathologically by widespread demyelination involving the basis pontis, and the tegmental structures. The condition is frequently associated with chronic alcoholism or the rapid correction of severe hyponatremia. The clinical picture varies from asymptomatic to coma. CPM should be suspected when an already seriously ill patient or alcoholic develops quadriplegia and signs of brainstem dysfunction. Computed tomography reveals characteristic low attenuation (Fig. 2.8) and MRI

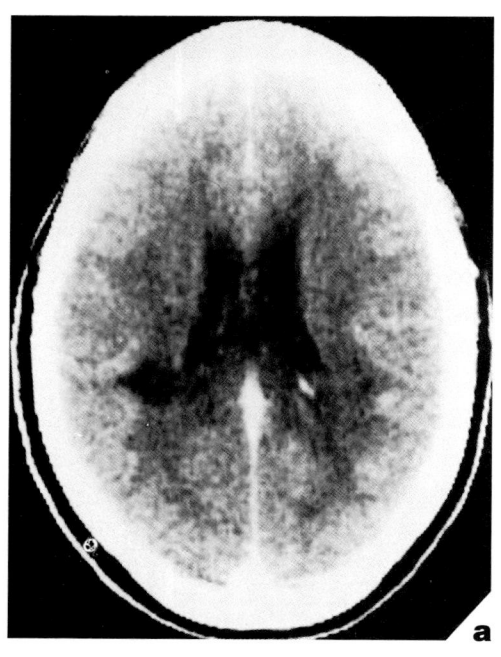
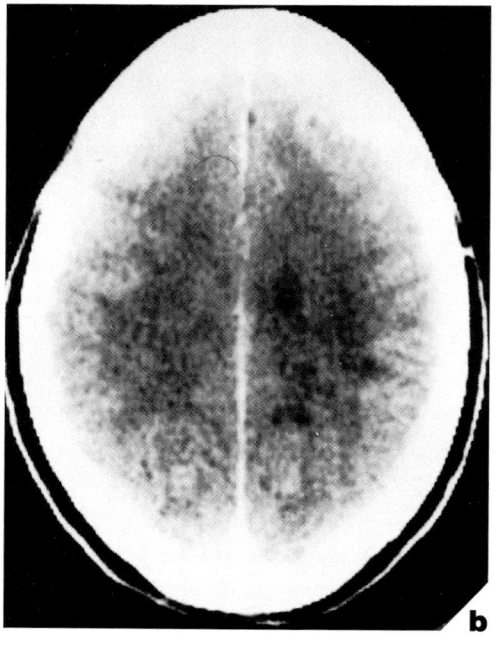

Figure 2.6
*Progressive multifocal leukoenceph-alopathy (PML). **a,b** Contrast-enhanced CT sections show small, nonenhancing areas of low attenuation in both central hemispheres.*

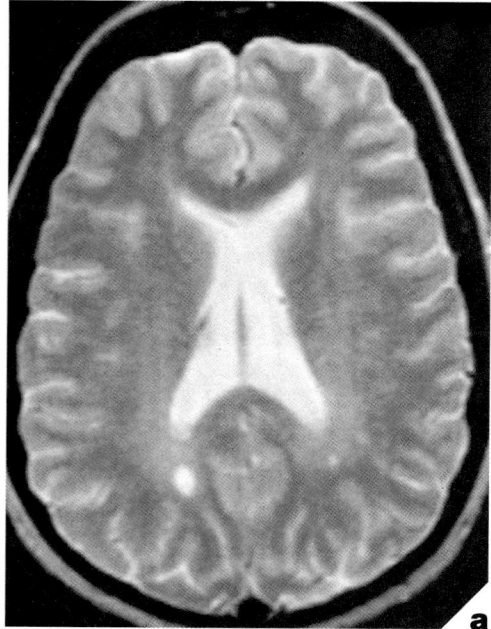
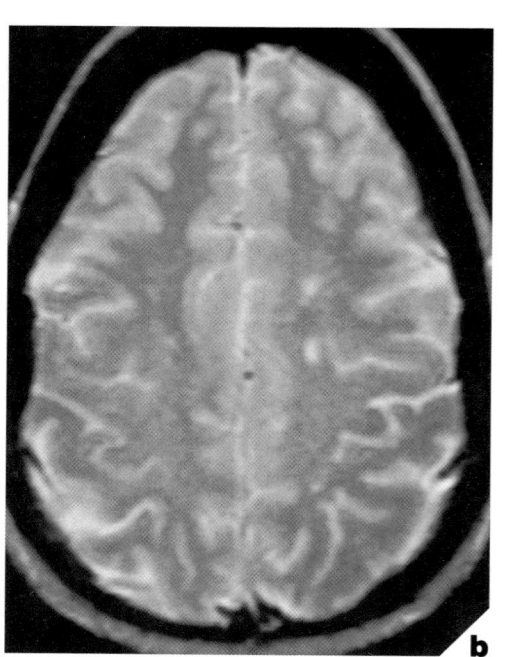

Figure 2.7
*Lyme disease. **a,b** T2-weighted MR images show multiple small bright foci of T2 signal abnormality in the deep white matter of both cerebral hemispheres.*

shows dark-T1, bright-T2 signal abnormality (Fig. 2.9) in the pons.

Ischemic Disorders

Most lesions in the cerebral white matter demonstrated on MRI are caused by vascular insults. Cerebral infarcts may be large and involve both grey and white matter structures, often in a wedge-shaped pattern and the infarct may follow the distribution of a cerebral artery. In contrast, an end-artery or arteriole occlusion may result in a lacunar infarct. Lacunes are usually smaller than 2 cm in diameter and typically occur in the cerebral white matter or in the basal ganglia. Lacunar infarcts may be the result of vascular thrombosis, embolic phenomena, or lipohyalinosis (fatty and fibrous infiltration) affecting nonanastomosing end-arteries. When acute, lacunar infarcts may be associated with some degree of edema and mass effect on the adjacent brain and ventricular system. Associated hemorrhage is rare. When old, lacunar infarcts may cavitate and fill with CSF.

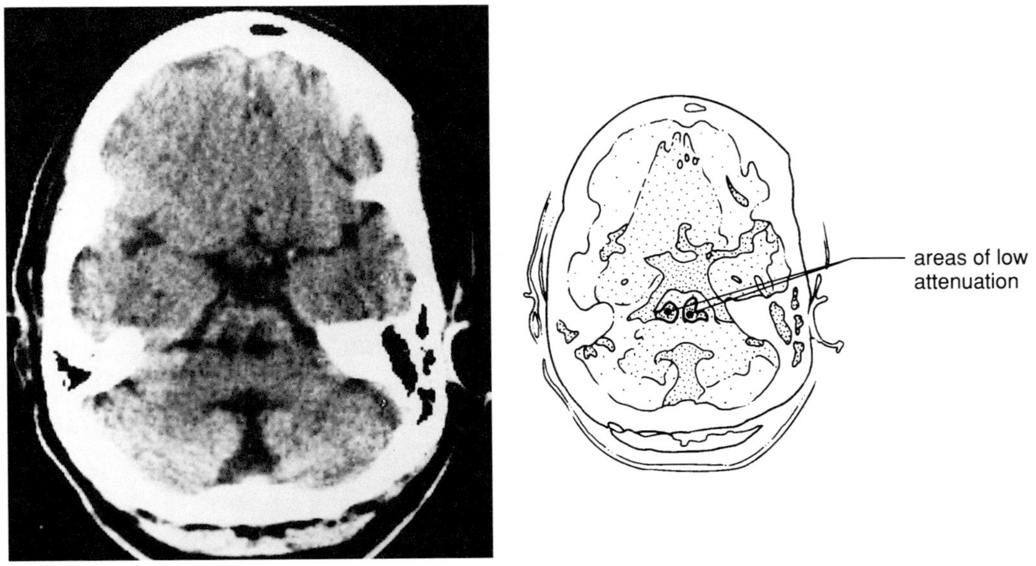

Figure 2.8
Central pontine myelinolysis (CPM). Axial CT reveals two low attenuation areas in the mid-pons.

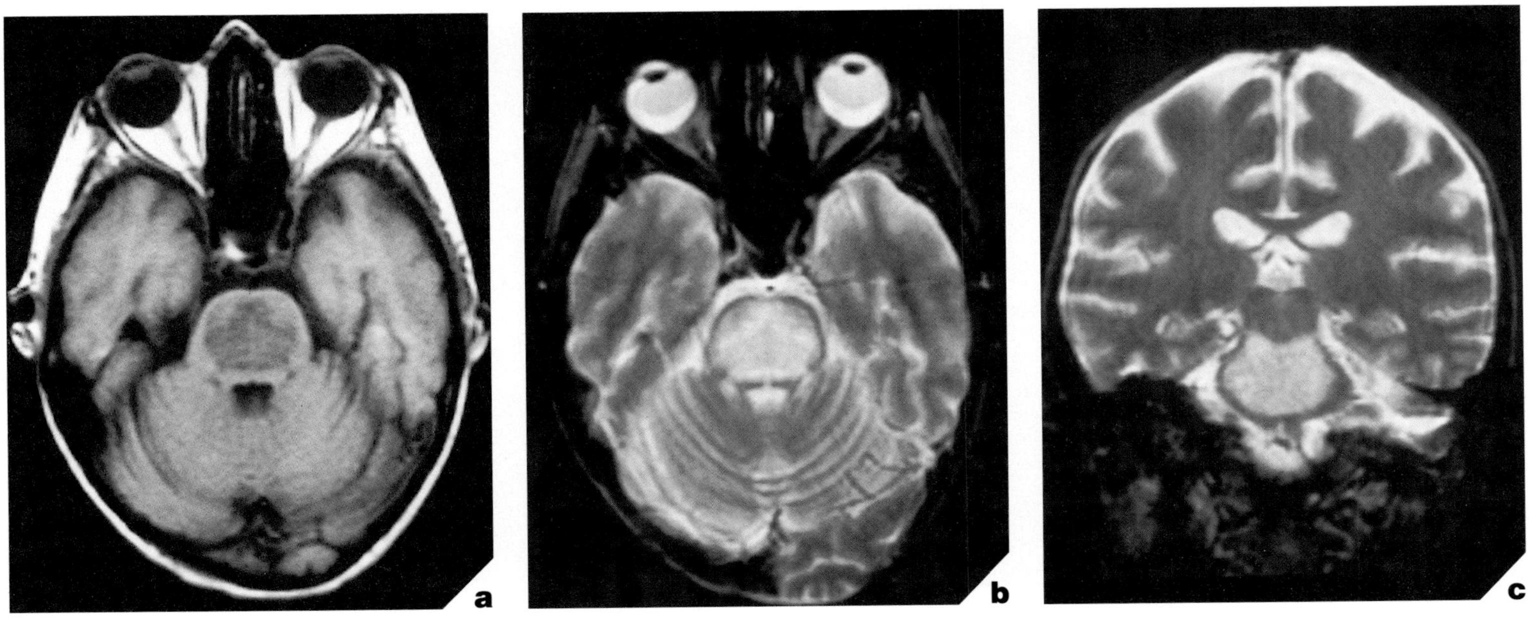

areas of low attenuation

Figure 2.9
*Central pontine myelinolysis (CPM). MRI demonstrates **a** dark-T1, **b,c** bright-T2 signal abnormality involving most of the pons.*

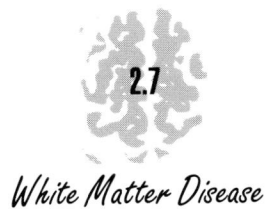

White Matter Disease

Risk factors for lacunar infarction include hypertension (most importantly), heart disease, diabetes mellitus, carotid artery disease, vasculitis, hypercoagulable states, and other conditions. CT shows a low dense, usually oval-shaped lesion. MRI often detects more lesions than CT, particularly in the middle and posterior fossa. Lacunar infarcts demonstrate dark-T1, bright-T2 signal characteristics.

Not all vascular-related insults to the brain result in frank cerebral infarction. Probably a majority of such insults result in degeneration of neurons and glia, without cavitation. Pathologically, there is gliosis, demyelination, myelin pallor, and the creation of small holes or sieves within the brain (etat criblet). These lesions are readily identified on MRI on the basis of their dark-T1, bright-T2 signal characteristics and are a common cause of the small bright foci seen on T2-weighted images in elderly patients (Fig. 2.10) (see Chapter 5). On CT these lesions are usually not identifiable individually, but demonstrate broad areas of periventricular low attenuation (Fig. 2.11). Superimposed true lacunar infarcts may be difficult to identify.

These lesions have been called degenerative microangiopathy, Binswanger's disease, subcortical arteriosclerotic encephalopathy, etc. Degenerative microangiopathy is a preferred general term since it does not imply an associated clinical state. Binswanger's disease should be reserved for describing a form of multiple-infarct dementia seen in hypertensive patients and caused by occlusive disease of the penetrating lenticulostriate and thalamoperforating arteries.

RADIATION AND CHEMOTHERAPY EFFECTS

Disseminated necrotizing leukoencephalopathy (DNL) is a severe demyelinating process which has been reported most often in patients receiving radiation and chemotherapy for leukemia. Methotrexate (given intrathecally or in high systemic doses) is the most commonly implicated drug. Similar findings may be seen in patients undergoing radiation therapy for primary and metastatic brain tumors (Fig. 2.12).

NEOPLASMS INVOLVING WHITE MATTER

Most primary and secondary neoplasms of the brain are not confined to the white matter and are usually readily distinguishable from true white matter disease. The vasogenic edema associated with neoplasms is often predominantly or exclusively within the white

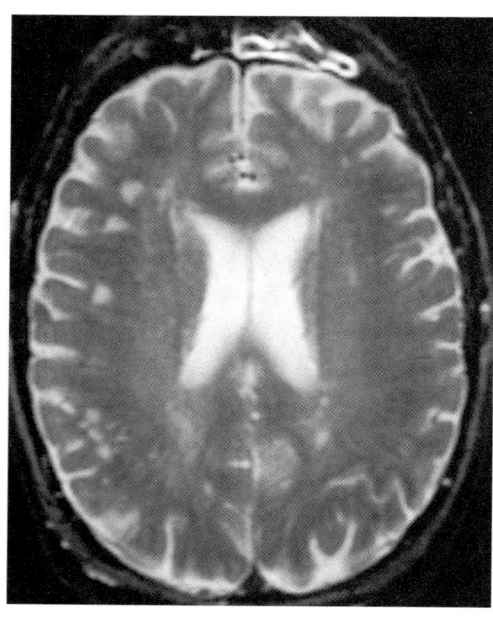

Figure 2.10
Degenerative microangiopathy. T2-weighted axial MR image shows several areas of subcortical hyperintensity. Note how the distribution differs from the periventricular predominance of multiple sclerosis plaques.

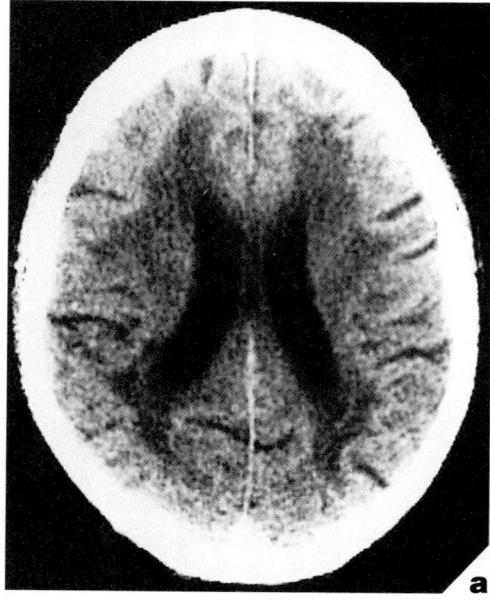
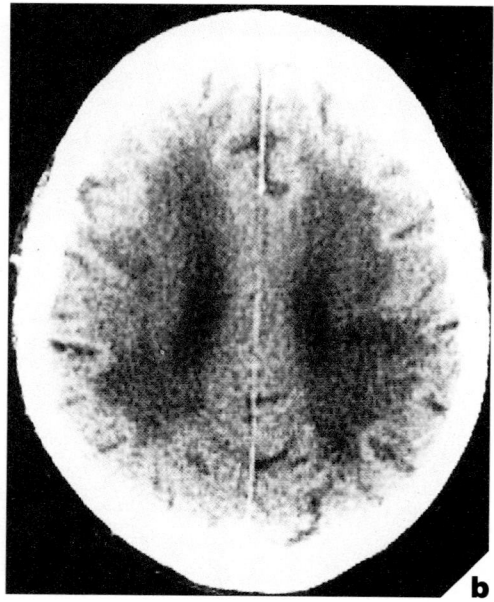

a

b

Figure 2.11
*Binswanger disease. **a,b** Broad areas of low attenuation are present in the white matter of both hemispheres in this demented, 63-year-old hypertensive man.*

matter, and has a distinctive appearance on CT and MRI (see Chapter 4). Due to hemodynamic factors, metastases occur most frequently at the cortico-medullary junction. CNS lymphoma may occasionally infiltrate exclusively through the white matter and mimic other white matter diseases on CT and MRI.

DYSMYELINATING DISEASES

Dysmyelinating diseases (leukodystrophies) are a result of failure to maintain or produce normal myelin. There are a large number of congenital disorders of metabolism which result in dysmyelinating disease. They typically present in infancy or early childhood with developmental retardation and other neurologic signs and symptoms. With few exceptions, they have similar CT and MR findings and thus close correlation with history, physical examination, and laboratory findings are necessary to distinguish these rare disorders from each other.

Adrenoleukodystrophy (Fig. 2.13) is a combination of Addison's disease and leukodystrophy. It is an X-linked recessive disorder and therefore affects mostly boys. The onset is typically between 4 and 8 years of age. Clinical signs of either the adrenal insuf-

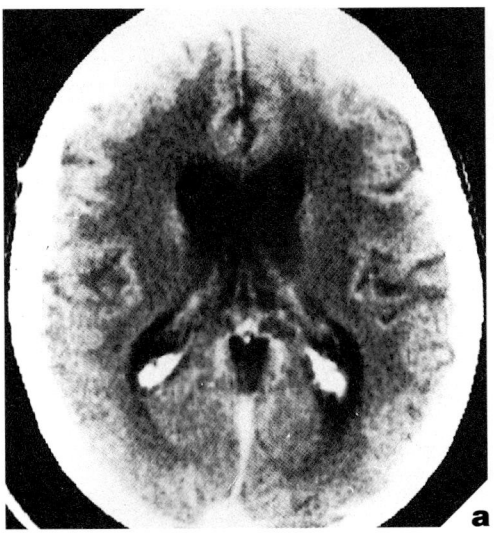 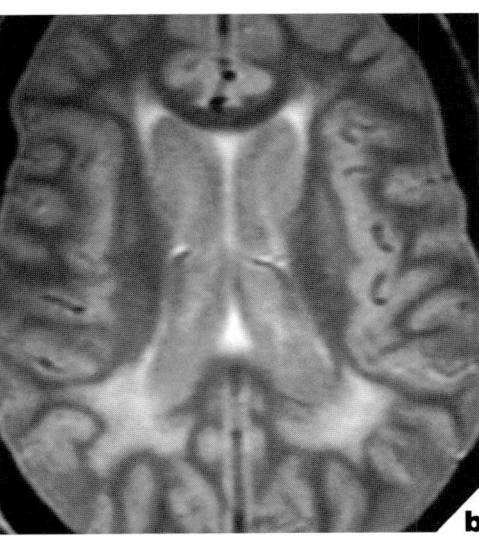 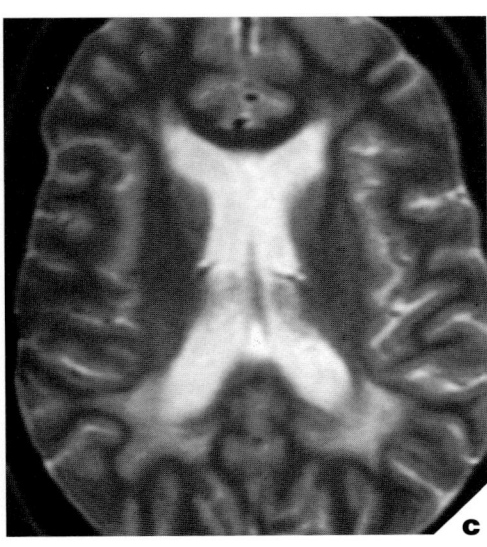

Figure 2.12
*Radiation necrosis. **a** Axial CT shows diffuse low attenuation in the hemispheric white matter bilaterally. **b,c** T2-weighted axial MR sections in another patient with radiation necrosis show high intensity in the deep frontal and periatrial white matter.*

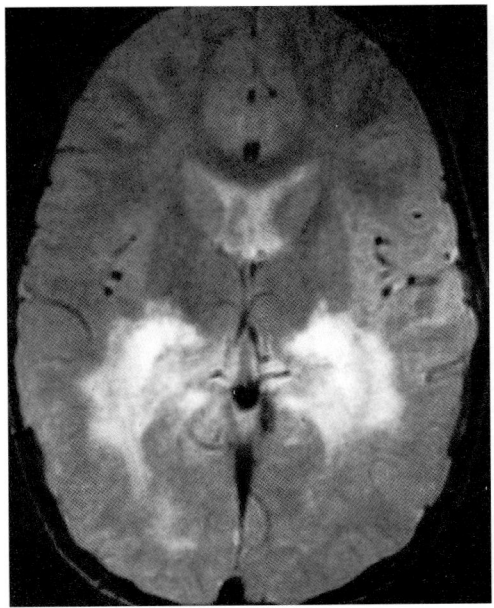 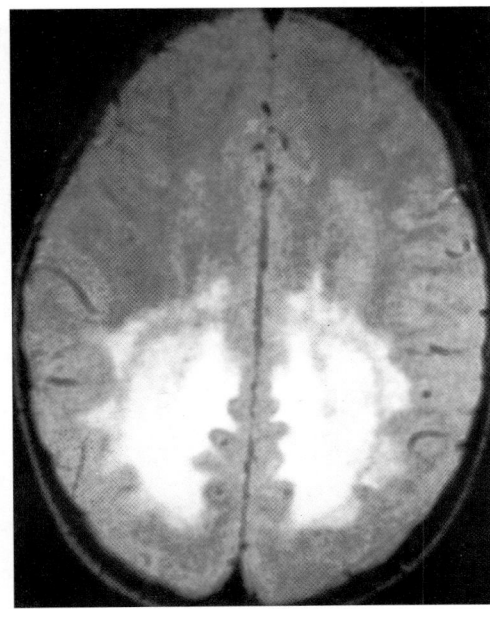

Figure 2.13
Adrenoleukodystrophy. T2-weighted axial images demonstrate symmetrical bright-T2 signal abnormality which is confined to the periatrial regions.

White Matter Disease

ficiency or the cerebral lesion may appear first. MRI shows confluent, symmetrical bright-T2 abnormal signal intensity in the white matter of the occipital and parietal lobes. CT shows low attenuation in these locations (Fig. 2.14). However, a sizable minority of patients show variations of this typical pattern.

Globoid cell leukodystrophy (Krabbe disease) is an autosomal recessive disorder usually manifested in infancy by generalized rigidity, loss of head control, vomiting, altered level of consciousness, and bouts of crying and hyperirritability. It is due to a deficiency of the enzyme galactocerebrosidase, which causes an accumulation of galactocerebroside, particularly in cerebral white matter. CT and MRI usually show symmetrical white matter lesions (Fig. 2.15).

Alexander's disease is a rare disease of unknown etiology. No familial incidence has been reported and no metabolic abnormality has yet been found. Widespread destruction of the white matter is usually most pronounced in the frontal regions (Fig. 2.16). The onset is in infancy with seizures, spasticity, and failure to thrive.

Canavan's disease (Fig. 2.17) is an autosomal recessive disease in which multiple small cysts develop in the white matter, either confined to the subcortical white matter, or diffuse. The brain develops a spongy

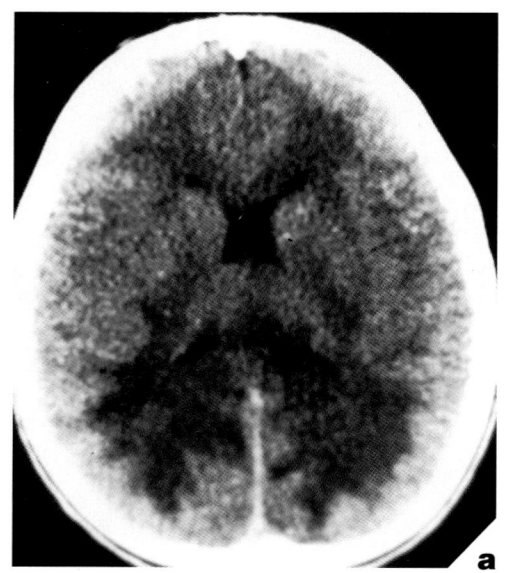
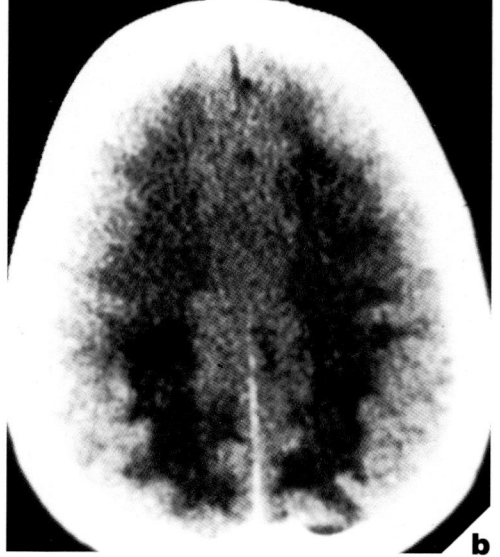

Figure 2.14

*Adrenoleukodystrophy (ALD). **a,b** CT images show decreased attenuation in the peri-atrial white matter.*

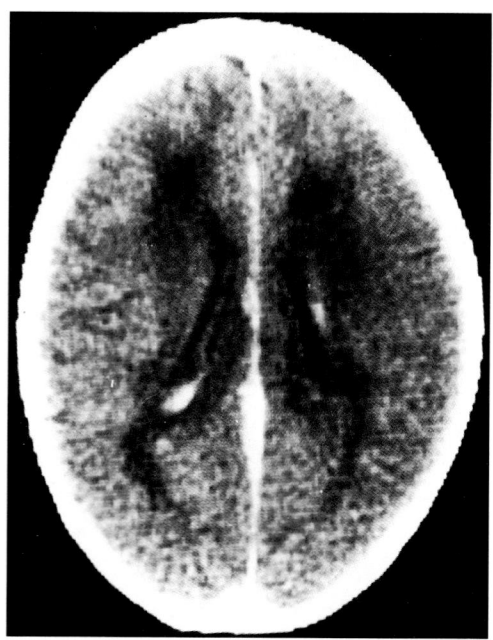
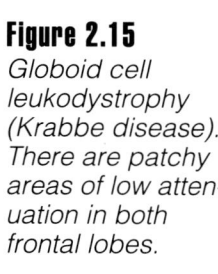

Figure 2.15

Globoid cell leukodystrophy (Krabbe disease). There are patchy areas of low attenuation in both frontal lobes.

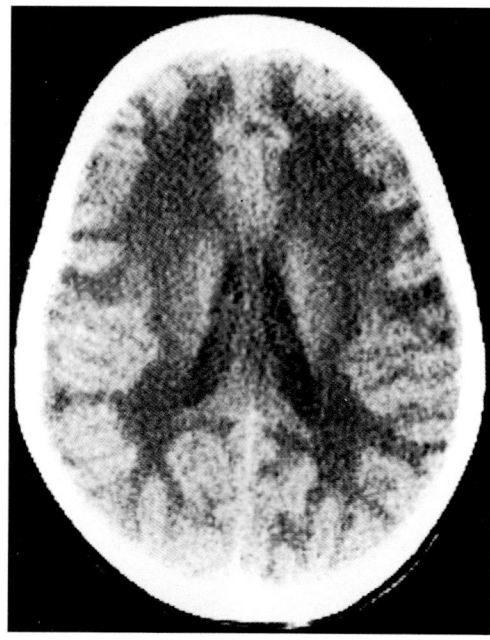

Figure 2.16

Alexander disease. Axial CT demonstrates severe, uniform low density throughout the white matter of both hemispheres. The changes are most severe in the frontal lobes.

consistency and this disorder has been termed *spongy degeneration.* As with the other leukodystrophies, bright-T2 signal is present in the involved portions of the brain. Canavan's and Alexander's diseases are the only two leukodystrophies that commonly cause megalencephaly.

Metachromatic leukodystrophy (Fig. 2.18) is one of the most common leukodystrophies; it is caused by decreased aryl sulfatase A. The white matter of the frontal lobes is typically involved prior to more posterior involvement. Characteristically, there is preservation of the subcortical "U" fibers.

Other metabolic disorders may result in leukodys-trophies. Lipid storage diseases may primarily affect cerebral white matter. Phenylketonuria has been shown to result in small bright foci of T2 signal abnormality in the peri-atrial white matter, bilaterally.

WALLERIAN DEGENERATION

Since its original description in the 19th Century by Waller of axonal degeneration in frog glossopharyngeal nerves, Wallerian degeneration is a term which has come to refer to any type of anterograde axonal degeneration in either the central or peripheral ner-

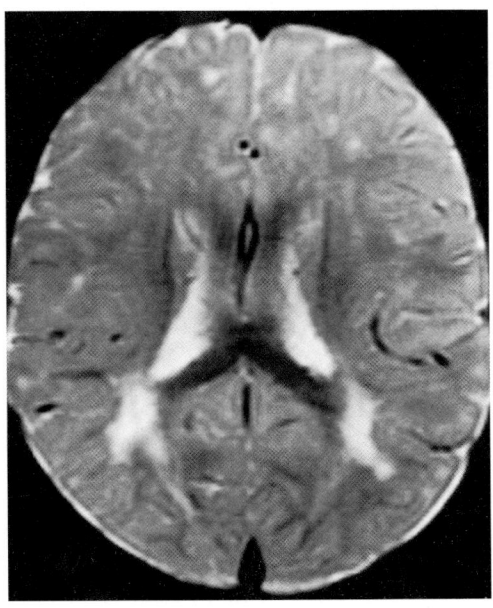
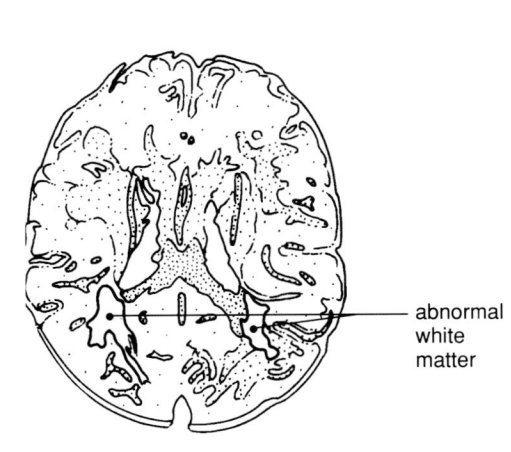

abnormal white matter

Figure 2.17
Canavan's disease. Axial T2-weighted image demonstrates symmetrical bright signal abnormality in the deep white matter adjacent to the postero-lateral angles of the lateral ventricles.

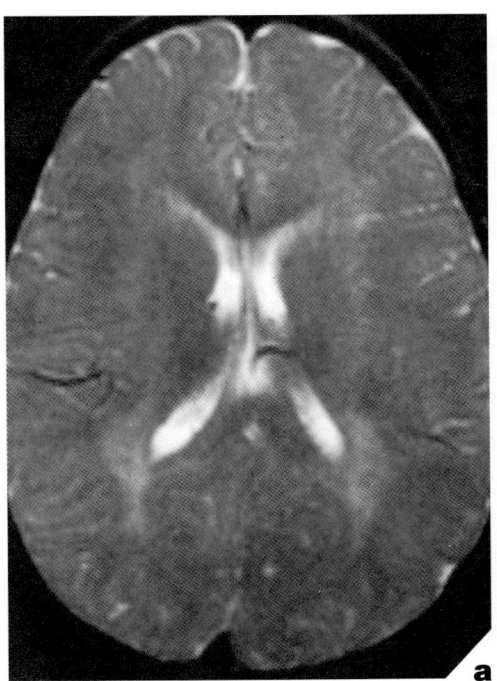
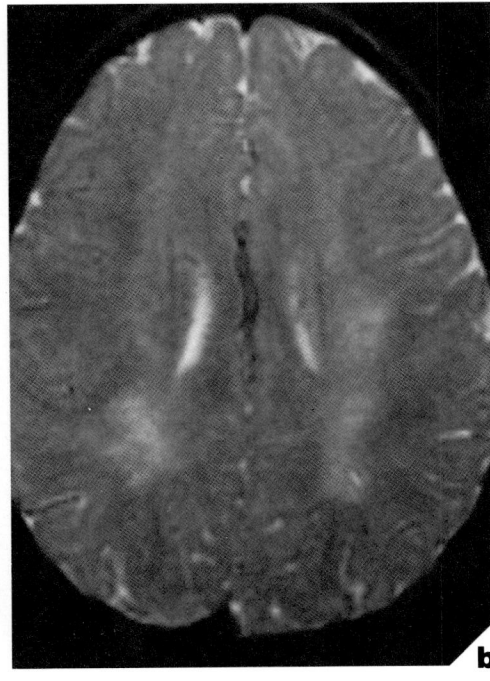

a b

Figure 2.18
Metachromatic leukodystrophy.
a,b *Axial T2-weighted images show symmetrical areas of slightly increased T2 signal in the deep white matter of both cerebral hemispheres. Note the preservation of normal signal intensity in the subcortical white matter ("u" fibers); this is characteristic of metachromatic leukodystrophy.*

White Matter Disease

vous system. It is most commonly seen in the brain following large, hemiplegic cerebral infarcts which involve the motor strip. A band of dark-T1, bright-T2 signal abnormality can be seen to originate in the infarct and extend caudally in the distribution of the cortico-spinal tract (Fig. 2.19). After 1 to 2 years, there is tissue loss visible in the ipsilateral pons, medulla and cerebral peduncle which may be visualized by CT or MRI (Fig. 2.20).

During the earliest phase of Wallerian degenera-

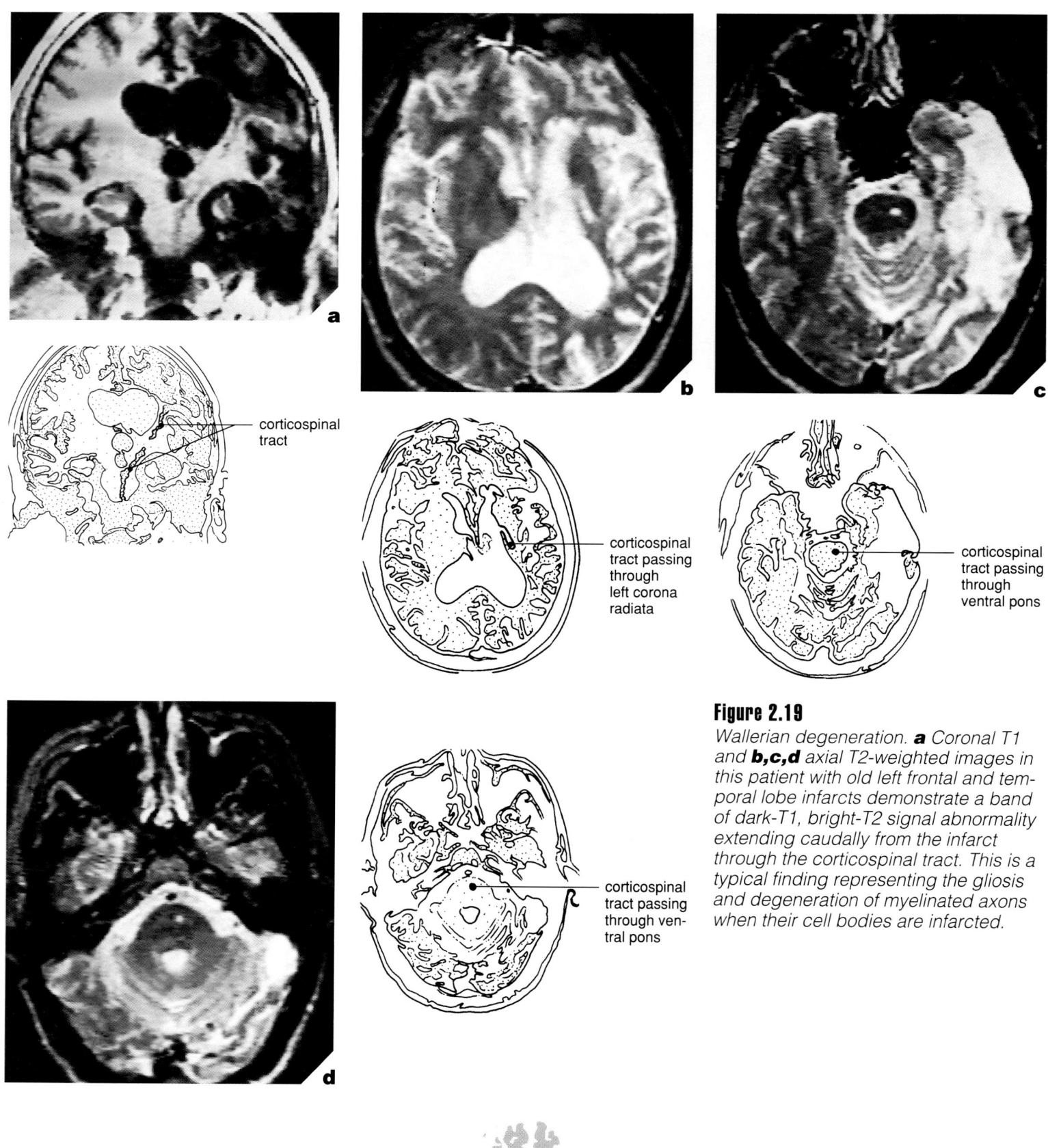

Figure 2.19

*Wallerian degeneration. **a** Coronal T1 and **b,c,d** axial T2-weighted images in this patient with old left frontal and temporal lobe infarcts demonstrate a band of dark-T1, bright-T2 signal abnormality extending caudally from the infarct through the corticospinal tract. This is a typical finding representing the gliosis and degeneration of myelinated axons when their cell bodies are infarcted.*

corticospinal tract

corticospinal tract passing through left corona radiata

corticospinal tract passing through ventral pons

corticospinal tract passing through ventral pons

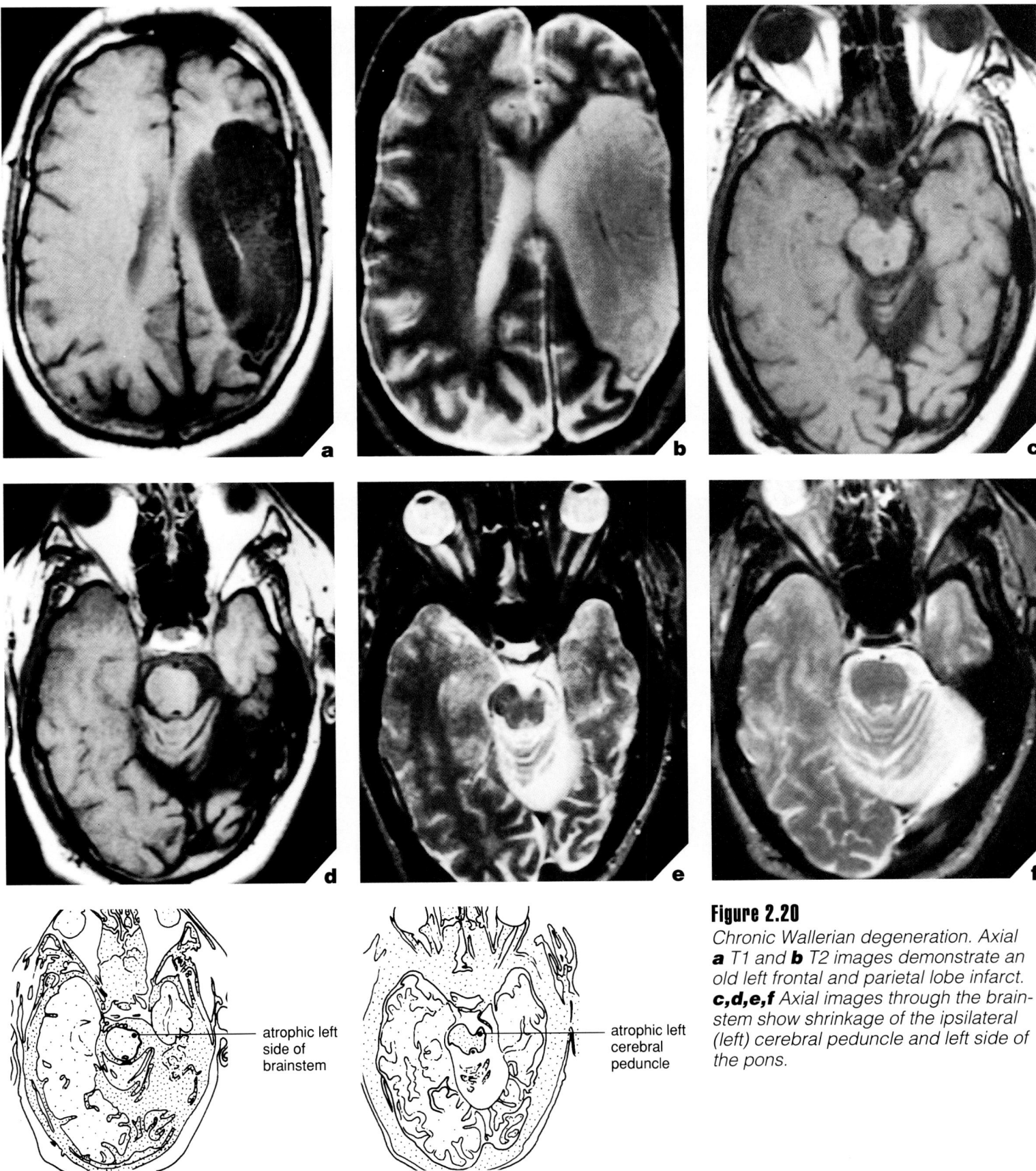

Figure 2.20

*Chronic Wallerian degeneration. Axial **a** T1 and **b** T2 images demonstrate an old left frontal and parietal lobe infarct. **c,d,e,f** Axial images through the brainstem show shrinkage of the ipsilateral (left) cerebral peduncle and left side of the pons.*

atrophic left side of brainstem

atrophic left cerebral peduncle

2.13

White Matter Disease

tion, the signal abnormality is dark on proton density weighted images (Fig. 2.21). This is believed to reflect specific, dynamic pathological processes occurring in the axons and their sheaths. The myelin proteins are first removed, leaving the myelin lipids intact. These are relatively hydrophobic and result in dark proton density signal abnormality until the myelin lipids themselves are removed, usually by 10 weeks.

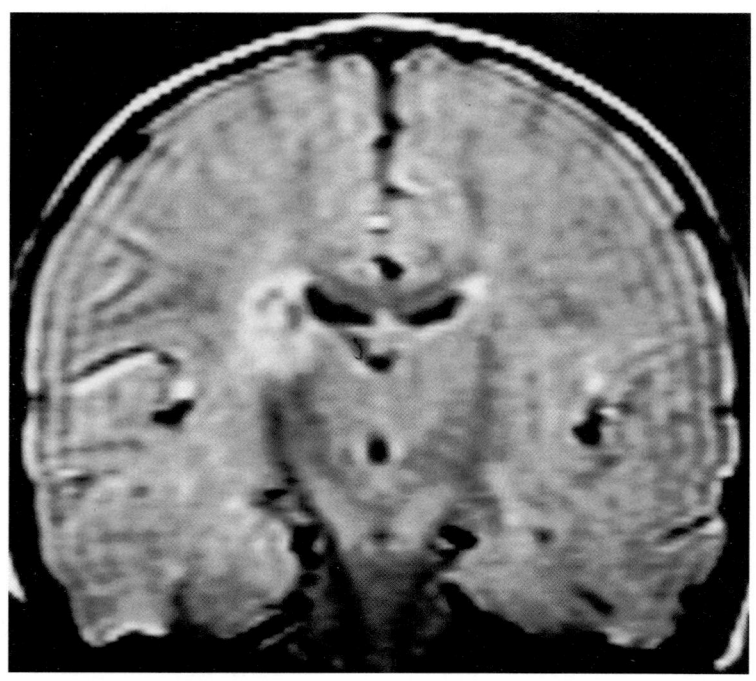
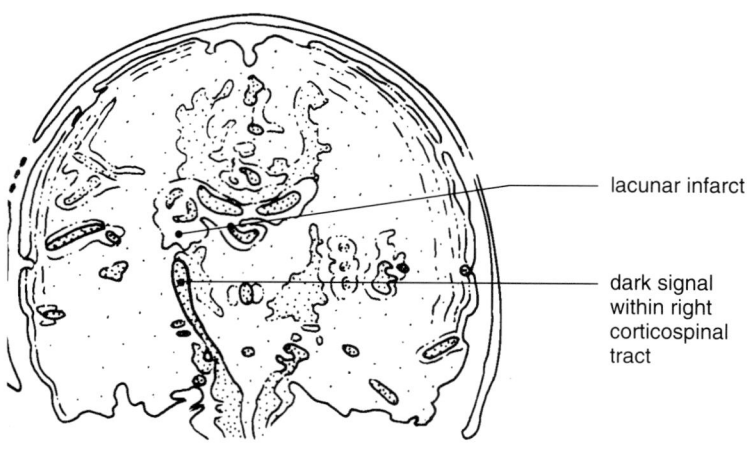

Figure 2.21

Subacute Wallerian degeneration. Proton density coronal MR image of a patient with a lacunar infarct in the right corona radiata also demonstrates dark signal abnormality in the right corticospinal tract due to destruction of the myelin proteins, leaving the myelin lipids intact. Compare with the normal slightly dark signal in the left corticospinal tract.

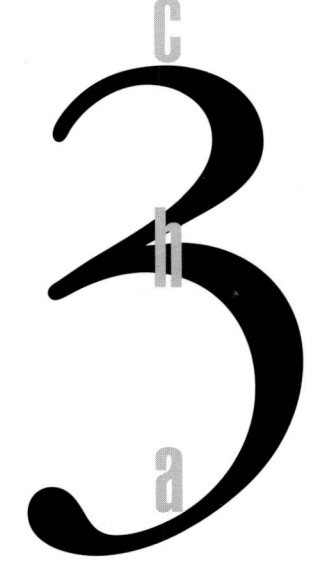

Chapter 3

Intracranial Inflammatory
Disease

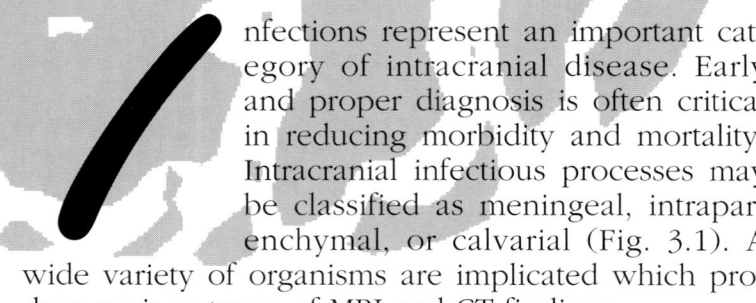

*i*nfections represent an important category of intracranial disease. Early and proper diagnosis is often critical in reducing morbidity and mortality. Intracranial infectious processes may be classified as meningeal, intraparenchymal, or calvarial (Fig. 3.1). A wide variety of organisms are implicated which produce various types of MRI and CT findings.

MENINGEAL INFECTIONS

Meningitis

Meningitis usually refers to inflammation of the piarachnoid (leptomeninges). Diagnosis depends on clinical signs and symptoms and examination of the cerebrospinal fluid. The role of imaging studies is to detect complications such as an associated parenchymal infection, empyema or hydrocephalus, and to evaluate the temporal bone and paranasal sinuses as potential sources of infection.

Pyogenic (or purulent) meningitis is often diffuse in nature because of the absence of anatomic barriers to its spread. The most common etiologic organisms are *Hemophilus influenzae*, *Neisseria meningitidis*, and *Streptococcus pneumoniae*, which in the aggregate account for 80% to 90% of all cases. In neonates, the main causes are *Streptococcus agalactiae* (Group B streptococcus) and *Escherichia coli*.

In the early stages, CT scans may be normal. MRI and noncontrast CT may reveal obliteration of the basal cisterns due to the presence of isodense pus. Contrast-enhanced CT and MRI often reveal abnormal enhancement of the meningeal surfaces of the brain (Fig. 3.2). This is due to the presence of vascular granulation tissue and incompetent blood–brain barrier in meningeal neovessels. However, this is not a consistent finding and its absence should not exclude the diagnosis of meningitis.

The main differential diagnosis is leptomeningeal carcinomatosis. This can have an appearance similar to that of meningeal infection on MRI and CT. Meningitis and carcinomatosis can usually be distinguished on clinical grounds and by examination of the CSF.

Granulomatous meningitis is characterized by a thick exudate in the subarachnoid space, most commonly at the base of the brain. The outlet foramina of the fourth ventricle are frequently blocked, result-

Classification of Intracranial Infections

I. Meningeal infections
   A. Meningitis (leptomeningitis)
   B. Subdural empyema
   C. Epidural empyema

II. Brain parenchymal infections
   A. Encephalitis
   B. Cerebritis
   C. Cerebral Abscess
   D. Ventriculitis

III. Osteomyelitis of the skull

Figure 3.1

Classification of intracranial infections.

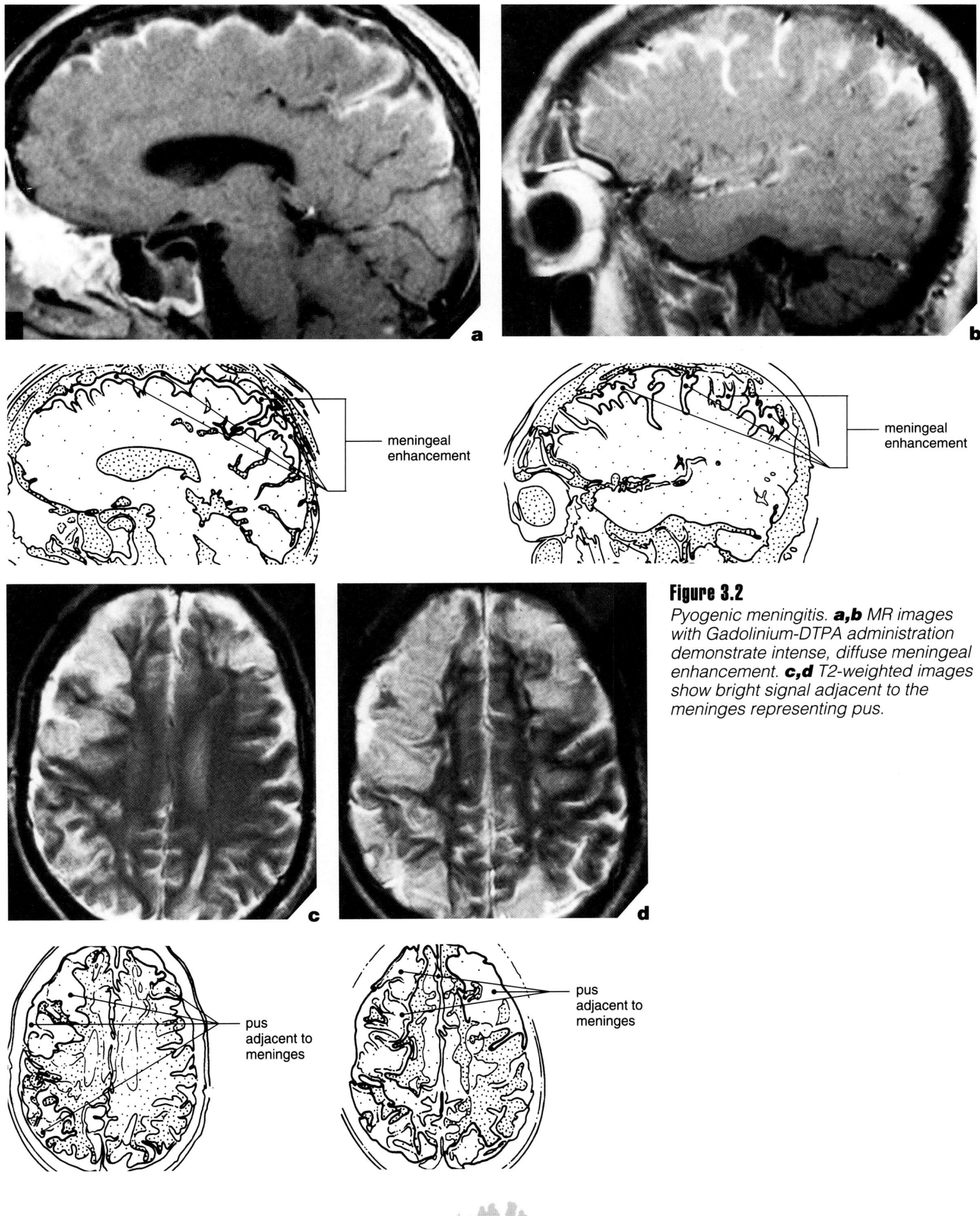

Figure 3.2

*Pyogenic meningitis. **a,b** MR images with Gadolinium-DTPA administration demonstrate intense, diffuse meningeal enhancement. **c,d** T2-weighted images show bright signal adjacent to the meninges representing pus.*

meningeal
enhancement

meningeal
enhancement

pus
adjacent to
meninges

pus
adjacent to
meninges

a

b

c

d

3.3

ing in hydrocephalus. The most common organism is *Mycobacterium tuberculosis* (Fig. 3.3). Occasionally, the thick granulomatous exudate may calcify (Fig. 3.4). Fungi that can cause granulomatous meningitis include coccidioides, cryptococcus, and blastomyces. Sarcoidosis may also cause a granulomatous meningitis.

Neonatal meningitis, particularly when associated with dehydration, may result in dural sinus thrombosis, usually involving the superior sagittal sinus (Fig. 3.5). The triangular-shaped clot is seen in silhouette by surrounding contrast material; this is termed the "delta" sign.

SUBDURAL EMPYEMA

Subdural empyema represents an infection of the subdural space. It most commonly arises from adjacent infection such as meningitis, paranasal sinusitis, otitis media, mastoiditis, calvarial osteomyelitis, wound infection, or penetrating trauma. The subdural space probably becomes infected by direct extension or by local hematogenous spread via bridging veins and dural venous sinuses. Often, a subdural empyema represents a neurosurgical emergency, as the infective process can spread readily to the cortical veins causing thrombophlebitis, venous infarction, intracranial hypertension, and death. Antibiotic therapy alone is usually ineffective; craniotomy, with removal of the infected membranes, may be necessary. However, subdural empyemas need to be distinguished from subdural effusions that are often associated with neonatal meningitis. It is difficult to reliably distinguish subdural empyema from subdural effusion unless the etiology of the subdural collection and the clinical history is known.

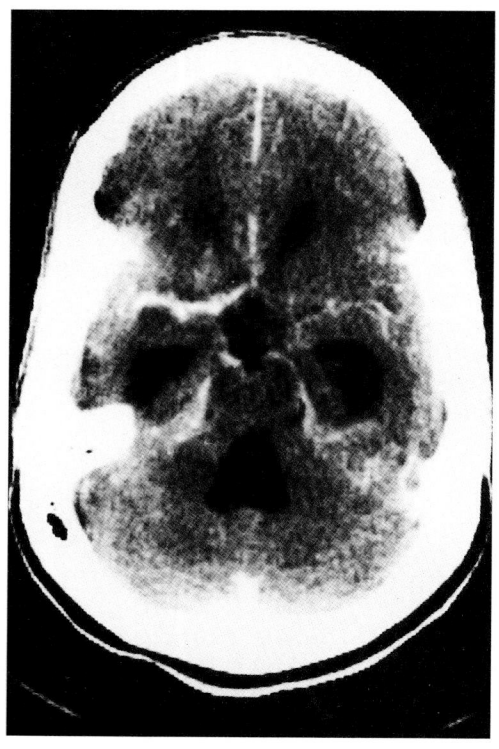

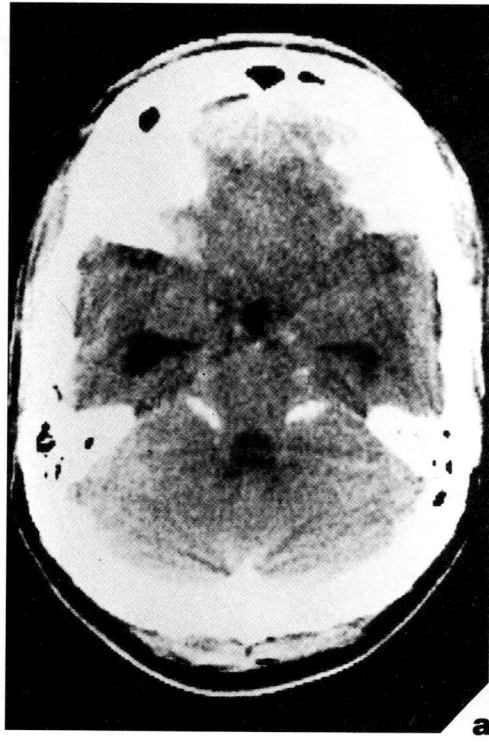

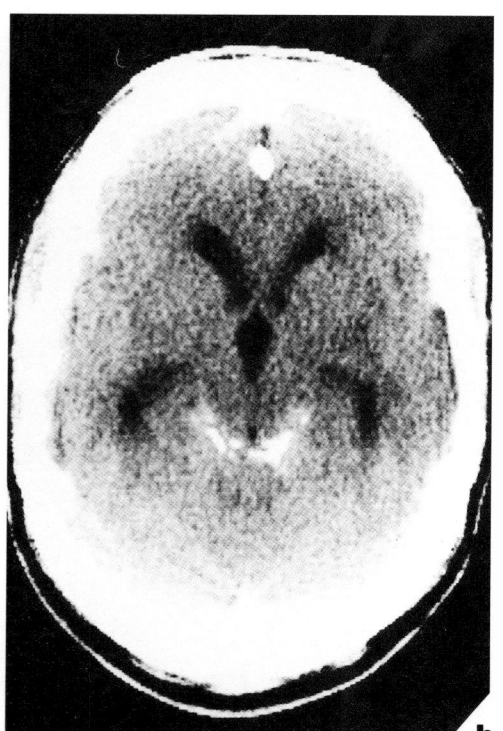

Figure 3.3

Tuberculous meningitis. A contrast-enhanced CT scan shows abnormal enhancement of the basal cisterns. There is hydrocephalus secondary to obstruction of the outlet foramina of the fourth ventricle.

Figure 3.4

Coccidioidal meningitis. **a,b** *Noncontrast scans show extensive calcifications in the basal cisterns.*

MRI and CT usually show a crescentic area of decreased attenuation adjacent to the inner table of the skull with an enhancing inner membrane. Coexistent subdural effusion and subdural empyema may occur (Fig. 3.6) and show different densities or signal intensities.

Epidural abscess or empyema usually develops as a sequelae of adjacent paranasal sinusitis, calvarial osteomyelitis, penetrating trauma, surgery, otitis media, mastoiditis, or congenital skull defects; occasionally,

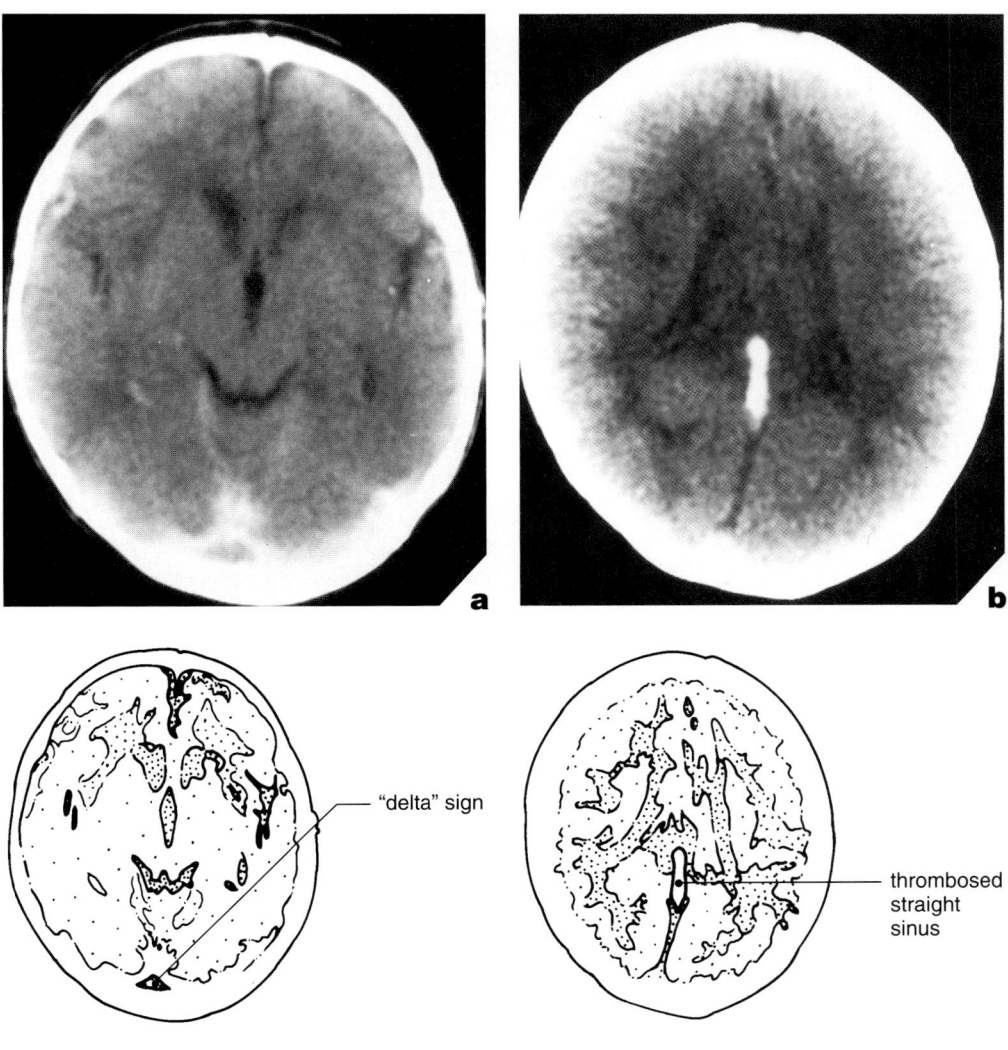

"delta" sign

thrombosed straight sinus

Figure 3.5

*Dural sinus thrombosis. **a** Contrast-enhanced CT scan in this 4-month-old with Hemophilus influenzae meningitis shows a triangular-shaped filling defect in the superior sagittal sinus (the "delta" sign).*

*This is characteristic of superior sagittal sinus thrombosis. **b** Unenhanced CT image shows increased density in the straight sinus representing thrombus.*

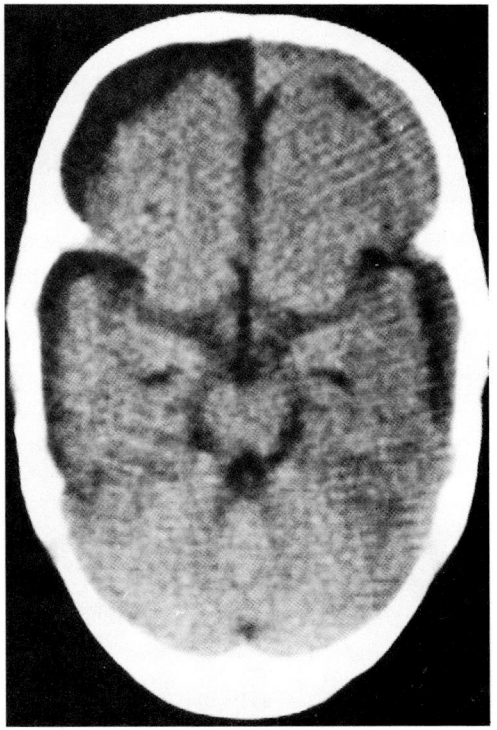

Figure 3.6

Subdural empyema and contralateral subdural effusion. A noncontrast CT section in a 6-month-old boy with Hemophilus influenzae meningitis and an abnormally increasing head circumference shows bilateral subdural fluid collections. On the right, the fluid is of CSF density; on the left, the collection is considerably denser. Pus was aspirated from the left side. Aspiration of the right subdural space yielded clear fluid consistent with a "sympathetic" effusion.

it is due to hematogenous spread. MRI and CT show an extra-axial collection adjacent to the inner table of the skull with an enhancing margin (Fig. 3.7). Unlike subdural empyema, the collection has a convex inner margin pointing toward the brain. These usually represent surgical emergencies.

PARENCHYMAL INFECTIONS OF THE BRAIN

Encephalitis

Encephalitis refers to a diffuse inflammatory process involving the brain. The disorder is usually either viral or toxic/metabolic in origin. Many viruses can cause central nervous system infection, including herpes simplex, cytomegalovirus, rubella and varicella (Fig. 3.8), among others.

Herpes simplex encephalitis (HSE) is the most common cause of nonepidemic encephalitis in the United States. HSE is caused by the type 1 virus in adults and the type 2 virus in the fetus and neonate. In type 2 HSE, early intrauterine infection results in severe brain destruction, microcephaly, and intracranial calcifications, similar to other TORCH syndromes.

When acquired in the neonatal period, HSE can result in extensive brain necrosis. MRI and CT reflect the pathological findings of diffuse cavitation of the brain, contrast enhancement of the cortical surfaces, and progressive cystic encephalomalacia and cortical calcification (Fig. 3.9).

In adults, infections with type I Herpes virus result in a necrotizing, rapidly disseminating encephalitis with a predilection for the temporal lobes (Fig. 3.10). CT shows low-attenuation zones involving the temporal and frontal lobes, frequently with abnormal contrast enhancement of the related brain surfaces (especially the nearby sylvian fissures). MRI shows signal abnormalities and abnormal enhancement in the same regions.

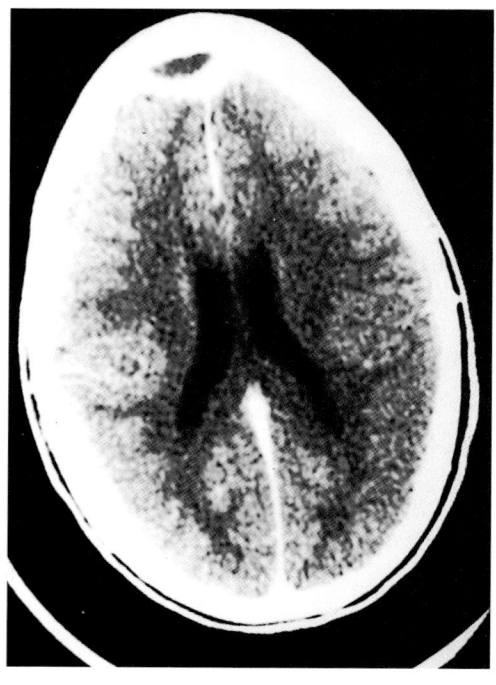 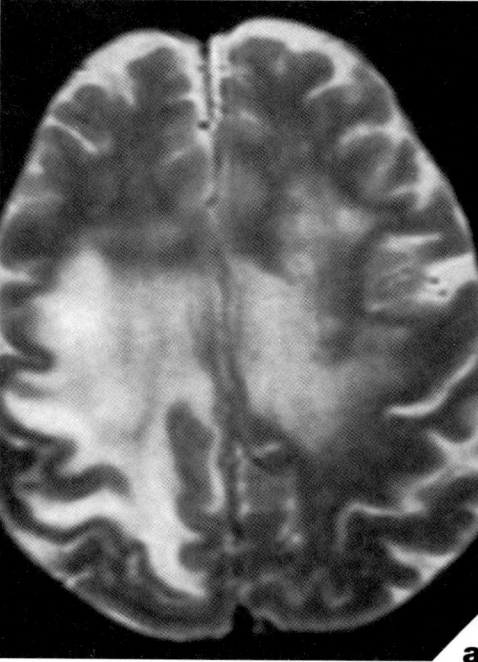 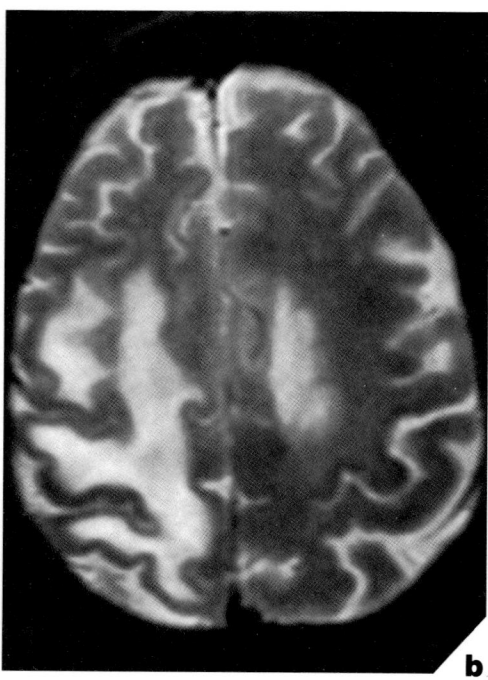

a

b

Figure 3.7

Epidural empyema. A contrast-enhanced CT in a 14-year-old boy with pansinusitis shows an epidural pus collection in the mid-frontal region. There is marked enhancement of the underlying meninges.

Figure 3.8

*Encephalitis. **a,b** DNA–viral encephalitis demonstrates diffuse areas of bright-T2 signal abnormality, largely confined to the white matter of the right parietal and posterior frontal lobes.*

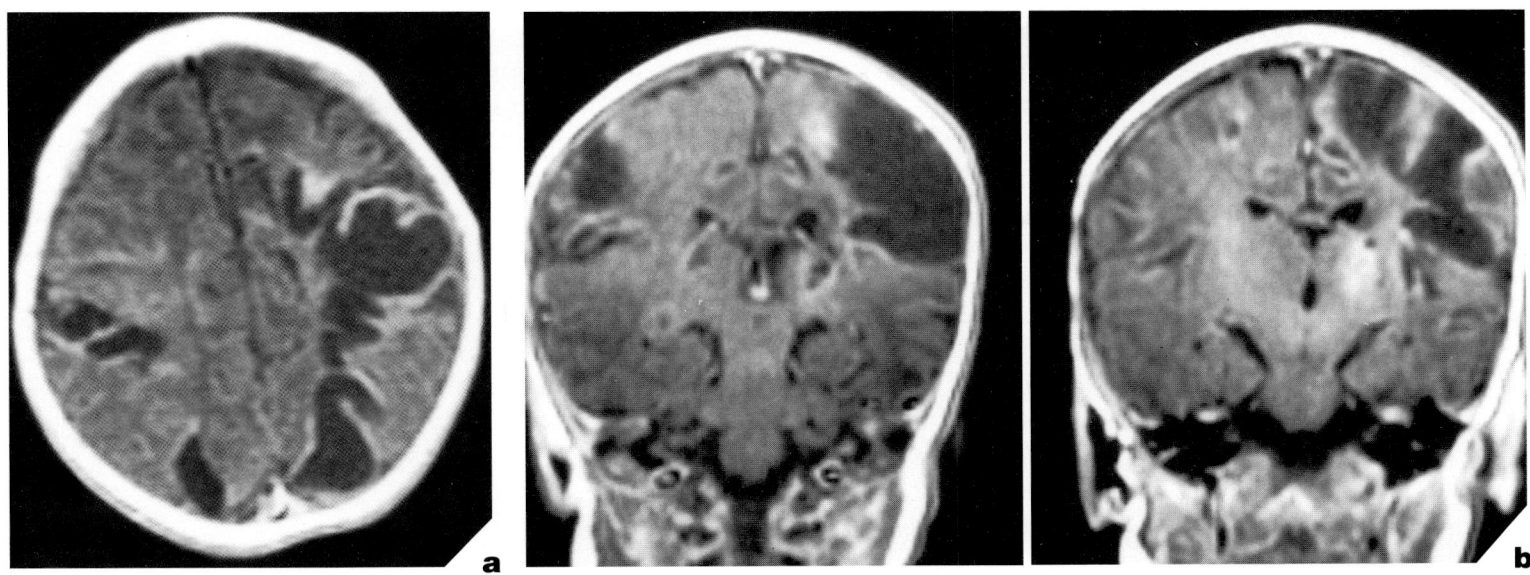

Figure 3.9

*Neonatal Herpes encephalitis. Gadolinium-enhanced **a** axial and **b** coronal T1-weighted MR images show extensive cavitary necrosis of brain parenchyma and areas of enhancement in this patient with resolving type II Herpes simplex encephalitis.*

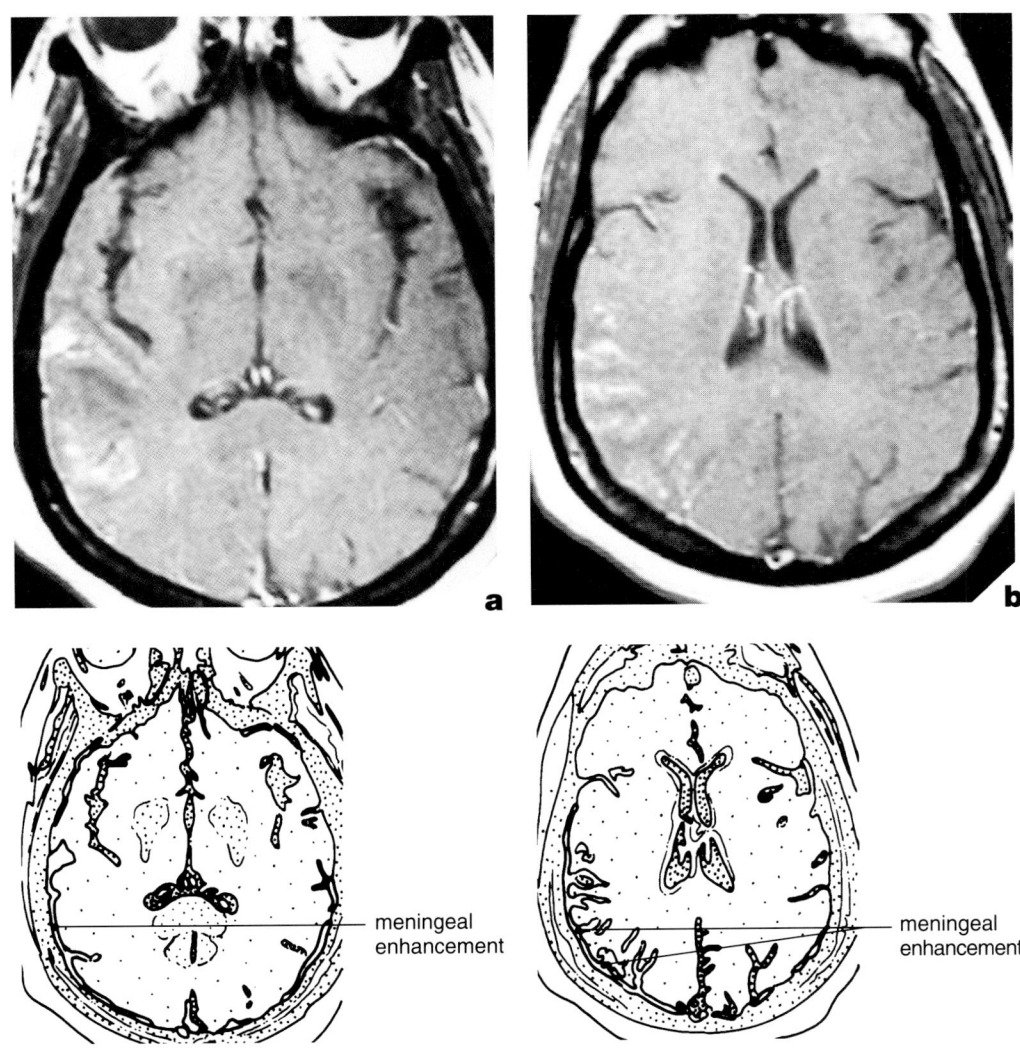

Figure 3.10

*Herpes encephalitis. **a,b** Contrast-enhanced axial MR scans show abnormal meningeal and parenchymal enhancement in the temporal and parietal lobes.*

meningeal
enhancement

meningeal
enhancement

Cerebritis and Cerebral Abscess

Cerebritis represents the earliest stage of a focal inflammatory process involving the brain. It is usually due to bacteria or fungi, and may progress to abscess formation. CT usually shows low density in the involved areas of the brain; often there is irregular contrast enhancement without sharply defined rings (Fig. 3.11). MRI demonstrates bright-T2 signal abnormality in the involved portion of the brain and is more sensitive to the early pathological changes than CT.

If not successfully treated medically, cerebritis is followed by a stage of encapsulation, which in turn leads to formation of a well-defined abscess wall (Fig. 3.12). Sequential CT or MRI scans can determine whether the process resolves with antibiotic therapy or progresses to form an abscess. In differentiating an abscess from an area of cerebritis, the most reliable finding is the presence of a well-formed ring configuration on contrast-enhanced MRI or CT (Fig. 3.13). Abscess cavities frequently have thinner walls medially than laterally, ostensibly because inflammation of white matter is associated with less tissue reaction than inflammation of gray matter (Fig. 3.14).

A granulomatous abscess may be quite irregular

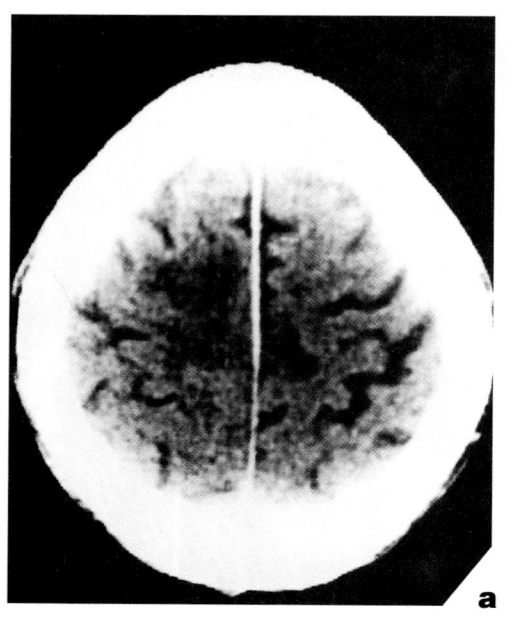
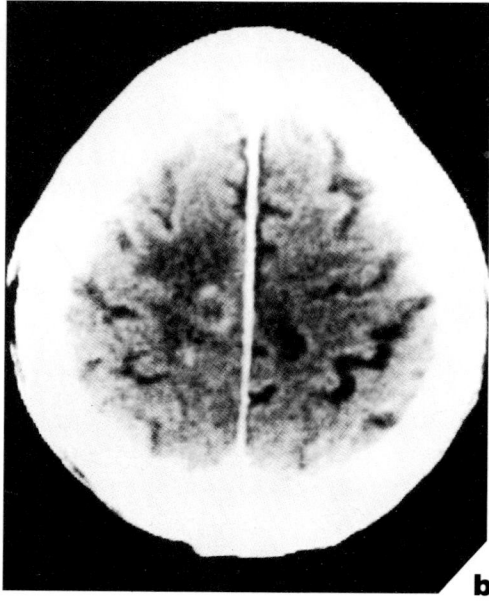

a

b

Figure 3.11

Cerebritis and cerebral abscess. **a** *Noncontrast CT scan demonstrates a poorly marginated area of decreased attenuation in the white matter of the right centrum semiovale;* **b** *following the intravenous administration of contrast medium, an ill-defined area of enhancement is demonstrated.*

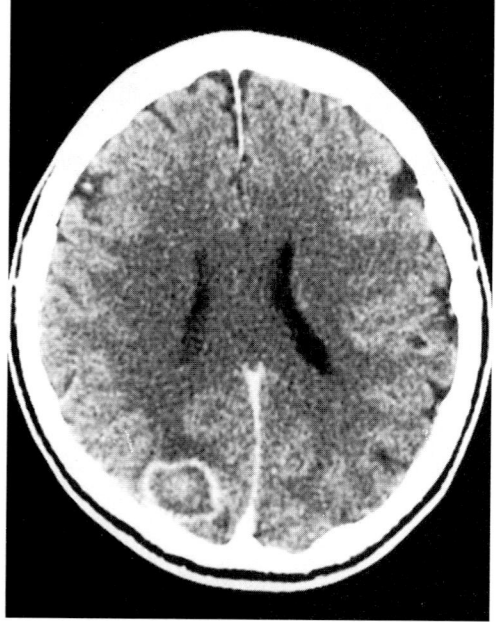
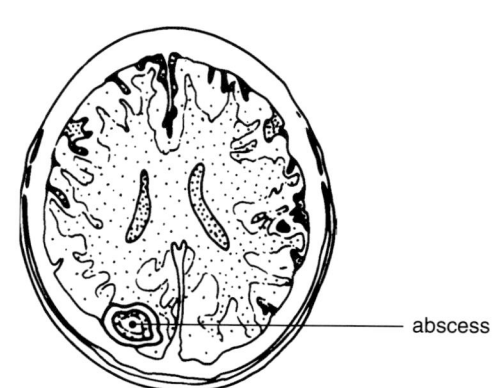

abscess

Figure 3.12

Cerebral abscess. Axial CT scan with contrast demonstrates a well-defined ring enhancement in this cerebral abscess caused by Staphylococcus Aureus.

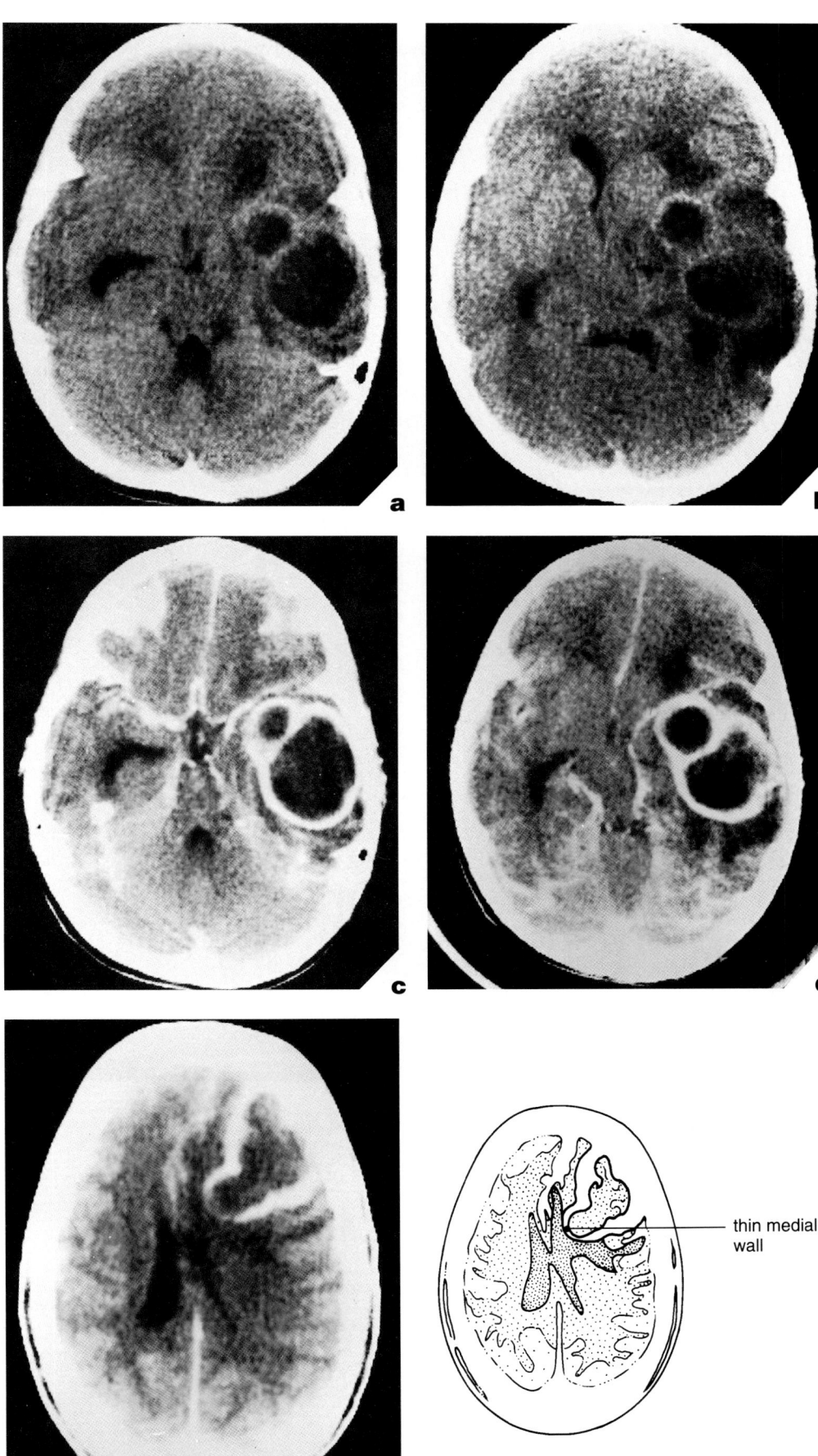

Figure 3.13

*Cerebral abscess. **a,b** Noncontrast and **c,d** contrast-enhanced scans show a multiloculated abscess in the left temporal lobe. There is marked mass effect with evidence of both transtentorial and subfalcine herniation. Well-formed rings of contrast enhancement are demonstrated.*

Figure 3.14

Cerebral abscess. The abscess wall is thinner medially than laterally, probably because there is less tissue reaction on the white matter side of the cavity than on the cortical side.

thin medial wall

and nodular and may resemble a neoplasm. Sarcoidosis (Fig. 3.15) represents one such form of this type of granulomatous collection. Tuberculosis may give rise to multiple small nodular lesions secondary to hematogenous dissemination—a striking appearance resembling miliary tuberculosis of the lungs (Fig. 3.16).

Disseminated intraparenchymal histoplasmosis (Fig. 3.17) often produces multiple ring-enhancing lesions scattered throughout the brain. These generally have little surrounding edema but are often initially confused with metastatic disease.

Occasionally, small punctate calcifications are discovered in the brain parenchyma (Fig. 3.18) without evidence of surrounding edema or mass effect. As in the chest, such calcifications are frequently a result of old granulomatous disease that may have been subclinical.

A variety of parasitic diseases affect the brain. Cysticercosis is caused by the pork tapeworm *Taenia solium*. In the United States, it is seen most often in immigrants and travelers from Latin America and the Caribbean. CT and MRI show multiple small, usually at least partly calcified, cysts scattered throughout the brain parenchyma and subarachnoid space. Toxoplasmosis is the most common opportunistic CNS infection in patients with the acquired immunodeficiency syndrome (AIDS) (Fig. 3.19). Congenital

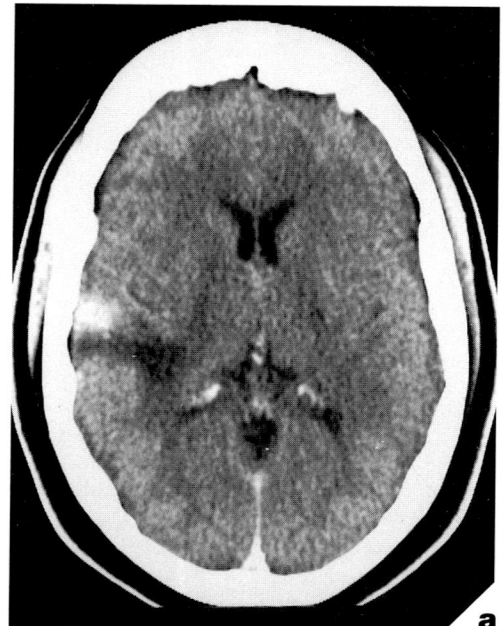

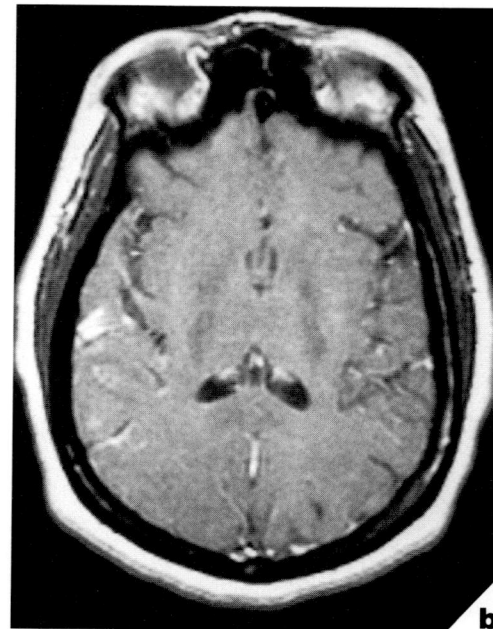

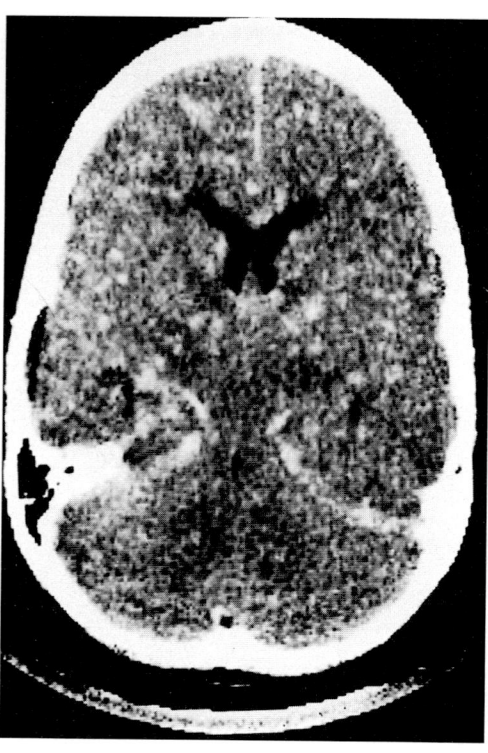

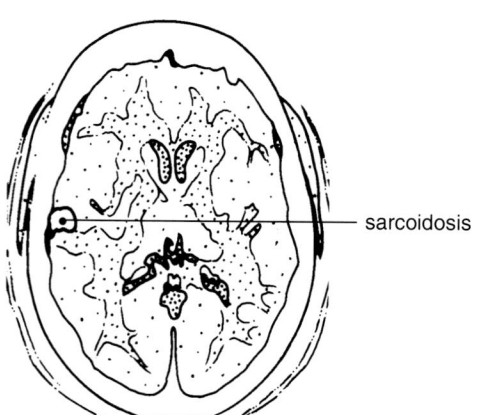

sarcoidosis

Figure 3.15
*Tuberculous abscess. **a** Contrast-enhanced CT and **b** MRI show nodular enhancement in the right sylvian region. This was proven at surgery to represent a tuberculous abscess. The patient had no evidence of pulmonary disease.*

Figure 3.16
"Miliary" tuberculosis. Numerous tiny areas of contrast enhancement are scattered throughout the brain.

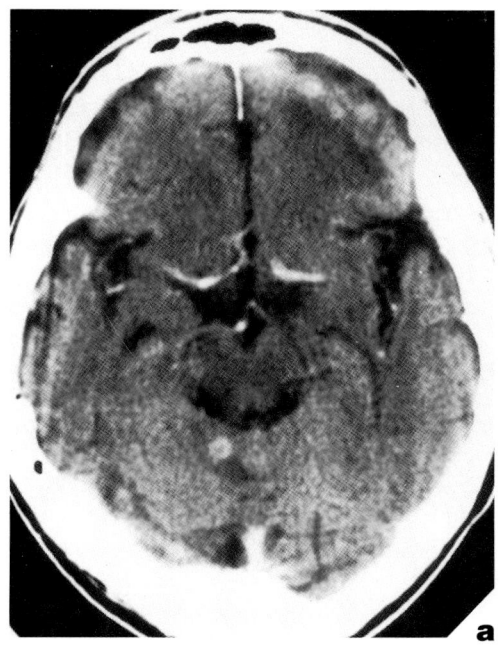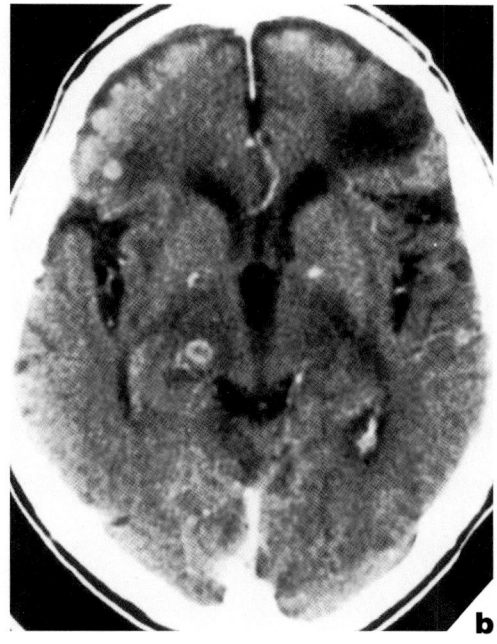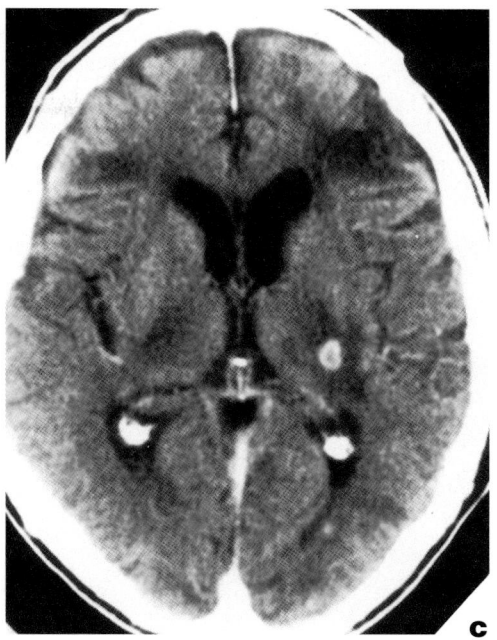

Figure 3.17

*Histoplasmosis of the brain. **a,b,c** Contrast-enhanced CT sections demonstrate numerous ring- and nodular-enhancing histoplasmosis abscesses. These are small and have rela-* *tively little surrounding edema. Incidentally demonstrated is an old watershed infarct in the left frontal lobe.*

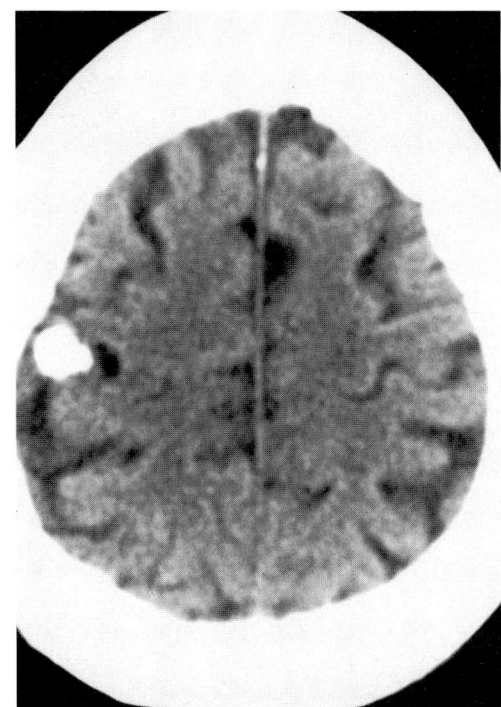

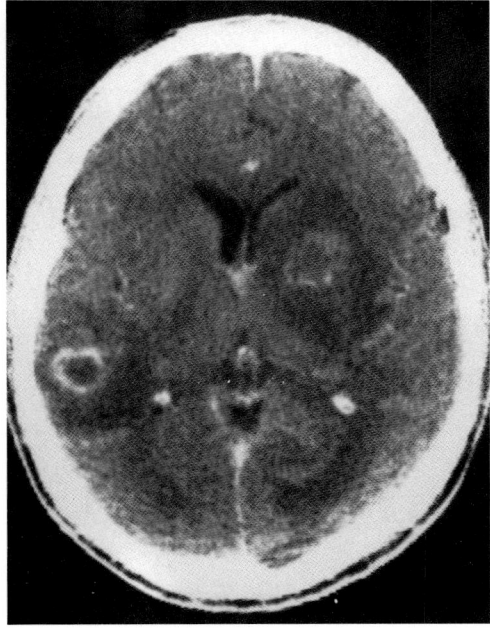

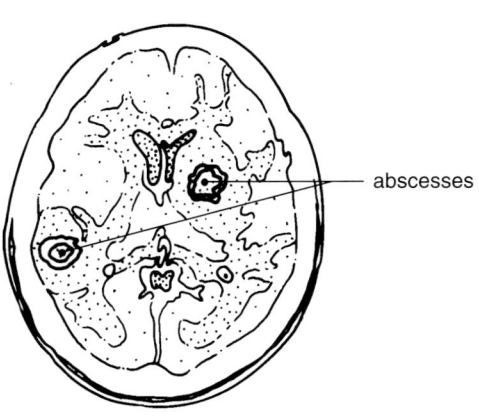

abscesses

Figure 3.19

Toxoplasmosis. A contrast-enhanced CT in this patient with AIDS shows two areas of ring enhancement with surrounding edema.

Figure 3.18

Tuberculoma. There is a nodular area of calcification within the posterior right frontal lobe cortex. This represents an old, burned-out abscess.

(fetal) toxoplasmosis (Fig. 3.20) and cytomegalovirus (Fig. 3.21) may result in widespread brain calcifications.

Pyogenic abscesses can occur in the sella turcica. The abscess appears as a low-density sellar or suprasellar mass with a rim of contrast enhancement on CT (Fig. 3.22). Clinical history is important since the CT or MRI appearance may be identical with that of other cystic pituitary masses.

Ventriculitis

Intraventricular inflammation may be secondary to a brain abscess adjacent to the subependymal region, or it may result from instrumentation, e.g., shunt tube placement. Ventriculitis is recognized on MRI and CT as an abnormal degree of enhancement of the ventricular lining (Fig. 3.23). As with meningeal enhancement caused by meningitis, the main differen-

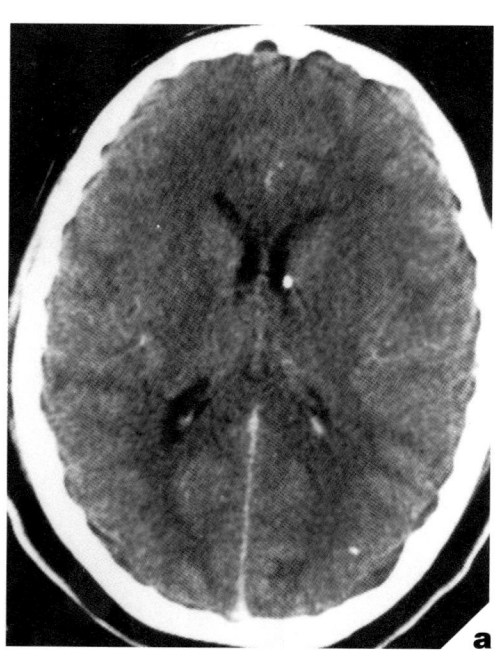 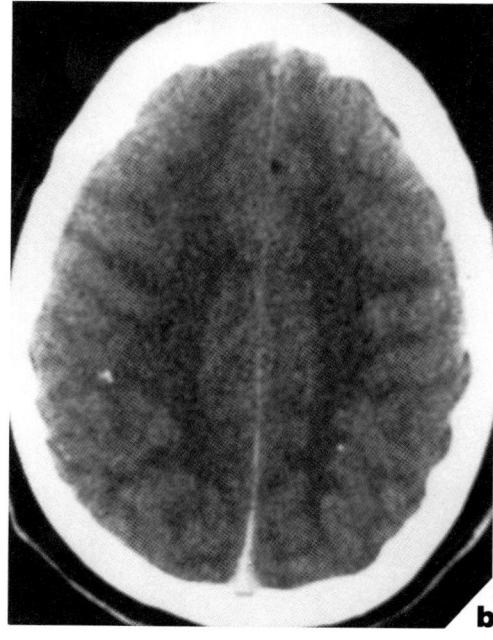 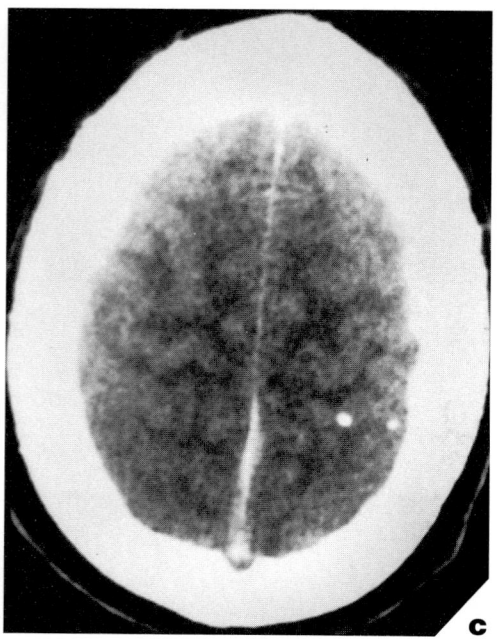

Figure 3.20

*Congenital toxoplasmosis. **a,b,c** Punctate calcifications are demonstrated in various locations in the brain.*

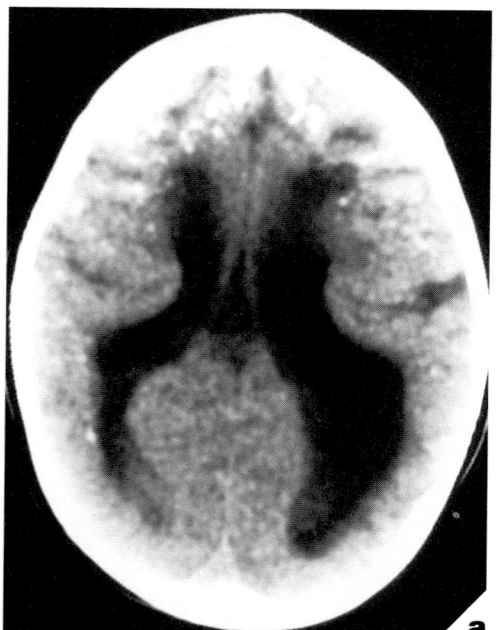 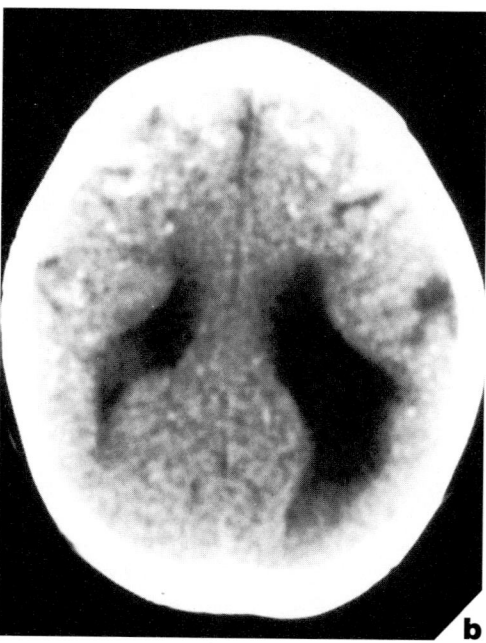

Figure 3.21

*Congenital cytomegalovirus. **a,b** Axial CT scans without contrast demonstrate innumerable, small intraparenchymal calcifications.*

tial diagnosis for ventriculitis includes neoplastic entities such as lymphoma or metastases.

OSTEOMYELITIS

Osteomyelitis most commonly involves the skull through direct extension from paranasal sinusitis (Fig. 3.24) or middle ear disease. Hematogenous spread may also occur, particularly in granulomatous disease such as syphilis. Complications such as epidural abscess and cortical vein or dural sinus thrombosis may occur. Computed tomography is superior to magnetic resonance imaging in providing detailed evaluation of the bony destruction. Bone scans are usually helpful here as well.

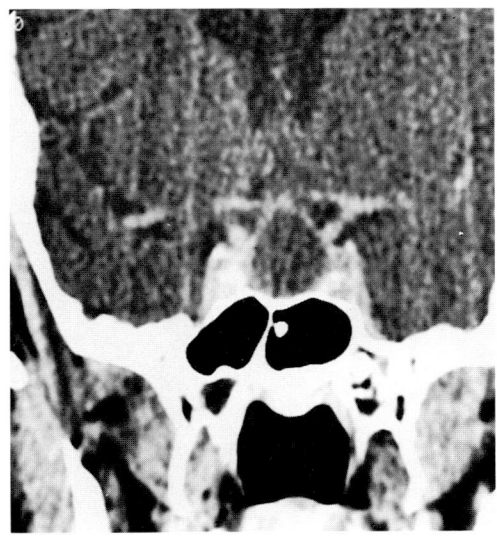

Figure 3.22
Pituitary abscess. This 60-year-old woman presented with headaches, fever, panhypopituitarism, and a bitemporal visual field defect. Contrast-enhanced coronal CT shows an area of ring enhancement in the sella turcica.

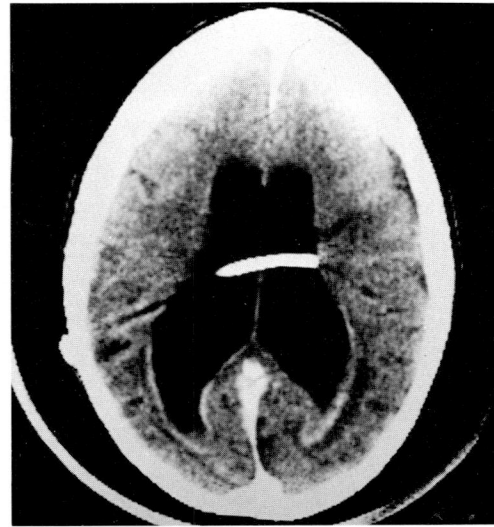

Figure 3.23
Ventriculitis. Axial CT section shows subependymal enhancement in both lateral ventricles. The patient had undergone ventriculoperitoneal shunting for hydrocephalus. Cultures of ventricular fluid yielded Pseudomonas aeruginosa.

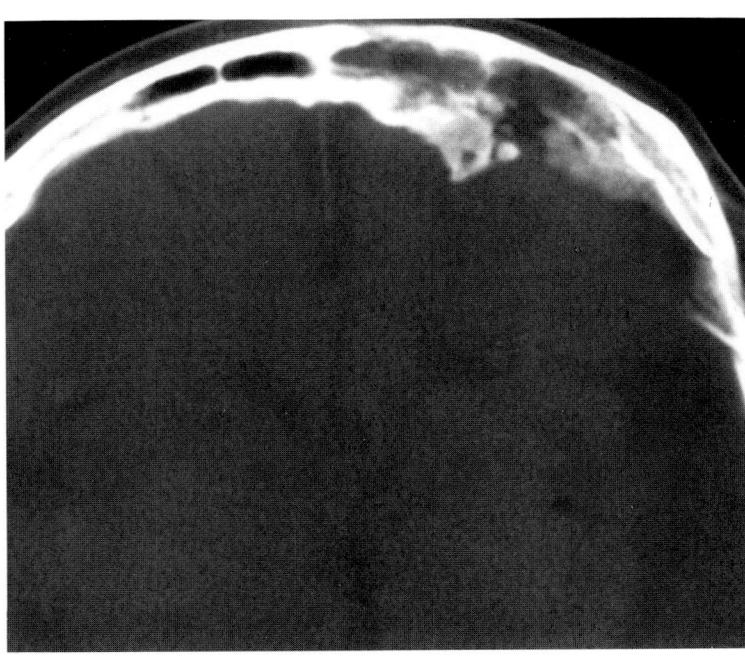

Figure 3.24
Osteomyelitis. There is destruction and fragmentation of the posterior wall of the left frontal sinus with associated sinus opacification.

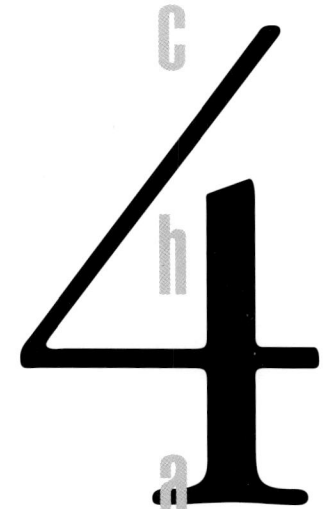

Chapter 4

Intracranial Neoplasms

he detection of intracranial neo-plasms by CT and MRI has had an in-estimable impact on the practice of neurology and neurosurgery. As ex-perience grows, the need for angio-graphic evaluation of intracranial neoplasms continues to decline. CT-guided stereotaxic biopsy has contributed to reduced mortality in the diagnosis of these lesions.

Various classifications of brain neoplasms are in widespread use. A particularly useful categorization is based both on cell type and location (Fig. 4.1). This scheme is useful in constructing a differential diagnosis based on radiological appearances.

Gliomas, metastases, and meningiomas comprise the majority of intracranial neoplasms. These three groups of neoplasms have certain specific appear-ances on CT and MRI which help limit the differential diagnosis. A number of tumors have a predilection for certain locations (e.g., intraventricular, sellar or parasellar, posterior fossa, pineal region), and a spe-cific differential diagnosis can be offered for tumors occurring at each of these sites. The patient's age at the time of presentation is an additional distinguish-ing factor. Many congenital neoplasms have unique radiological features.

GLIOMAS AND PRIMARY CNS LYMPHOMA

Astrocytoma and Glioblastoma Multiforme

Both of these terms refer to neoplasms of the astro-cyte. Kernohan has divided the tumors into grades I–IV, grade I being the least malignant (well differen-tiated), grade IV the most anaplastic. A later classif-ication by Russell and Rubinstein simply uses the terms *astrocytoma* (equivalent to Kernohan grade 1), *malignant astrocytoma* (Kernohan grade II), and *glioblastoma multiforme* (Kernohan grades III and IV).

The CT and MRI findings vary with the tumor grade. Low-grade astrocytomas are characterized by infiltration of the brain parenchyma with minimal mass effect relative to the size of the lesion, and little or no contrast enhancement. On CT (Fig. 4.2a), the lesion is hypodense with respect to normal brain; on MRI (Fig. 4.2b) there is dark-T1, bright-T2 signal ab-normality, often larger than the area of abnormal density on CT. Some low-grade astrocytomas are truly cystic and contain fluid. The presence of a tumor nodule may be the only clue that differentiates a cystic astrocytoma from other fluid-filled collections (e.g., abscess). Some neoplasms that are quite low in density may appear to be solid on gross inspection at surgery; histologic examination in such cases reveals numerous microscopic cysts. The term *microcystic astrocytoma* has been applied to characterize this morphologic pattern.

Grade II gliomas (malignant astrocytomas) (Fig. 4.3) demonstrate mild to moderate contrast enhance-ment, increasing edema and are more "space-occupy-ing" than infiltrative. They are intermediate in aggres-siveness between a low-grade astrocytoma and glio-blastoma multiforme.

Glioblastoma multiforme is a very malignant, rap-idly growing tumor. Rapid tumor growth leads to central necrosis. Computed tomography and mag-netic resonance imaging (Fig. 4.4) generally exhibit a large, inhomogeneous mass with poorly defined mar-gins, a central hypodense/hypointense area (Fig. 4.5), and a large amount of surrounding edema (Fig. 4.6). Typically, there is nodular, intense contrast enhance-ment that forms a thick, irregular ring. The size of a glioblastoma multiforme at the time of clinical pre-sentation is often a function of the tumor's location. Gliomas in the frontal regions tend to be more clini-cally "silent" than lesions in the motor strip. The de-gree of mass effect and midline shift also have impor-tant clinical significance. Seizures, headache, and loss of function are common modes of presentation for gliomas of any type.

Growth along white matter tracts often occurs. A large bilateral glioma that crosses from one hemi-sphere to the other via the corpus callosum ("butter-fly" glioblastoma) has a very characteristic appear-ance on MRI and CT (Fig. 4.7).

Figure 4.1
Classification of intracranial neoplasms.

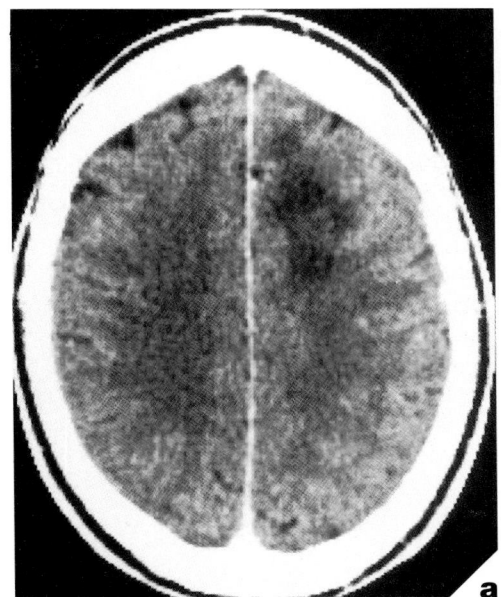

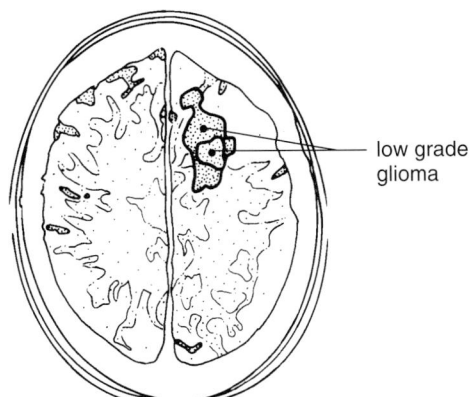

low grade
glioma

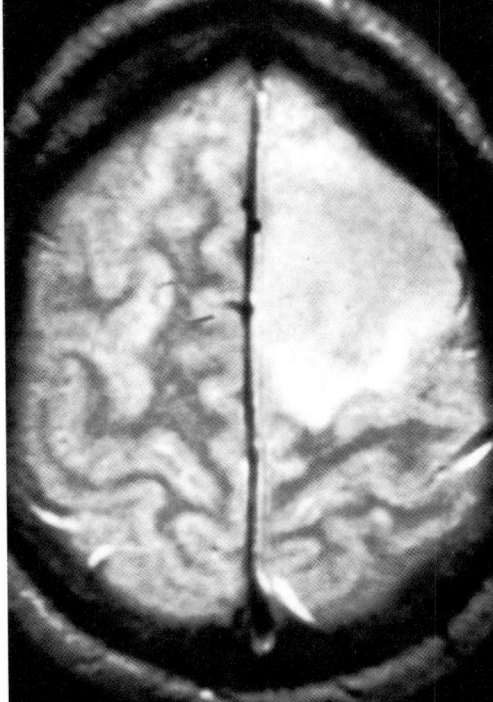

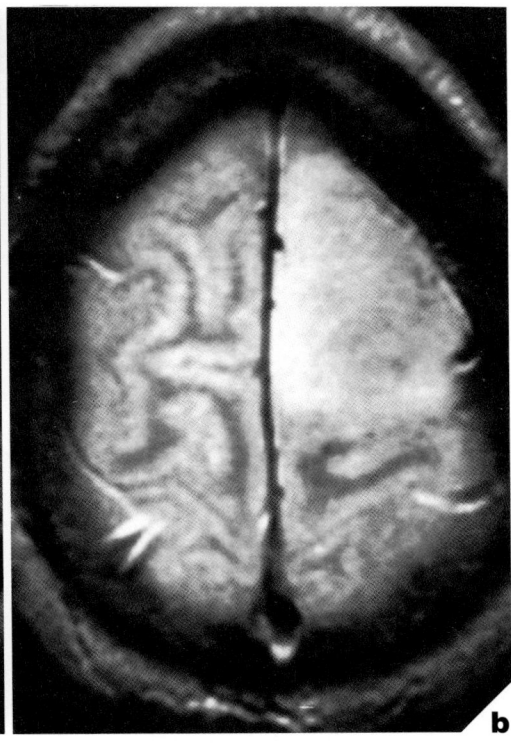

Figure 4.2

Low grade astrocytoma. **a** *CT scan shows an indistinct area of decreased attenuation in the deep white matter of the anterior left frontal lobe.* **b** *MRI of the same patient shows an area of bright-T2 signal abnormality which is greater in size than the corresponding area of decreased attenuation on CT. This is due to the greater ability of MRI to detect edema and other changes in water content than CT.*

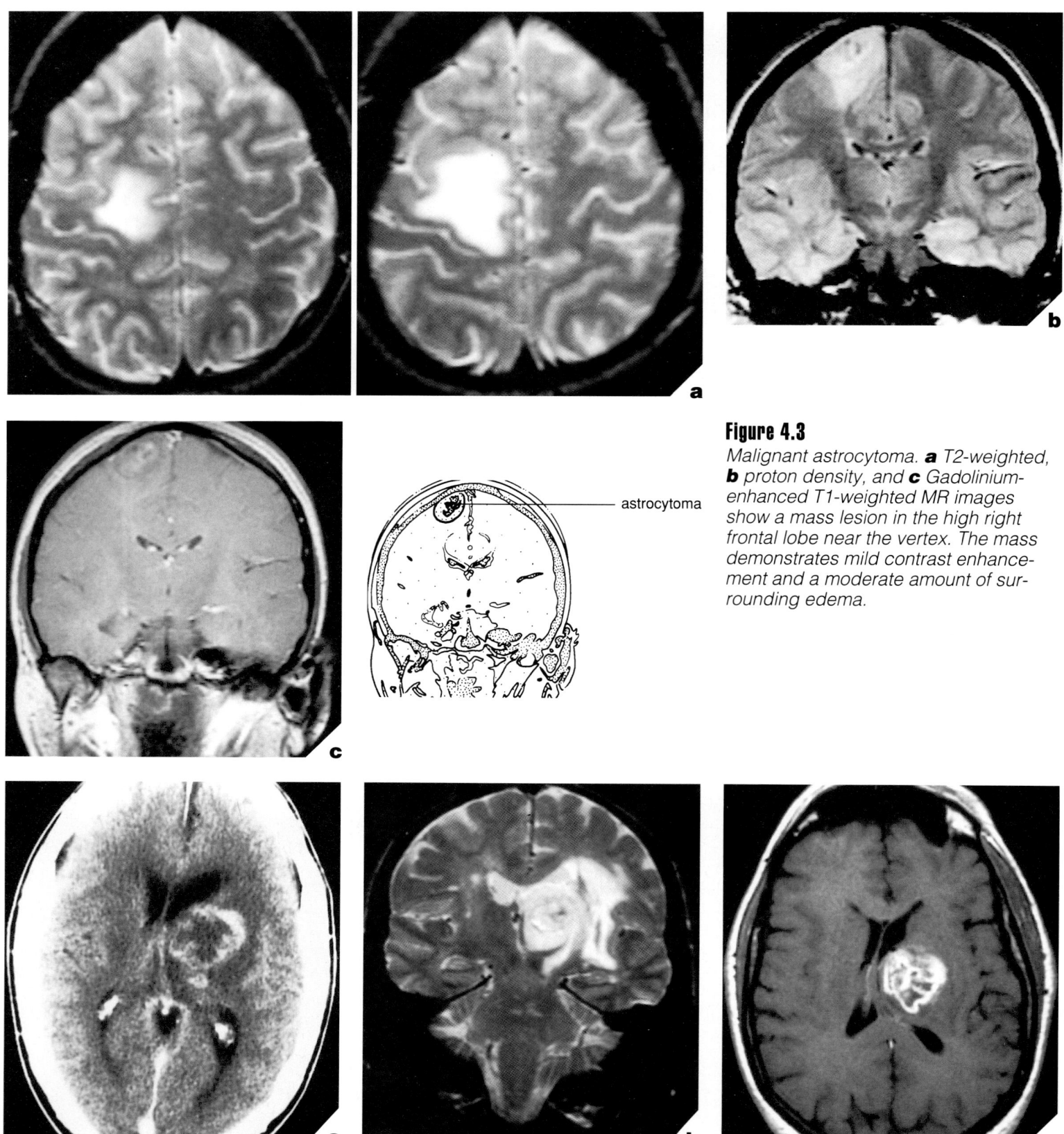

Figure 4.3

*Malignant astrocytoma. **a** T2-weighted, **b** proton density, and **c** Gadolinium-enhanced T1-weighted MR images show a mass lesion in the high right frontal lobe near the vertex. The mass demonstrates mild contrast enhancement and a moderate amount of surrounding edema.*

astrocytoma

Figure 4.4

*Glioblastoma multiforme. **a** CT and **b,c** MRI show a large, left thalamic mass with poorly defined, irregular margins. There is compression of the adjacent left lateral ventricle and midline shift from left to right. The mass shows bright-T2 signal abnormality (**b**) typical for nonhemorrhagic and noncalcified gliomas. Contrast enhancement is seen on both CT (**a**) and MRI (**c**).*

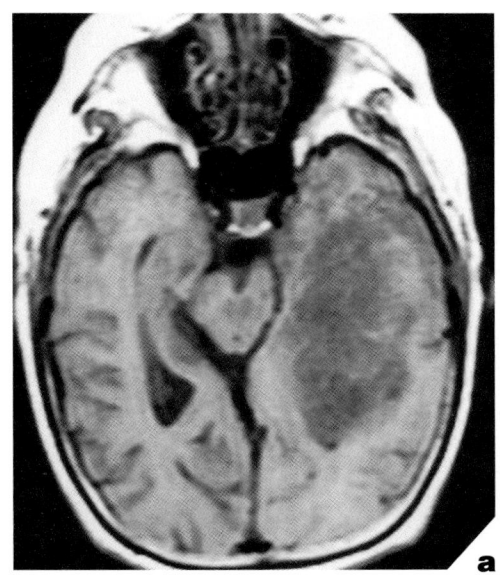 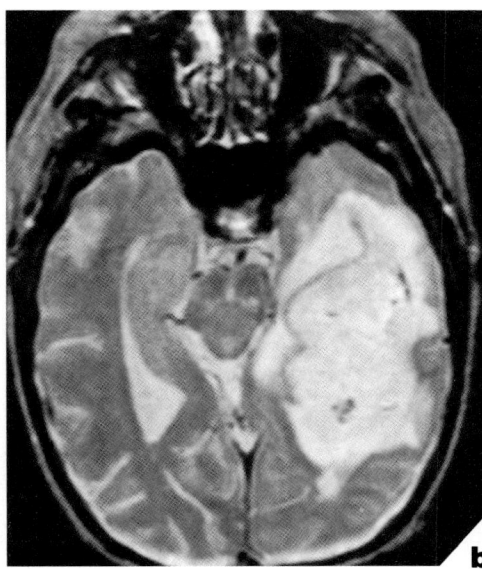 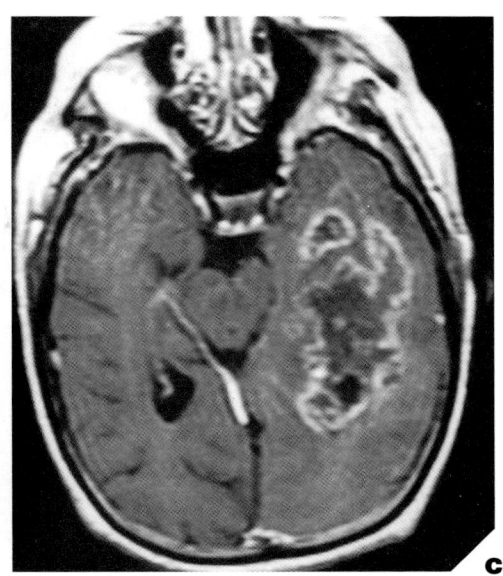

Figure 4.5

Glioblastoma multiforme. Unenhanced a T1, b T2, and c Gadolinium-enhanced T1-weighted MR images show an irregular mass, with ill-defined margins and central necrosis. Note the compression of the left cerebral peduncle.

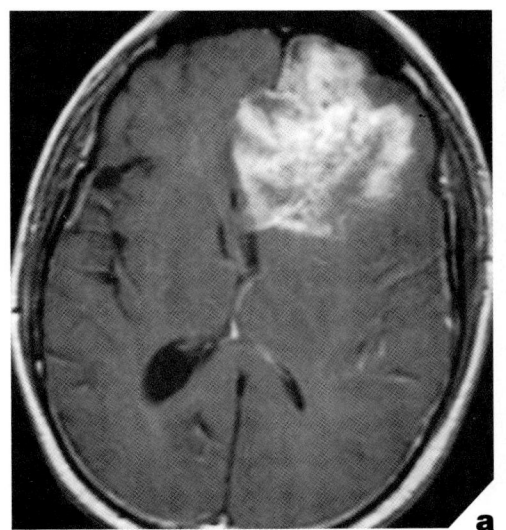 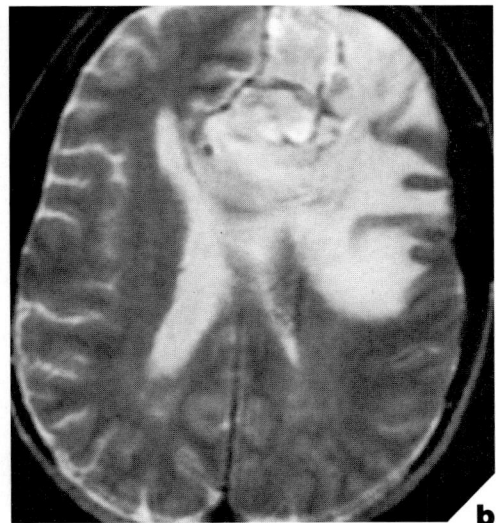

Figure 4.6

Glioblastoma multiforme. a Gadolinium-enhanced MR scan demonstrates a large, irregularly enhancing mass in the left frontal lobe with a tremendous amount of surrounding edema best appreciated on the b T2-weighted scan. T2-weighted images are usually unable to accurately distinguish edema from neoplasm.

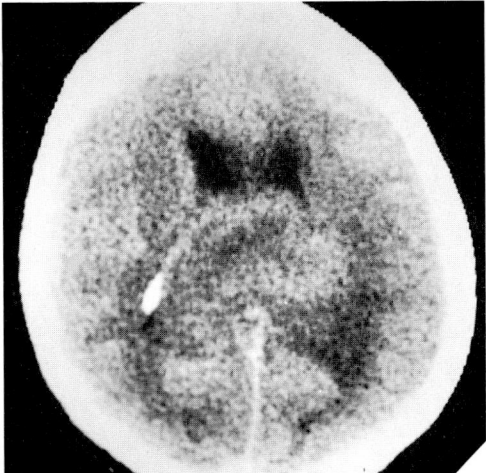 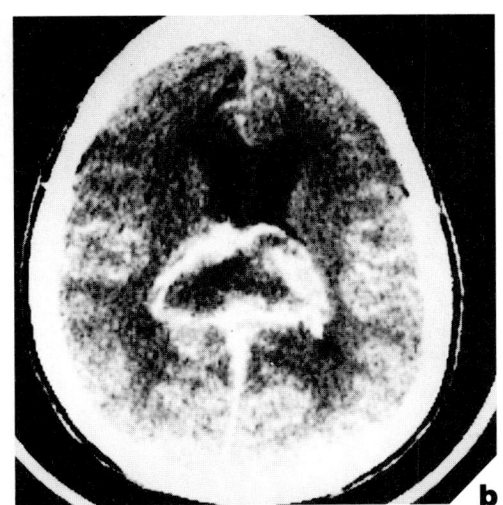

Figure 4.7

"Butterfly" glioblastoma of corpus callosum. A large mass is demonstrated in the splenium of the corpus callosum on these CT sections obtained a without and b with intravenous contrast material. There is intense ring enhancement.

Oligodendroglioma

Oligodendrogliomas are relatively uncommon tumors, representing approximately 5% of cerebral gliomas. Many also contain other glial cell types and are regarded as "mixed". Unlike astrocystomas, they frequently calcify. In addition, they tend to occupy a peripheral location in the brain, particularly in the frontal and temporal lobes. As with tumors in the astrocyte series, there is a spectrum of malignancy of oligodendrogliomas, which correlates with the degree of anaplasia, necrosis, cellularity, and vascularity. However, most oligodendrogliomas are relatively slow-growing neoplasms and therefore often attain a large size before causing symptoms.

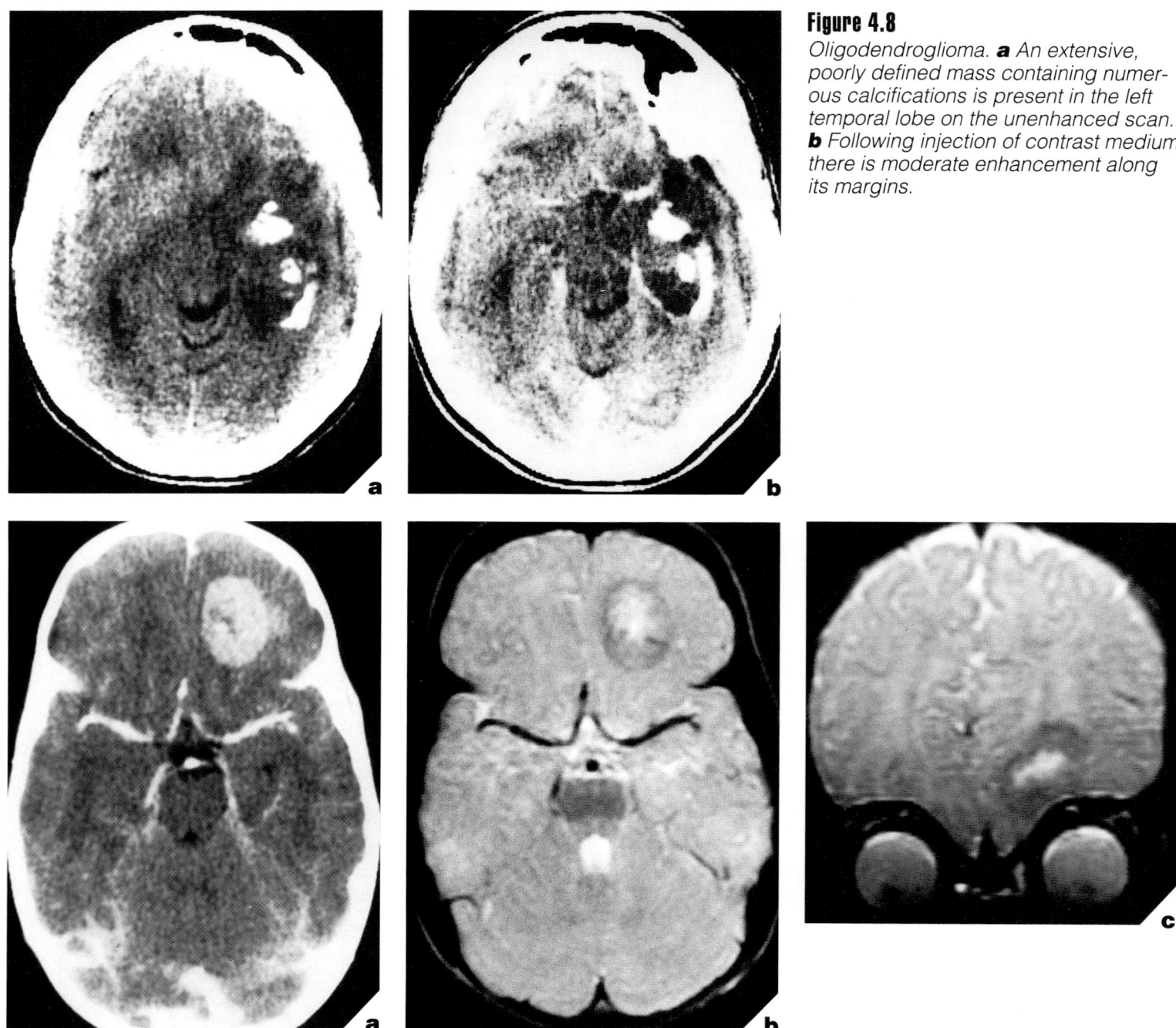

Figure 4.8

*Oligodendroglioma. **a** An extensive, poorly defined mass containing numerous calcifications is present in the left temporal lobe on the unenhanced scan. **b** Following injection of contrast medium there is moderate enhancement along its margins.*

Figure 4.9

*Primitive neuroectodermal tumor. **a** Contrast-enhanced CT and **b,c** noncontrast T2-weighted MR images of this two-year-old child show an oval-shaped, enhancing, intra-axial mass in the inferior left frontal lobe. At surgery, this mass was found to represent a primitive neuroectodermal tumor, the cerebral neuroblastoma. The densely cellular nature of this lesion probably accounts for the mixed signal intensity on the MR images.*

Oligodendrogliomas appear on CT (Fig. 4.8) as large, irregular, heterogeneous masses. Calcification is generally identified. There may be mild contrast enhancement.

years of life. Like medulloblastomas, they typically have dense cellularity and may be hyperdense on unenhanced CT scans. Contrast enhancement is variable.

Primitive Neuroectodermal Tumor (PNET)

Primitive neuroectodermal tumor (PNET) actually refers to a group of pediatric brain tumors. These tumors arise from primitive or undifferentiated neuroepithelial cells. The most common type of PNET is the cerebellar medulloblastoma, which will be considered later in this chapter since it is generally classified with posterior fossa tumors. Another type of PNET is the cerebral neuroblastoma (Fig. 4.9). This tumor usually develops during the first few

Ganglioglioma

This is a rare, relatively benign, slow-growing tumor that usually occurs in adolescents and young adults. The tumor is composed of a combination of ganglion cells and glial stromal elements. Most of these affect the cerebrum, particularly the temporal lobes.

Gangliogliomas may be solid or cystic and are typically well demarcated. They typically show calcification on CT. Most show some degree of enhancement with iodinated contrast or Gadolinium (Fig. 4.10).

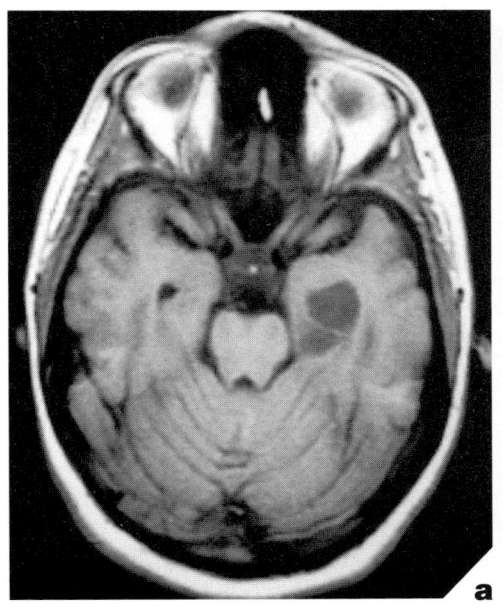
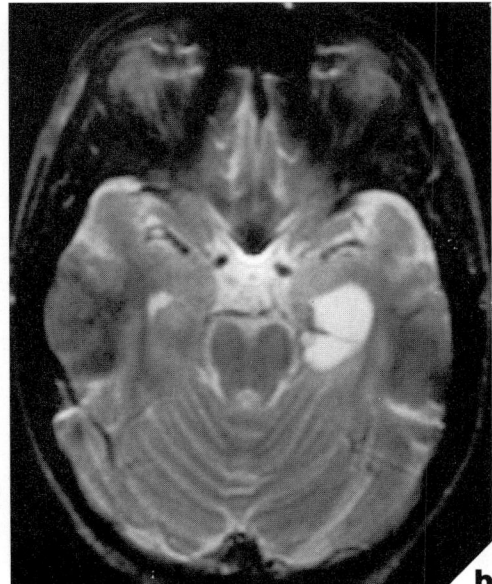
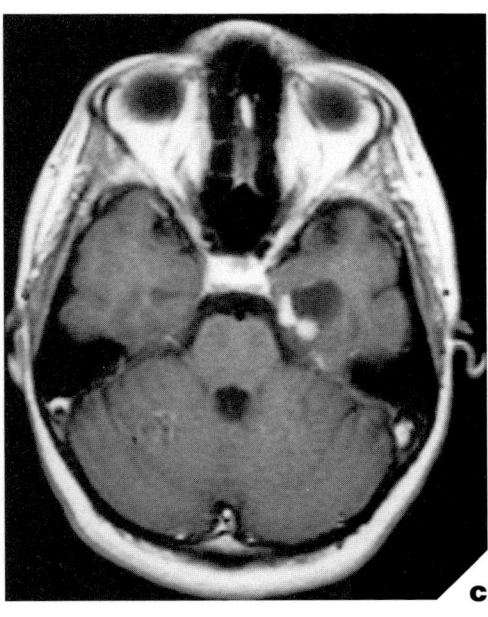
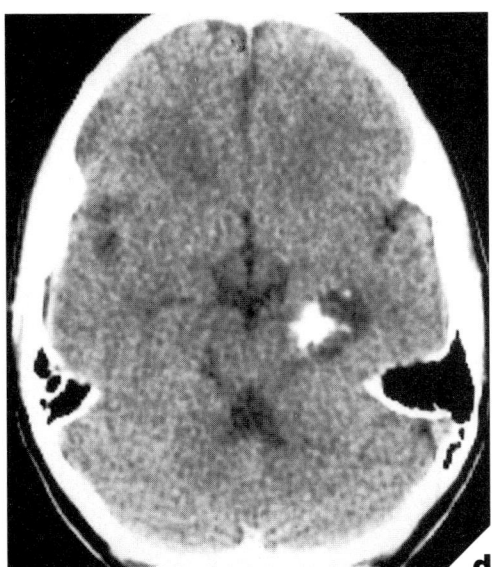

Figure 4.10

*Ganglioglioma. **a** T1, **b** T2, and **c** Gadolinium-enhanced T1-weighted images show a well-demarcated cystic mass in the left temporal lobe with some enhancement along its medial wall. **d** Unenhanced CT shows calcification. These findings are typical of a ganglioglioma.*

Gliosarcoma

These unusual tumors have both glial and sarcomatous elements. Radiologic differentiation from glioblastoma is difficult or impossible (Fig. 4.11).

Ependymoma

Ependymomas are gliomas which most commonly occur in children. Most are infratentorial and therefore are discussed in greater detail later in this chapter. When they arise from the ependymal cells lining the lateral ventricles, they frequently have calcifications and may invade deep into the brain (Fig. 4.12).

Primary Cerebral Lymphoma

Primary central nervous system lymphoma (also called reticulum cell sarcoma or microglioma) fre-

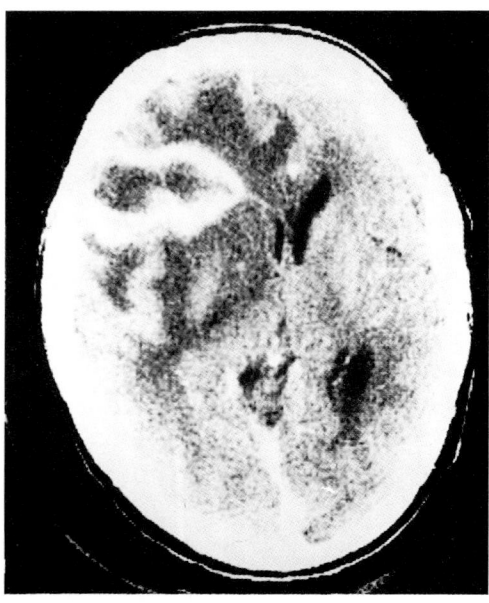

Figure 4.11
Gliosarcoma. Axial CT section with contrast enhancement shows a very irregular area of enhancement in the right frontal lobe with a central area of necrosis. There is a large amount of surrounding edema, mass effect and subfalcine herniation.

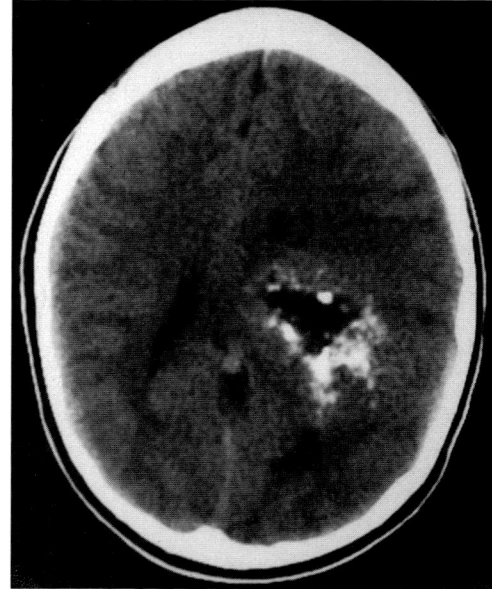

Figure 4.12
Ependymoma. Axial CT section without contrast material reveals a mass in the left parietal lobe which contains numerous foci of calcification.

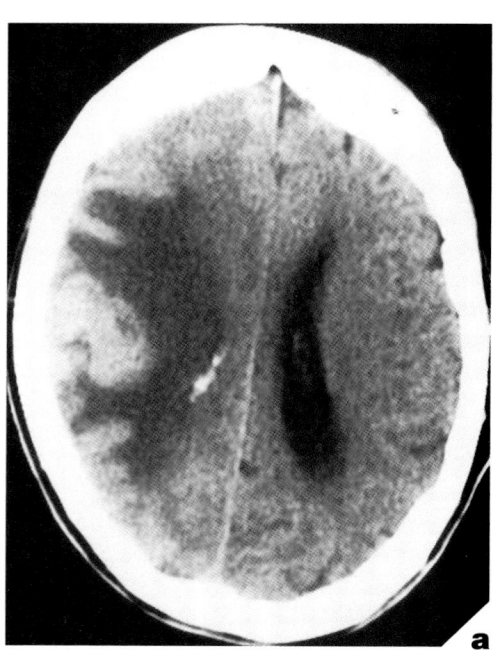 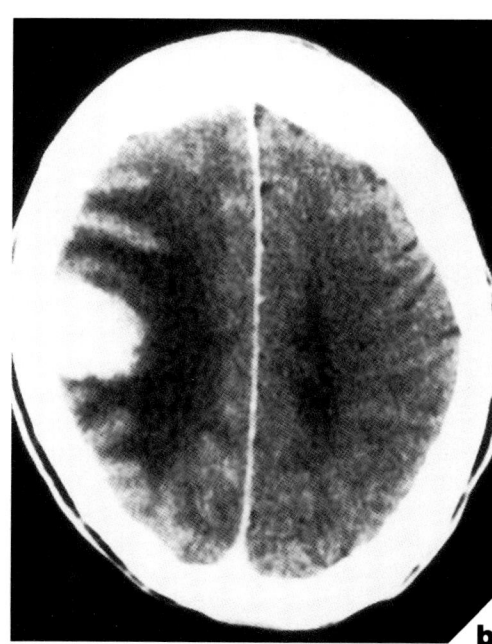

Figure 4.13
*Primary lymphoma of brain. **a** Unenhanced CT shows a slightly hyperdense mass with surrounding edema. **b** Post-contrast scan shows homogeneous enhancement.*

quently affects the basal ganglia and thalamus; the tumor may extend subependymally or along the corpus callosum. The incidence of lymphoma is markedly increased in patients undergoing immunosuppressive therapy and in patients with acquired immunodeficiency syndrome (AIDS). CT typically shows one or more isodense or slightly hyperdense masses (Fig. 4.13) which are typically dark on T1 and bright on T2 MR images. Characteristically, peritumoral edema and mass effect is minimal (Fig. 4.14). The masses usually enhance homogeneously without evidence of central necrosis. Lymphomas associated with AIDS are often atypical in enhancement characteristics and location. They are usually very difficult to distinguish from toxoplasmosis infection. CNS lymphoma (Fig. 4.15) may predominantly involve the meninges.

Esthesioneuroblastoma

An esthesioneuroblastoma (Fig. 4.16) is a tumor arising in the region of the cribiform plate which involves the olfactory nerves and is also called an olfactory neuroblastoma. It typically extends both inferiorly into the nasal cavity and superiorly into the anterior cranial fossa. These tumors show dark-T1, bright-T2 signal characteristics and usually readily enhance with Gadolinium-DTPA administration. CT may show erosion of the cribiform plate.

METASTASES

The most common sites of origin for brain metastases (Fig. 4.17) are malignancies of the lung, breast, kidney, colon, and skin (melanoma). With any type of metasta-

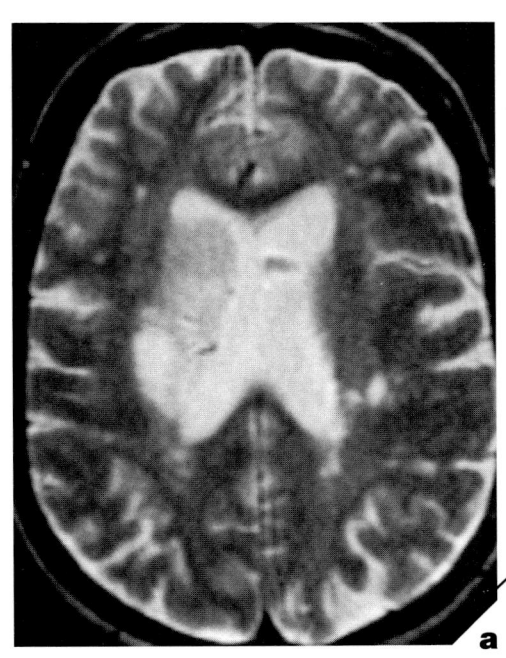

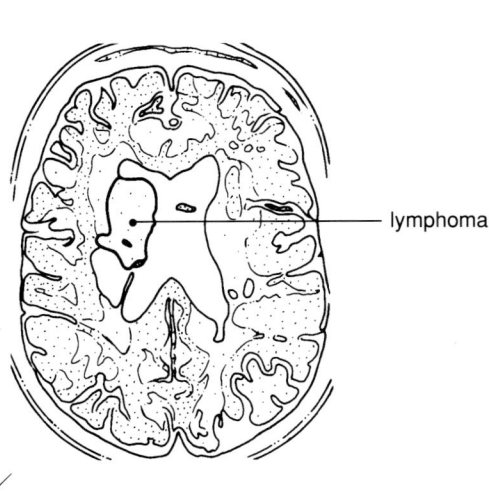
lymphoma

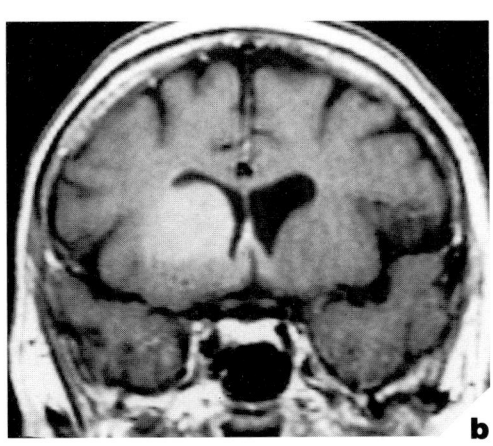

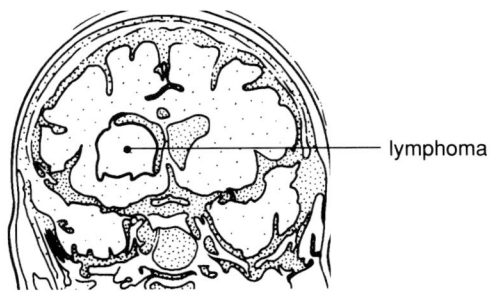
lymphoma

Figure 4.14

*Primary lymphoma of brain. **a** T2 and **b** Gadolinium-enhanced T1-weighted MR images show a mass infiltrating the right basal ganglia. This is a characteris-* *tic location for primary cerebral lymphoma. Homogeneous enhancement is demonstrated with a paucity of associated edema and mass effect.*

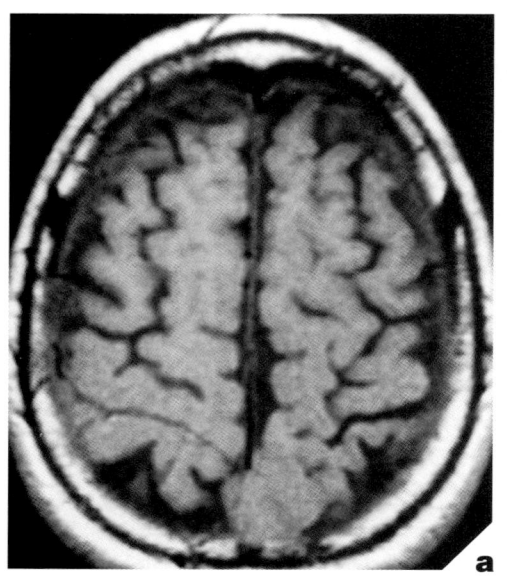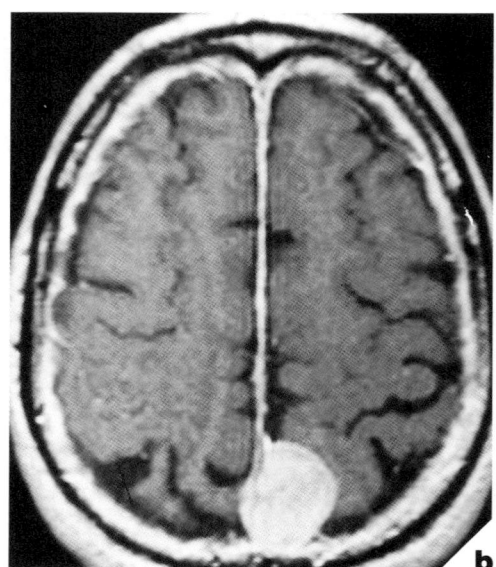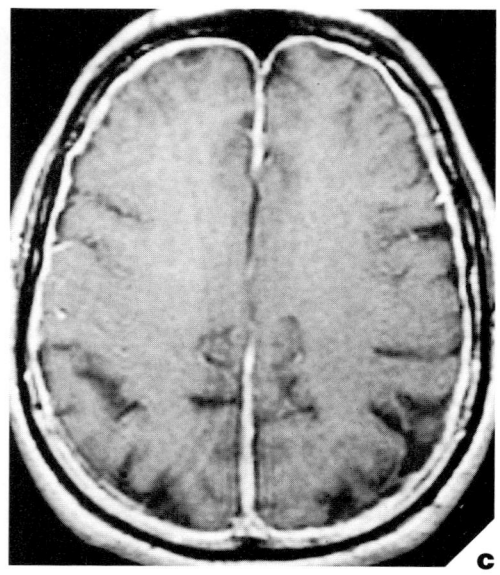

Figure 4.15

*Dural lymphoma. **a** Unenhanced and **b,c** Gadolinium-enhanced T1-weighted images show a homogeneously enhancing mass attached to the left side of the posterior portion of the falx cerebri. There is striking enhancement of all of the meningeal surfaces. This was proven at surgery to represent dural lymphoma.*

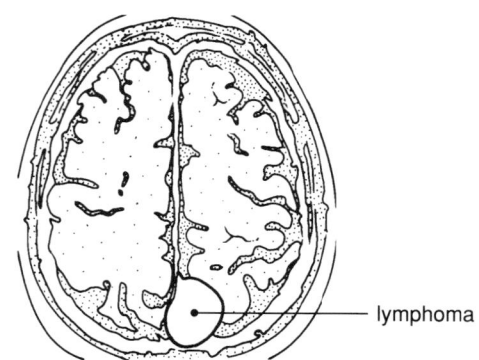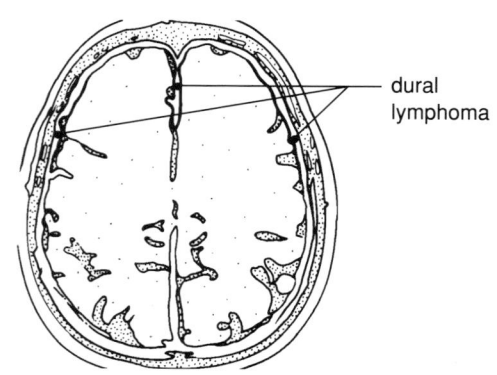

lymphoma

dural lymphoma

Figure 4.16

*Esthesioneuro-blastoma. **a,b** Gadolinium-DTPA enhanced MR images show a large, enhancing mass extending from the cribiform plate inferiorly into the nasal cavity and superiorly into the right side of the anterior cranial fossa.*

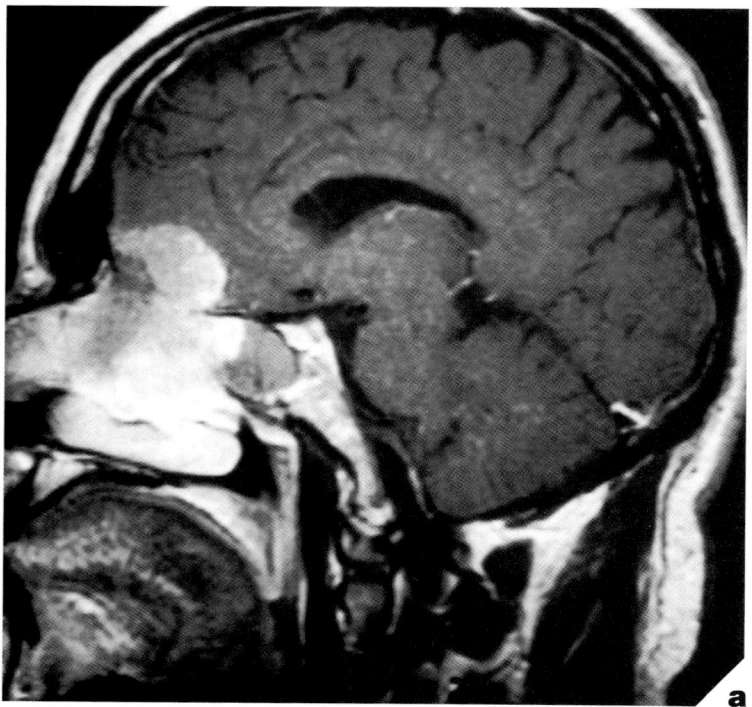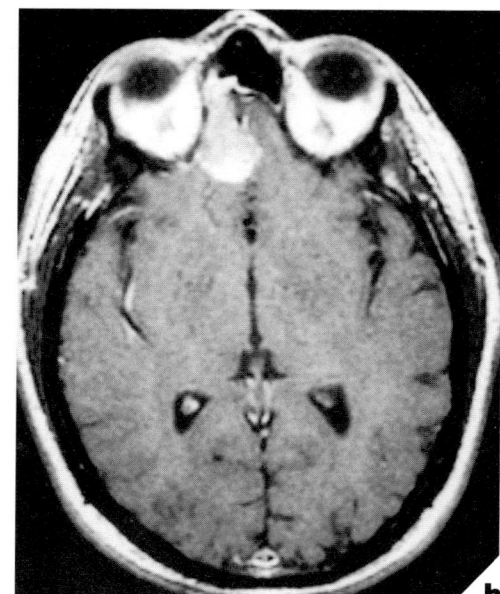

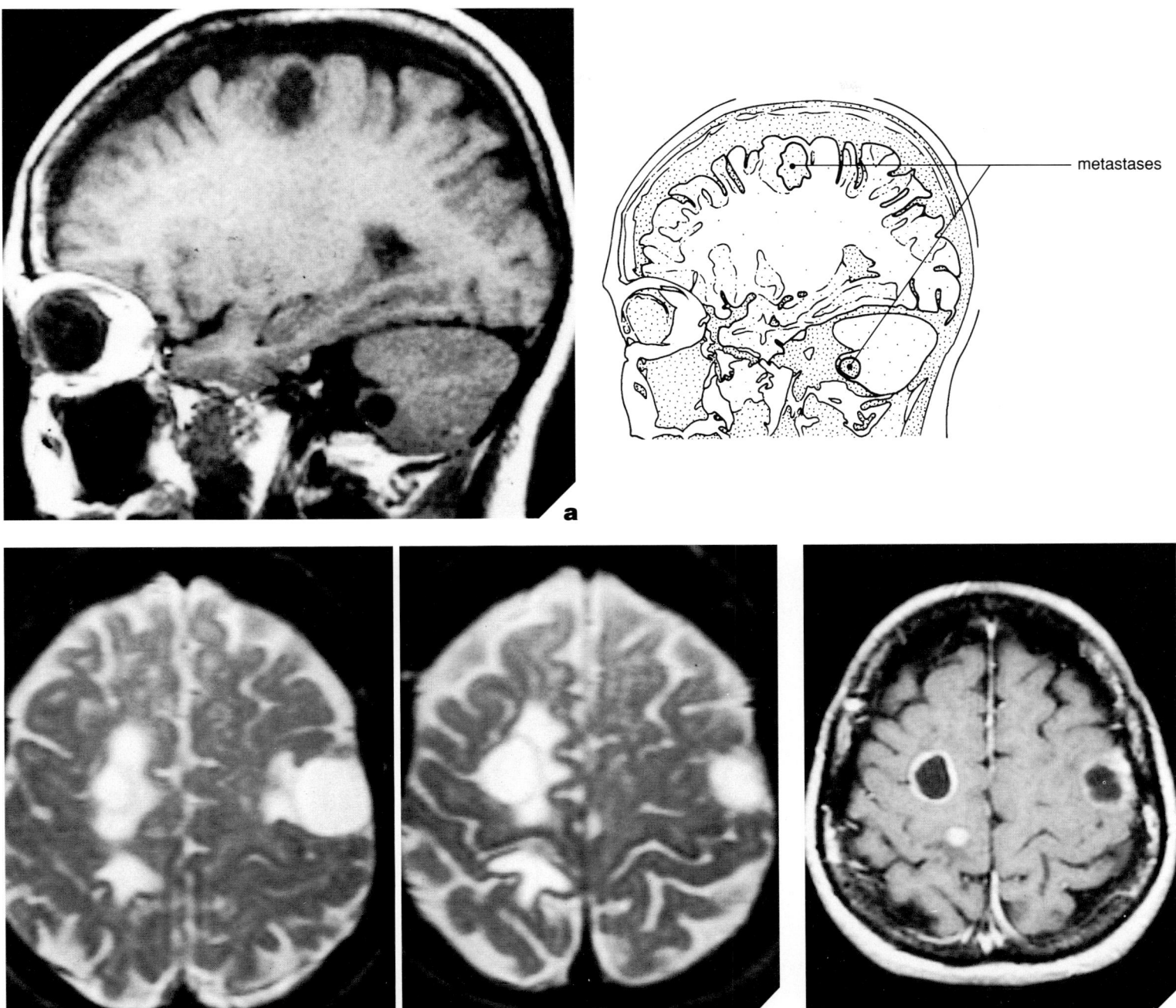

metastases

Figure 4.17

*Widespread metastases from breast carcinoma. **a** T1, **b** T2, and **c** Gadolinium-enhanced T1-weighted images demonstrate multiple nodular and ring-enhancing lesions in the cerebrum and cerebellum with surrounding edema. Typical dark-T1, bright-T2 signal abnormality is demonstrated in these non-hemorrhagic lesions.*

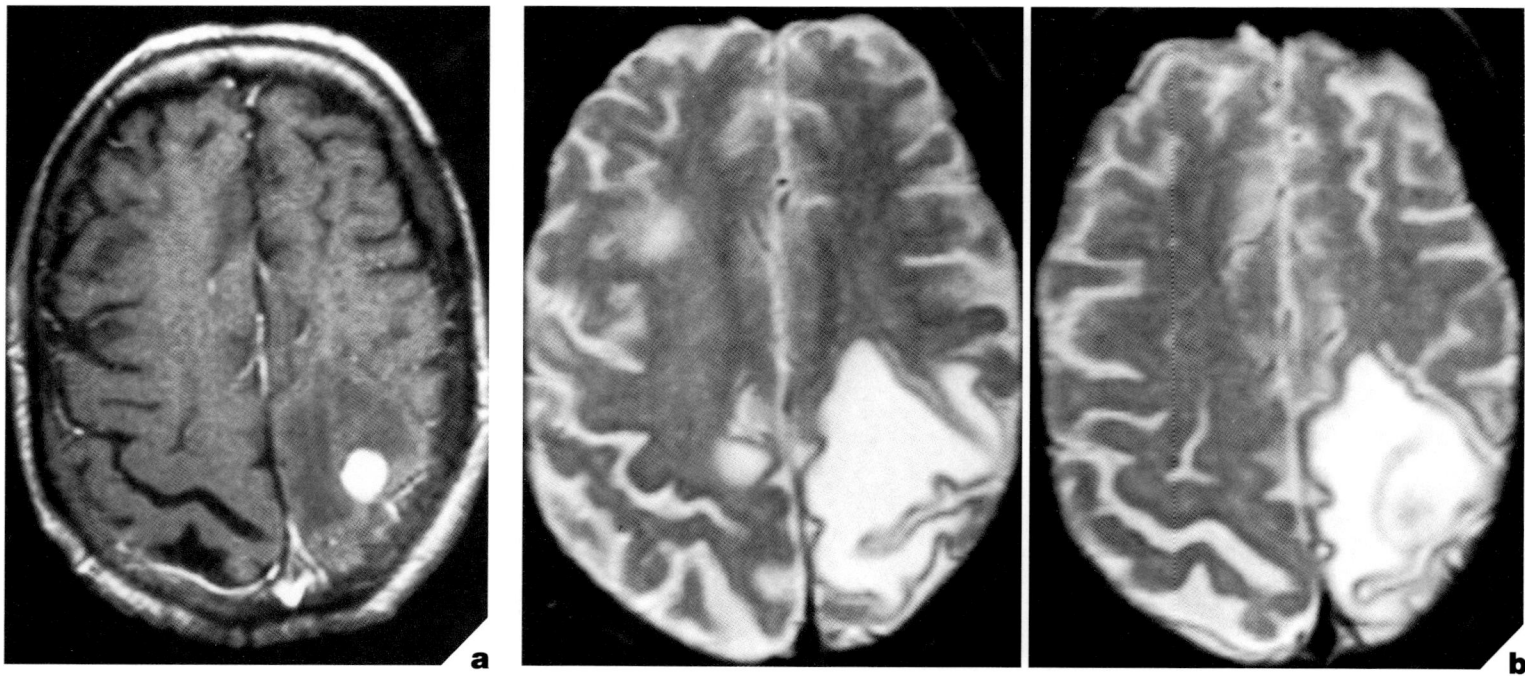

Figure 4.18

Brain metastasis from squamous cell carcinoma of the lung. ***a*** *Gadolinium-enhanced T1-weighted image shows a small*

area of nodular enhancement in the high left parietal lobe with ***b*** *a large amount of edema best seen on T2-weighted images.*

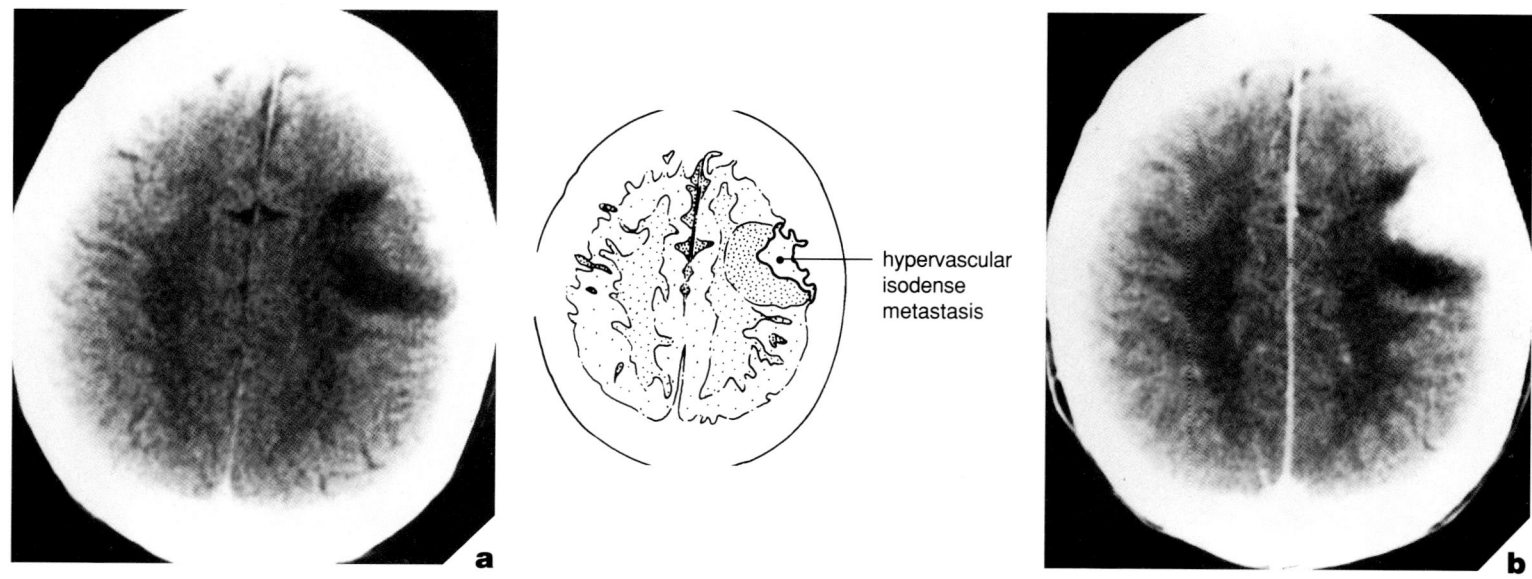

hypervascular
isodense
metastasis

Figure 4.19

Isodense metastasis from renal cell carcinoma. ***a*** *The dense cellularity and hypervascularity of renal cell carcinoma metastases often result in isodense or hyperdense appearances on*

unenhanced CT. ***b*** *There is intense contrast enhancement, typical of a hypervascular metastasis.*

sis to the brain, there is a proportionally larger amount of edema compared to the size of the actual mass (Fig. 4.18) than seen with primary brain tumors. Larger lesions often demonstrate ring enhancement due to central necrosis. A solitary metastasis to the brain may be surgically resectable; however, there are often numerous metastases at the time of presentation. On a noncontrast CT scan the density of a metastatic deposit depends on the degree of cellularity, vascularity, and the presence of hemorrhage or calcification (Fig. 4.19).

Mucinous carcinoma of the gastrointestinal (GI) tract frequently gives rise to hemorrhagic metastatic deposits (Fig. 4.20). Metastatic disease from the rectosigmoid and prostate typically involves the posterior fossa since the tumor cells travel cephalad through

Batson's vertebral venous plexus (Fig. 4.21). Bleeding is commonly seen with metastatic melanoma (Fig. 4.22) and choriocarcinoma (Fig. 4.23). Prostate metastases to the brain are rare (Fig. 4.24). Infrequently, metastases may involve the corpus callosum (Fig. 4.25) and may be confused with glioblastoma multiforme or multiple sclerosis. Occasionally there is direct invasion of the brain by primary skull or even scalp neoplasms (Fig. 4.26).

MULTIPLE MYELOMA

Multiple myeloma frequently causes numerous areas of destruction in the calvarium. This is identified as

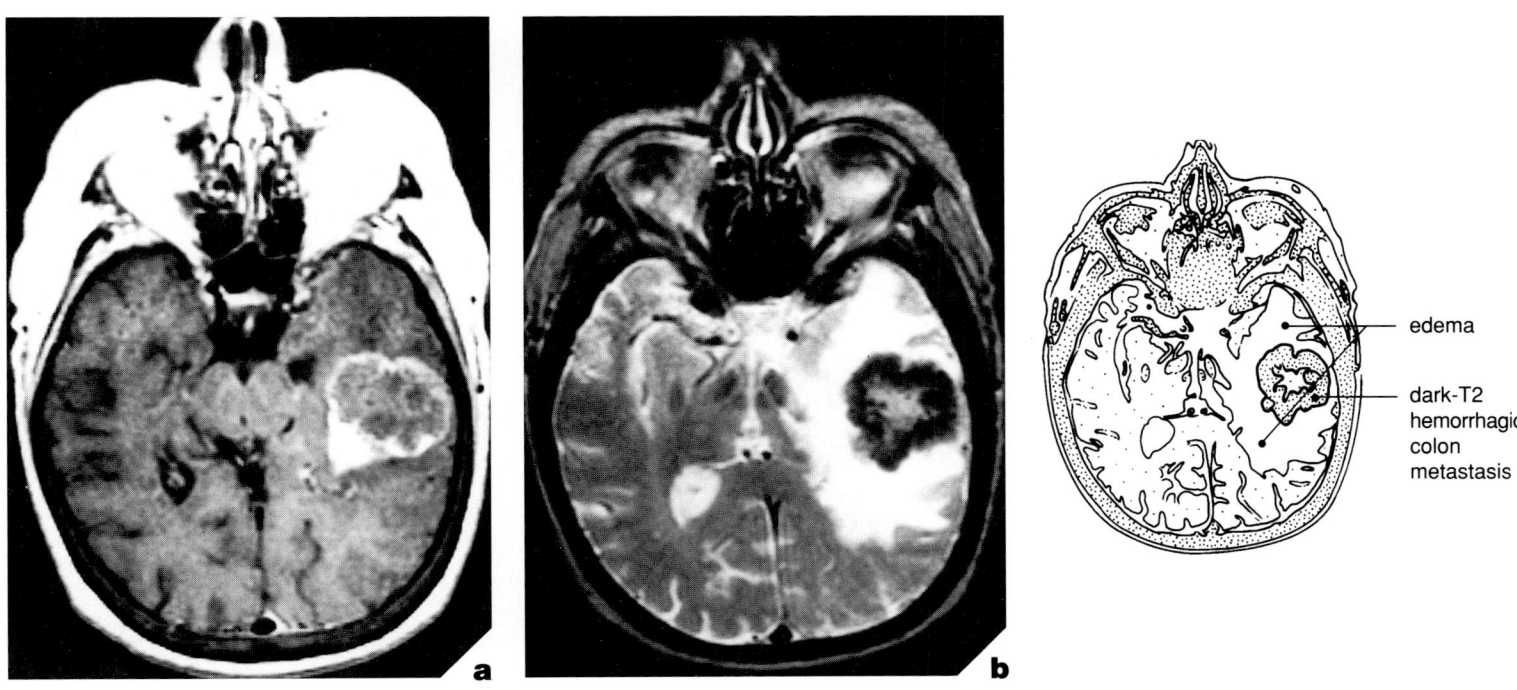

Figure 4.20

*Hemorrhagic metastasis from colon carcinoma. **a** This irregular, ring-enhancing left temporal lobe mass demonstrates* **b** *dark-T2 signal in its wall, indicating old hemorrhage. There is a large amount of surrounding edema.*

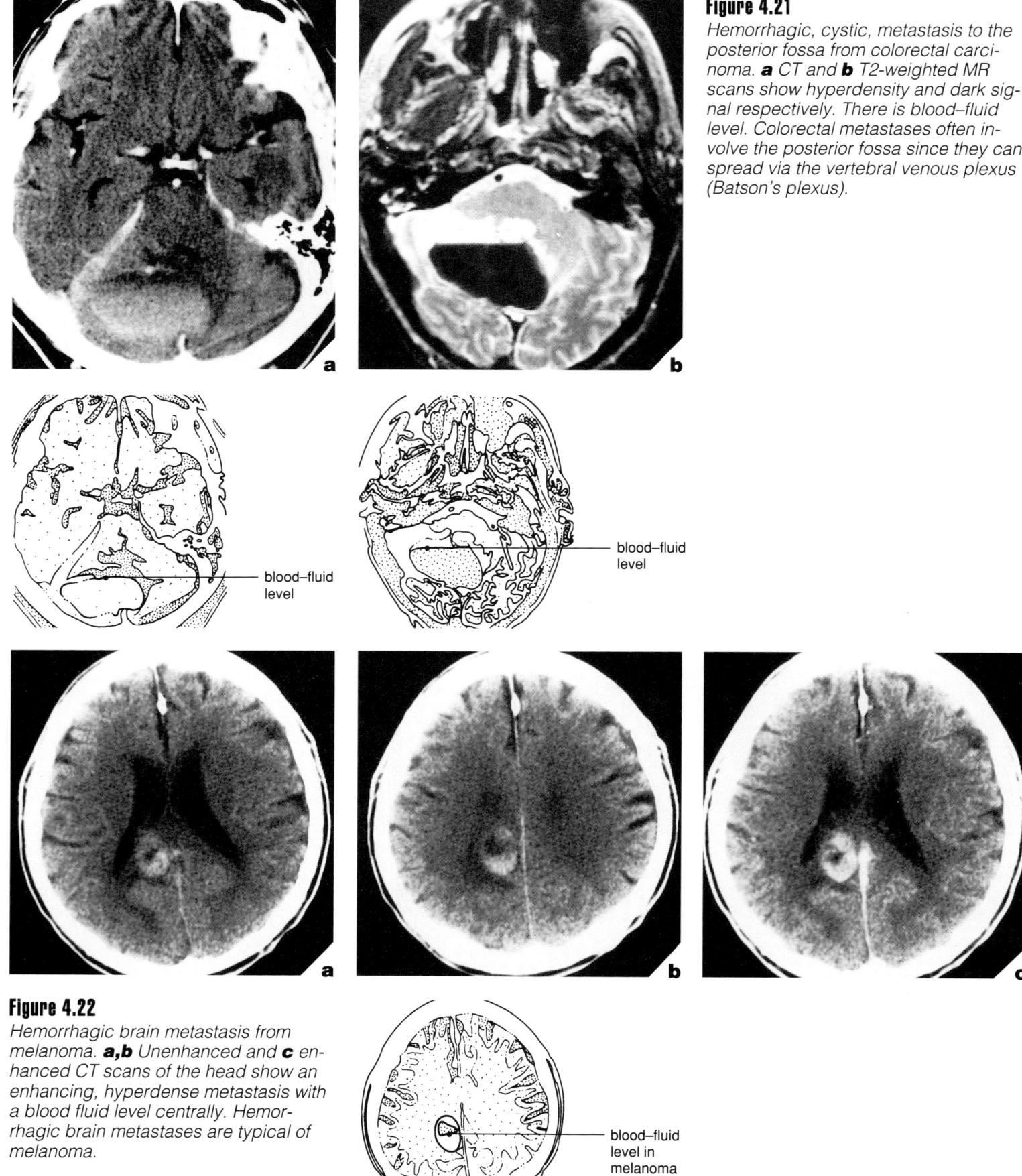

Figure 4.21

*Hemorrhagic, cystic, metastasis to the posterior fossa from colorectal carcinoma. **a** CT and **b** T2-weighted MR scans show hyperdensity and dark signal respectively. There is blood–fluid level. Colorectal metastases often involve the posterior fossa since they can spread via the vertebral venous plexus (Batson's plexus).*

blood–fluid level

blood–fluid level

Figure 4.22

*Hemorrhagic brain metastasis from melanoma. **a,b** Unenhanced and **c** enhanced CT scans of the head show an enhancing, hyperdense metastasis with a blood fluid level centrally. Hemorrhagic brain metastases are typical of melanoma.*

blood–fluid level in melanoma metastasis

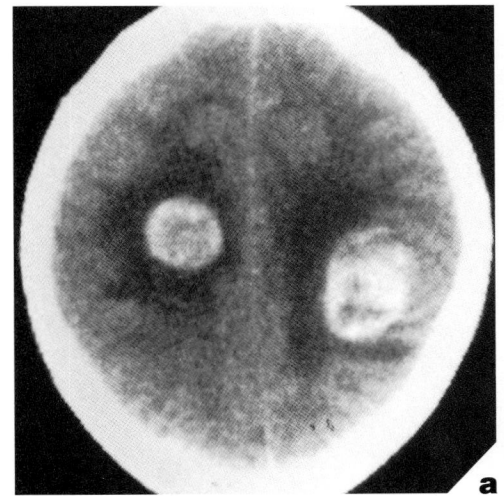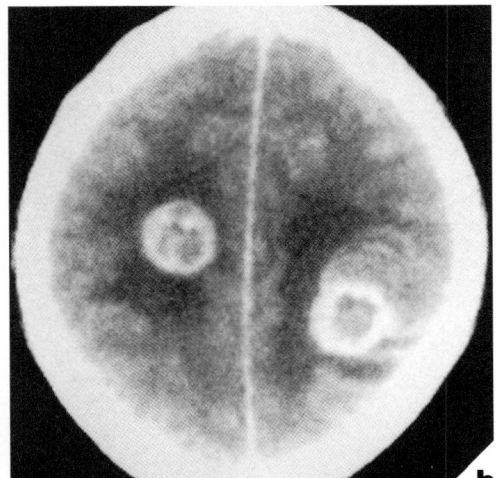

Figure 4.23

*Hemorrhagic brain metastases from choriocarcinoma. **a** Unenhanced and **b** enhanced CT scans of the head in this woman with a history of molar pregnancy show two hyperdense, hemorrhagic metastases.*

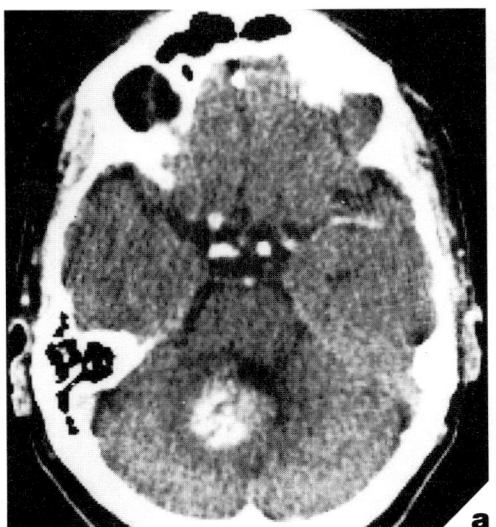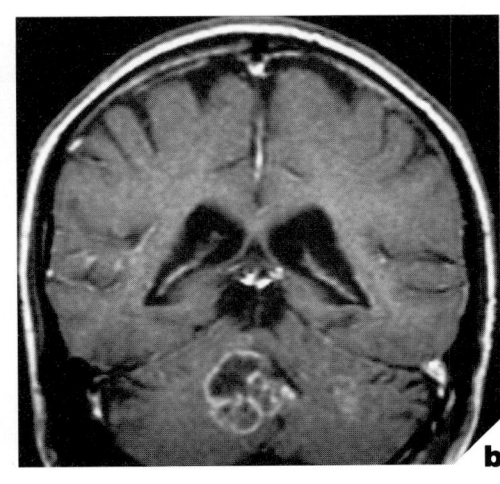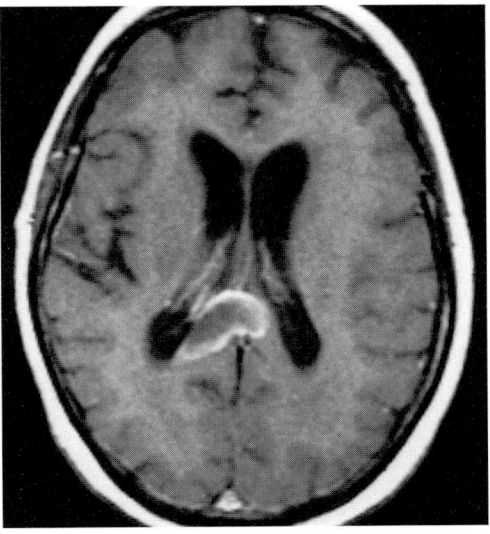

Figure 4.24

*Metastasis to the brain from prostate carcinoma. Contrast-enhanced **a** CT and **b** MRI in this elderly man with known prostate carcinoma show an enhancing mass in the right cerebellar hemisphere compressing the fourth ventricle.*

Figure 4.25

Corpus callosum metastasis. This T1-weighted MR image shows a ring enhancing mass in the splenium of the corpus callosum which at surgery was found to represent a metastasis from lung carcinoma.

Figure 4.26

Direct invasion of the brain by skin tumor. Gadolinium-enhanced T1-weighted image shows abnormal enhancement of the right side of the cerebellum and right side of the occipital bone due to direct invasion by basal cell carcinoma of the scalp.

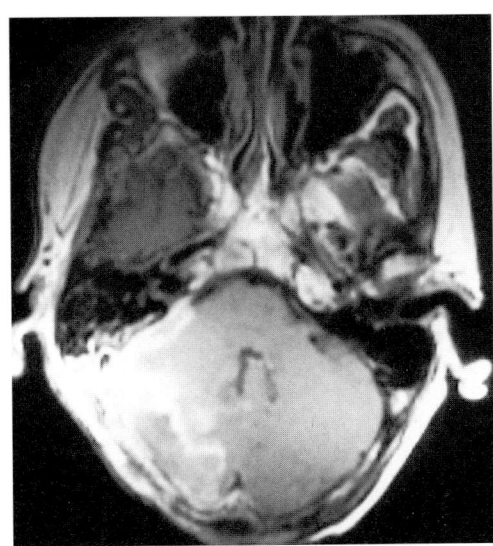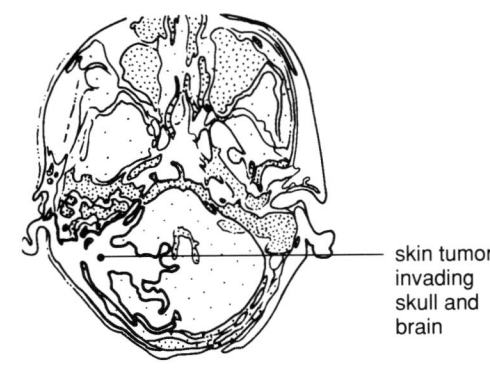

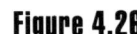 skin tumor invading skull and brain

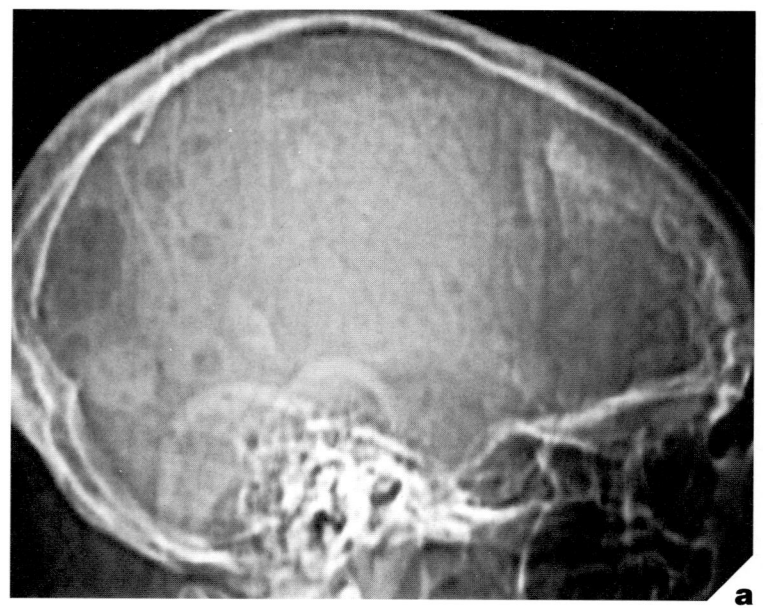

Figure 4.27

Multiple myeloma to the calvarium. ***a*** *CT scout film and* ***b*** *bone windows show numerous lytic defects, the hallmark of multiple myeloma.*

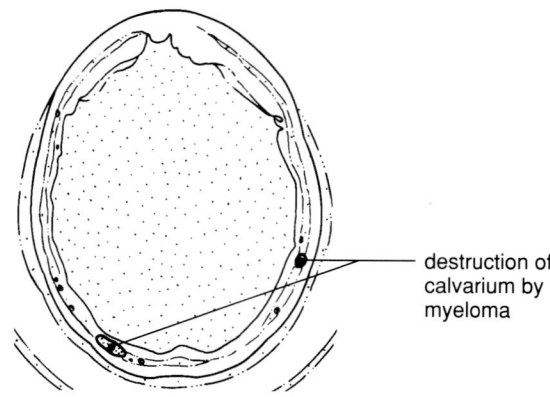

destruction of calvarium by myeloma

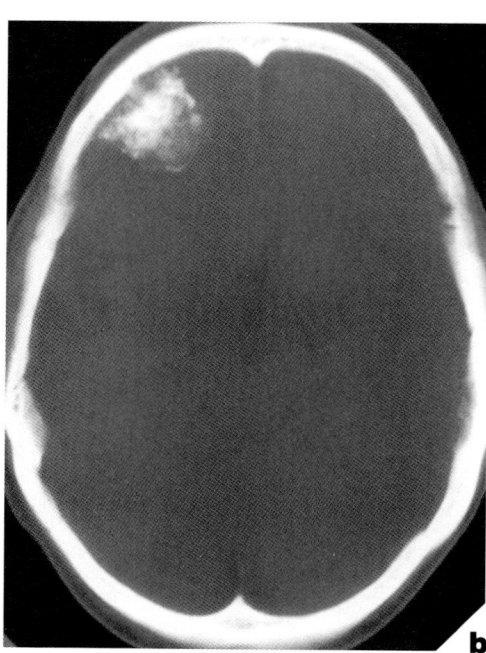

Figure 4.28

Calcified meningioma. ***a*** *Unenhanced CT scan with* ***b*** *bone windows show a heavily calcified anterior cranial fossa mass attached to the dura in the right frontal region.*

"punched-out" lytic lesions on skull films and CT (Fig. 4.27). Laboratory findings, including bone marrow studies are often necessary for confirmation.

MENINGIOMA

Meningiomas constitute about 15% of all intracranial tumors. They are primary tumors of the meninges and are therefore not brain tumors. Like other masses outside the brain (but inside the cranium), they are termed *extra-axial*. Meningiomas are often completely resectable and must be distinguished preoperatively from *intra-axial* tumors. Fortunately, CT, MRI and angiographic features are usually specific.

The noncontrast CT scan usually demonstrates a mass that is homogeneously isodense or hyperdense with respect to brain. The hyperdensity is probably due to the presence of psamommatous calcifications. Occasionally, there are nodular areas of calcification (Fig. 4.28); sometimes the entire meningioma may be densely calcified. Following intravenous injection of contrast material, there is usually dense, homogeneous enhancement (Fig. 4.29). The amount of surrounding edema is usually slight.

Meningiomas frequently involve the adjacent skull (Fig. 4.30). There may be direct invasion by the meningioma or there may be a reactive-type of hyperostosis, which is quite characteristic.

MRI typically shows intense enhancement with Gadolinium. This is fortunate since meningiomas are often isointense to brain on unenhanced T1 and T2 MR images (Fig. 4.31). However, some meningiomas are hyperintense on T2 images (Fig. 4.32) and might be confused with an intra-axial mass.

Angiography may be very specific in separating meningiomas from intra-axial brain tumors. Lesions in or near the cranial vertex usually have a prominent arterial supply (Fig. 4.33) via the middle meningeal artery, a branch of the internal maxillary branch of the external carotid artery. Selective external carotid artery or internal maxillary artery injections (Fig. 4.34) also show marked enhancement and blush. Typically, the tumor blush becomes apparent quite early in the injection and persists through the venous phase. Except in extremely aggressive meningiomas, early venous drainage is uncommon.

Meningiomas usually occur in typical locations. Sphenoid wing (Fig. 4.35) meningiomas may extend into the orbit. Optic sheath meningiomas (Fig. 4.36) typically result in thickening and "tram-track" enhancement of the optic nerve's coverings. The optic nerve otherwise is not involved.

Hemangiopericytoma

Hemangiopericytomas (Fig. 4.37) are rare lesions which are sometimes classified as *angioblastic meningiomas*. They have a tendency to recur and invade the brain. They may undergo malignant degeneration to fibrosarcoma. On CT and MRI, hemangiopericytomas resemble meningiomas in location, but they typically demonstrate invasion of the brain and/or considerable edema and mass effect.

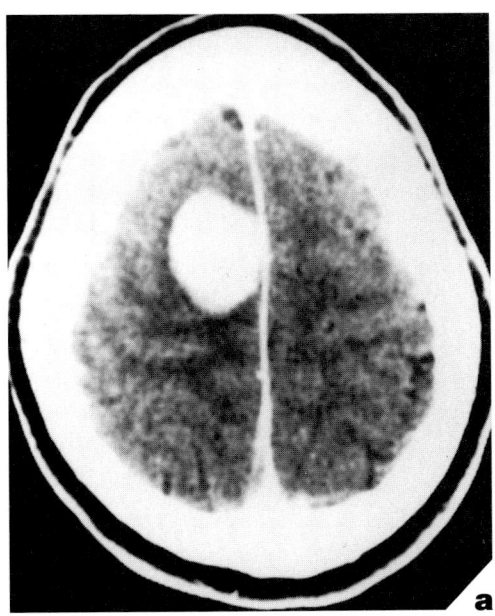

a

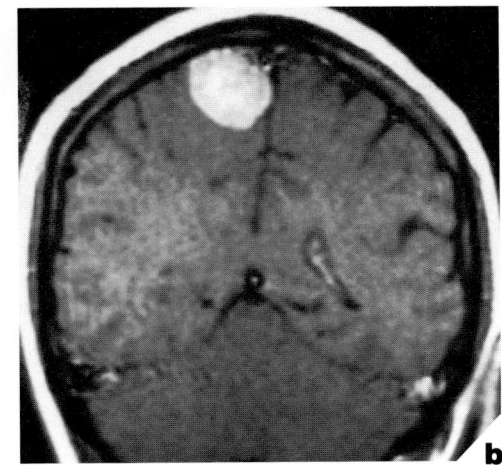

b

Figure 4.29

*Vertex meningioma. Contrast-enhanced **a** CT and **b** MR scans show homogeneous, intense enhancement within this small meningioma. There is no associated brain edema. The attachment of the lesion to the dura, including the falx cerebri, is well demonstrated.*

4.17

Intracranial Neoplasms

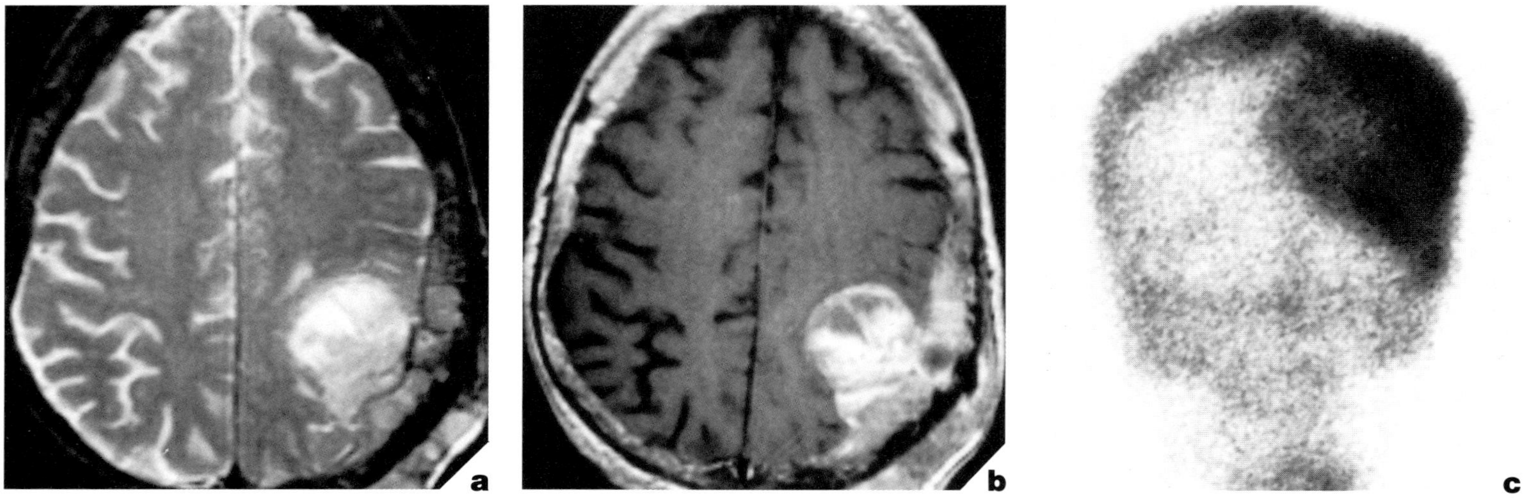

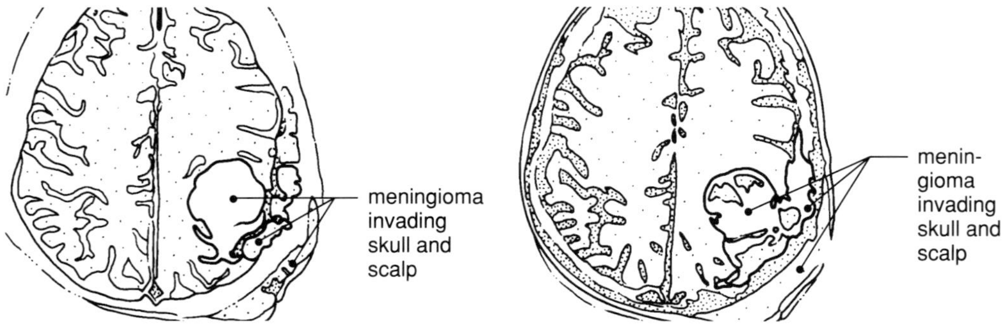

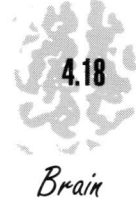

Figure 4.30

Meningioma with adjacent hyperostosis. **a** *Unenhanced T2-weighted and* **b** *Gadolinium-enhanced T1-weighted MR scans and* **c** *bone scan show marked abnormality of the left parietal bone and scalp overlying a meningioma.*

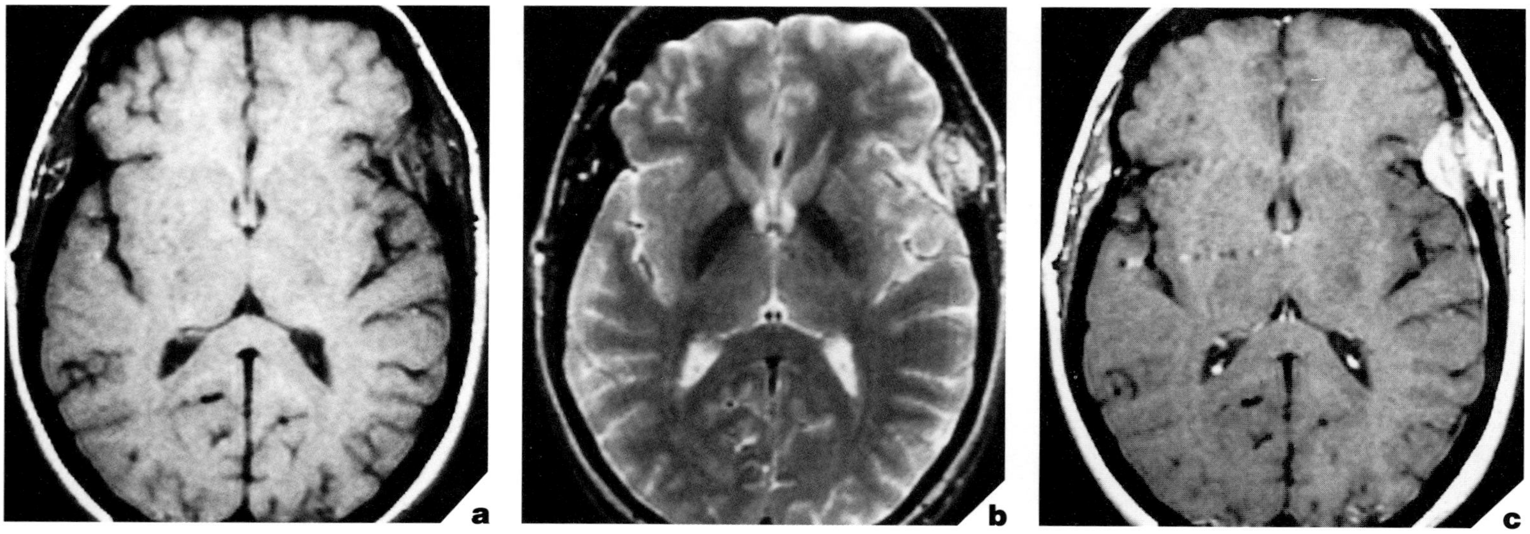

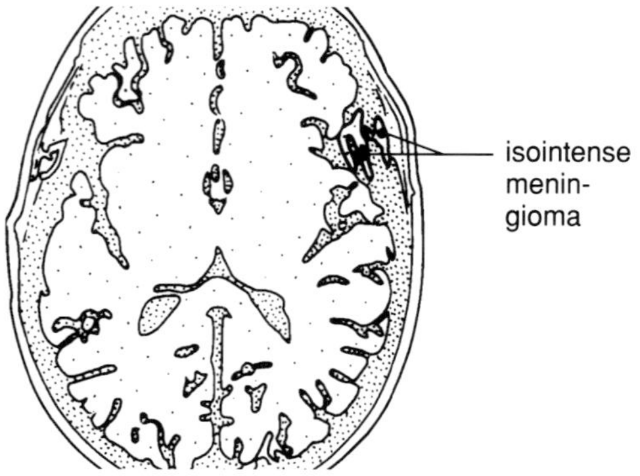

meningioma invading skull and scalp

meningioma invading skull and scalp

Figure 4.31

Isointense meningioma. **a** *T1 and* **b** *T2 sequences show an abnormal mass in the left pterionic region which is difficult to delineate since it is isointense to the surrounding brain. Following the intravenous administration of* **c** *Gadolinium-DTPA, there is intense enhancement of the meningioma, providing excellent definition of its size and extent. Note the calvarial invasion.*

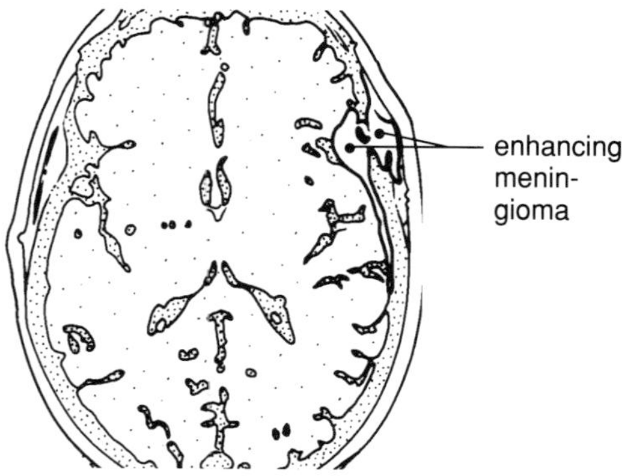

isointense meningioma

enhancing meningioma

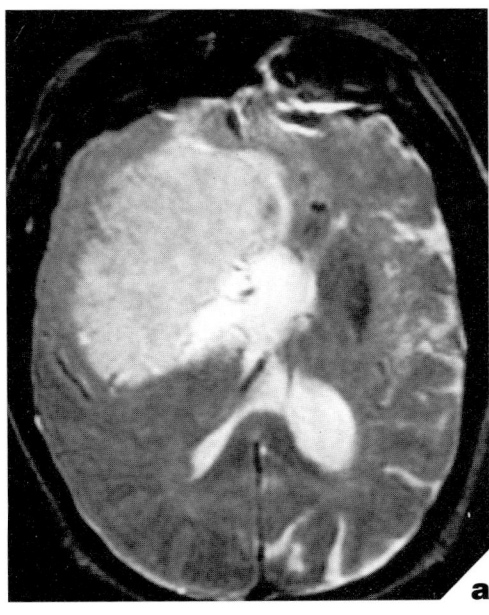

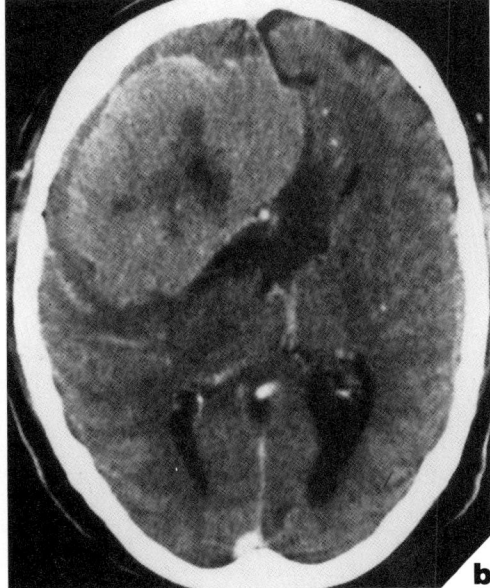

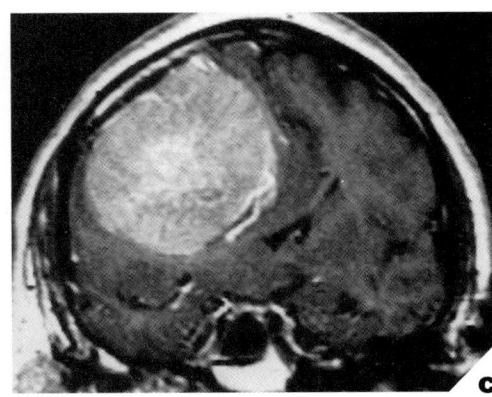

Figure 4.32

*Hyperintense meningioma. **a** T2-weighted axial MR image shows a hyperintense mass resulting in marked compression of the brain and ventricles and subfalcian herniation. Contrast-enhanced **b** CT and **c** MR images show moderate enhancement.*

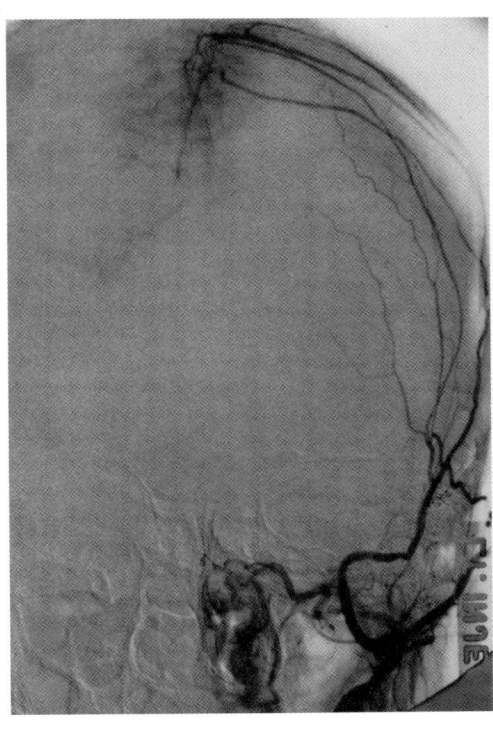

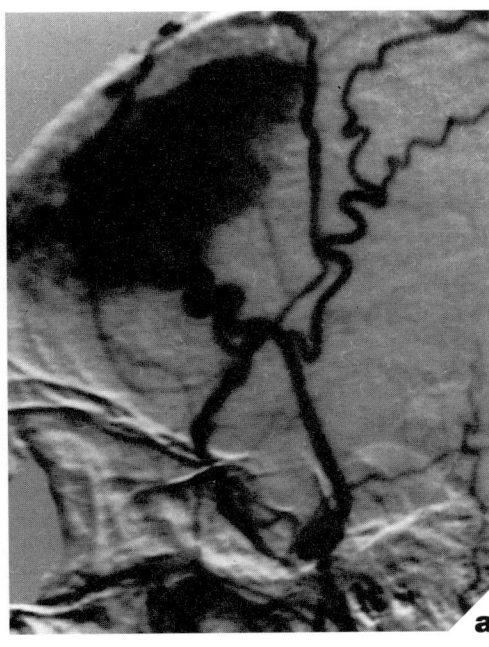

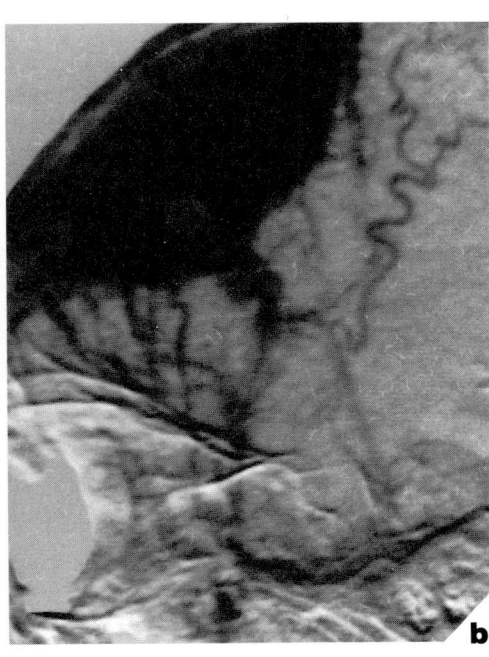

Figure 4.34

*Demonstration of meningioma angiographic blush. **a,b** Lateral digital subtraction images show prominent middle* *meningeal artery branches and early, intense tumor blush which persisted into the venous phase.*

Figure 4.33

Vertex meningioma. Selective left external carotid artery injection shows marked prominence and enlargement of middle meningeal artery branches and an enhancing mass at the cranial vertex.

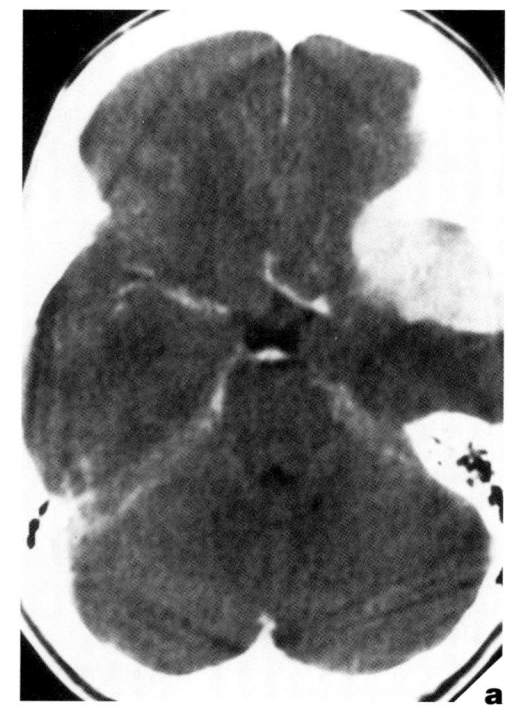

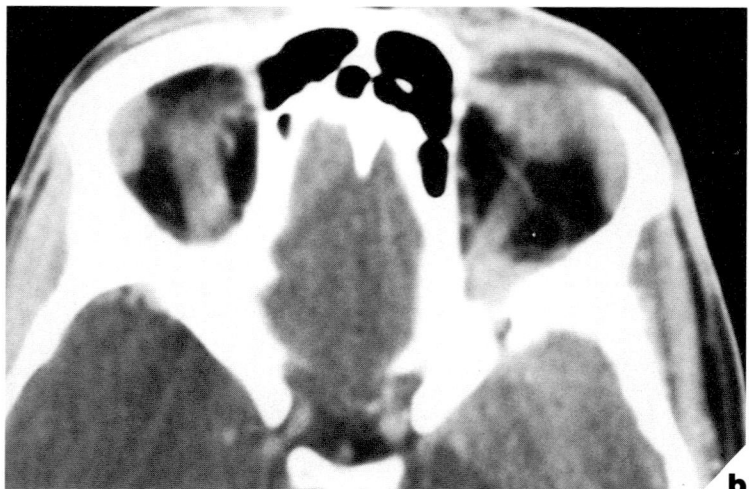

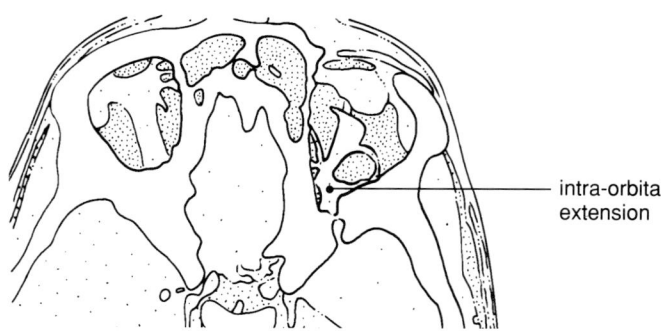

intra-orbital extension

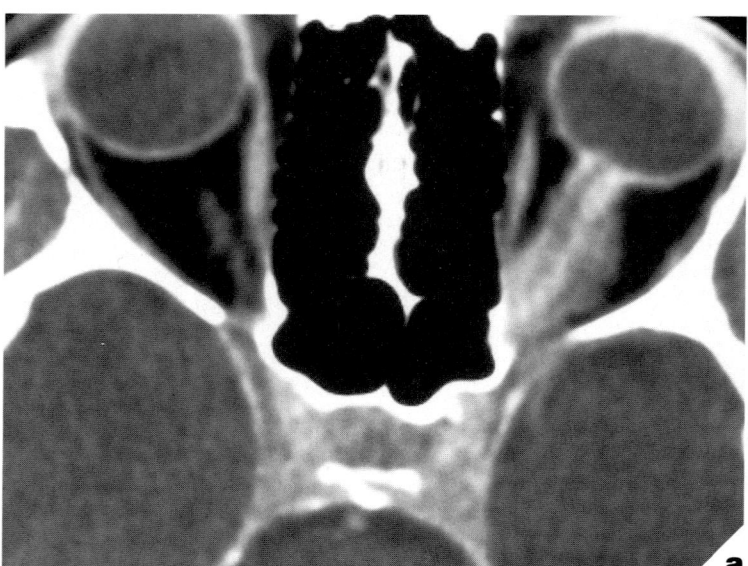

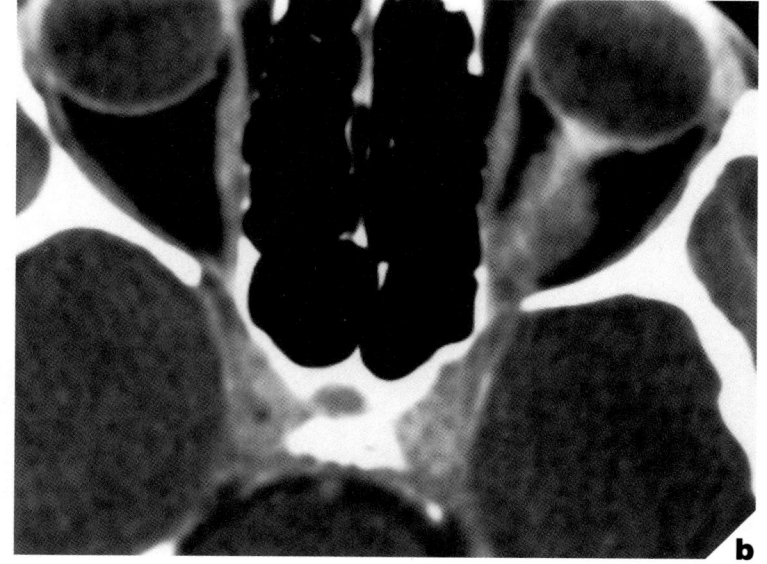

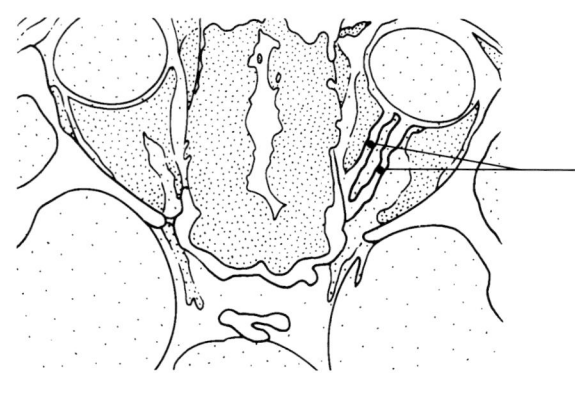

"tram-track" parallel linear enhancement in sheath of optic nerve

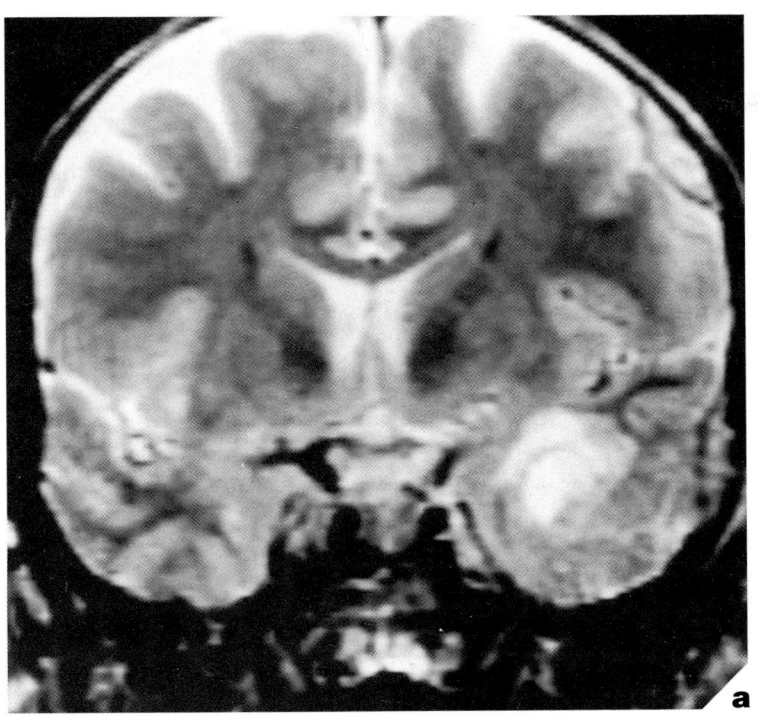

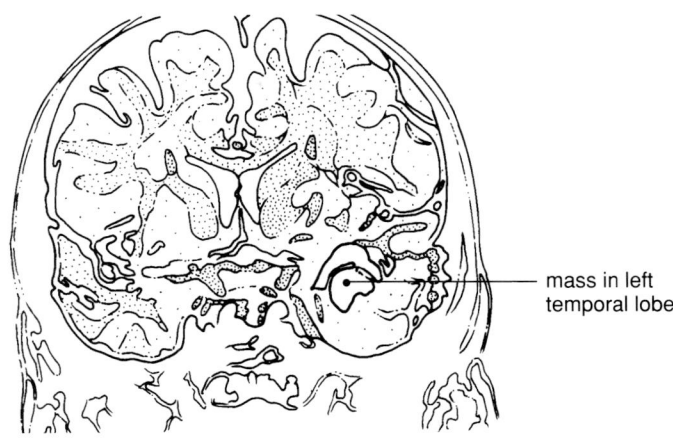

mass in left
temporal lobe

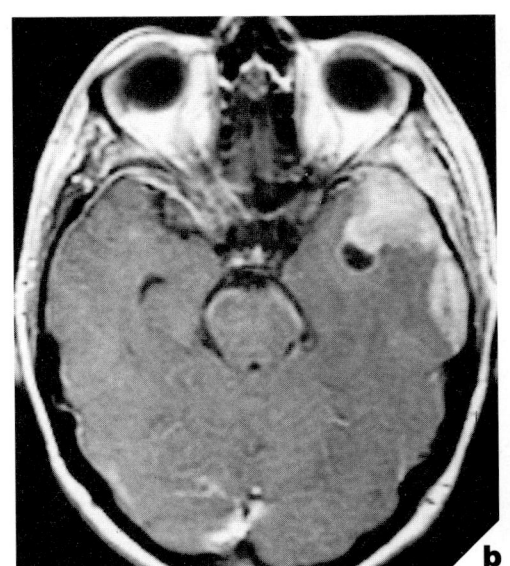

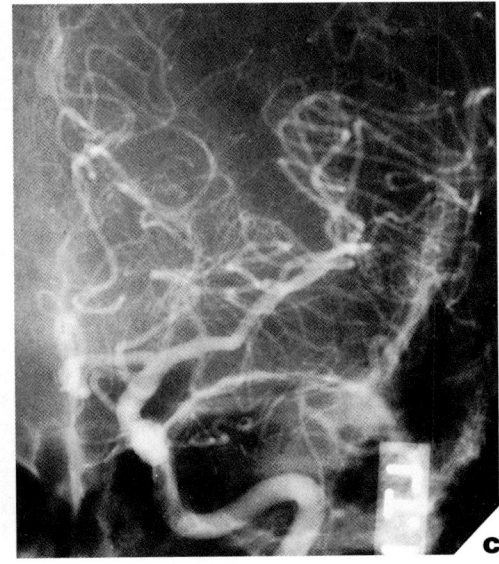

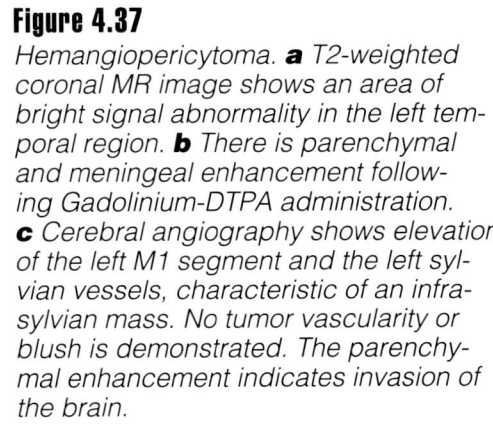

Figure 4.37

Hemangiopericytoma. **a** *T2-weighted coronal MR image shows an area of bright signal abnormality in the left temporal region.* **b** *There is parenchymal and meningeal enhancement following Gadolinium-DTPA administration.* **c** *Cerebral angiography shows elevation of the left M1 segment and the left sylvian vessels, characteristic of an infrasylvian mass. No tumor vascularity or blush is demonstrated. The parenchymal enhancement indicates invasion of the brain.*

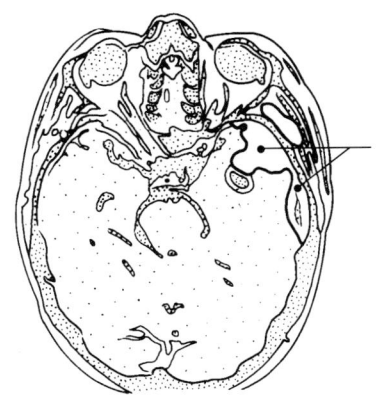

parenchymal
and
meningeal
enhancement

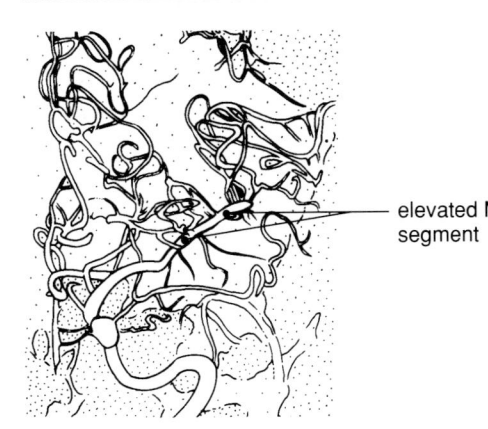

elevated M1
segment

INTRAVENTRICULAR TUMORS

Intraventricular tumors are considered separately because of their distinctive radiologic appearance and their potential for resectability. Ependymomas will be discussed with posterior fossa tumors.

Colloid Cyst

Another name for this benign tumor is *neuroepithelial cyst*. Colloid cysts are believed to arise in the primitive neuroepithelium where the choroid plexus, paraphysis, and the roof of the third ventricle are formed. They are characteristically located just behind the foramina of Monro near the roof of the third ventricle. The CT findings are distinctive. Noncontrast scans show a sharply circumscribed, usually high-density lesion in the anterior/superior third ventricle (Fig. 4.38). There may be slight contrast enhancement. Because of their strategic location, colloid cysts may obstruct one or both foramina of Monro, causing hydrocephalus. When small, they often cause only partial, transitory obstruction of the lateral ventricles. This causes headaches, which are characteristically relieved by rotating movements of the head.

Choroid Plexus Papilloma

Choroid plexus papillomas are most commonly encountered during the first decade of life, usually in infancy. The tumor typically arises in the lateral ventricle. Hydrocephalus secondary to overproduction of cerebrospinal fluid (CSF) may occur. In most instances, however, the hydrocephalus associated with a choroid plexus papilloma is due to mechanical obstruction of the CSF pathways by the tumor or by hemorrhage.

Computed tomography shows a homogeneous, lobulated, isodense or hyperdense intraventricular mass. Contrast-enhanced scans frequently show intense, homogeneous enhancement of the tumor. Magnetic resonance imaging (Fig. 4.39) with its multiplanar capabilities, is also an excellent method of imaging these lesions.

Intraventricular Meningioma

Intraventricular meningiomas are rare tumors that occur most commonly in the atrium of the lateral ventricles and much less frequently in the third or fourth ventricle. The tumor is thought to arise from rests of meningeal tissue formed by folding of the dural tube. The appearance on MRI and CT is similar to that of meningiomas at other sites, i.e., hyperdensity, isointensity and intense, homogeneous enhancement. Meningiomas in the atrium of a lateral ventricle often obstruct CSF flow from the ipsilateral temporal horn, leading to the so-called "trapped" temporal horn (Fig. 4.40).

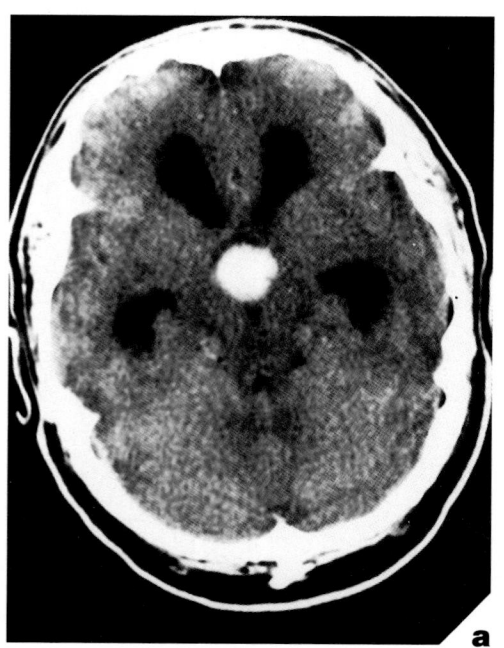
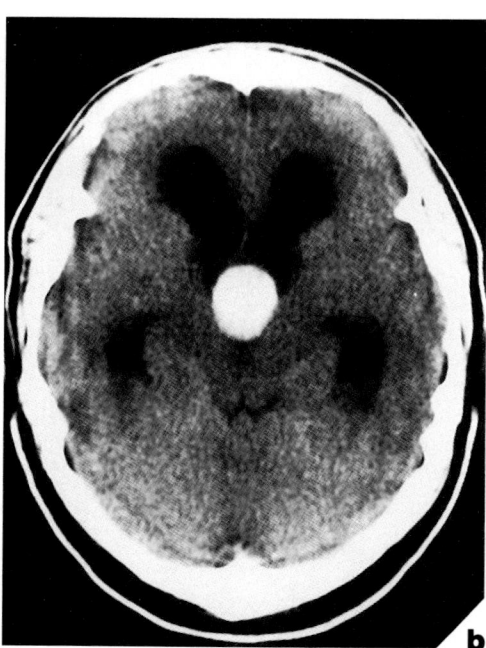

Figure 4.38
*Colloid cyst. **a,b** Unenhanced axial CT images demonstrate a large, hyperdense mass in the anterior third ventricle which results in obstruction of the lateral ventricles.*

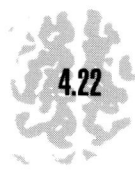

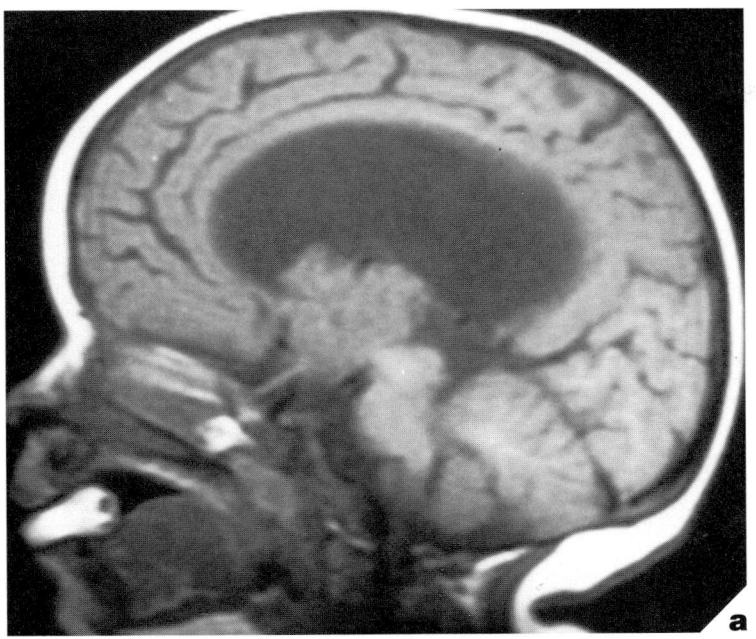

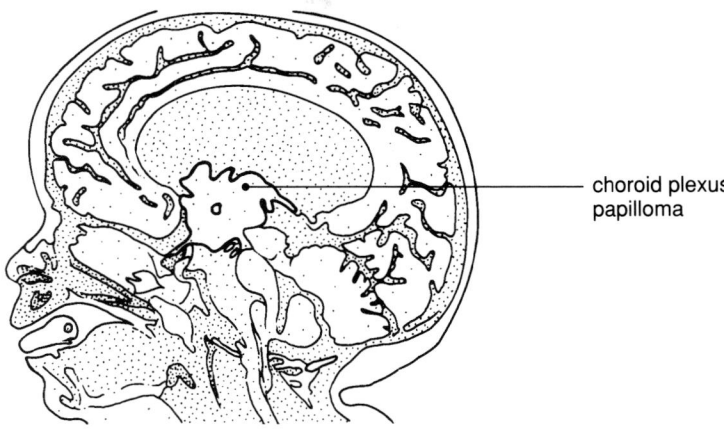

choroid plexus papilloma

Figure 4.39

Choroid plexus papilloma of the third ventricle. ***a*** *Sagittal and* ***b*** *axial T1-weighted images demonstrate a lobulated mass in the third ventricle extending into the right frontal horn.* ***c*** *The mass is isointense to the surrounding CSF on this T2-weighted image. The lesion obstructs the third ventricle and produces hydrocephalus.*

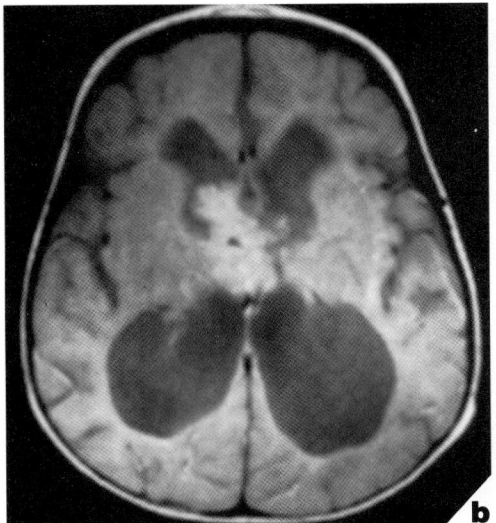

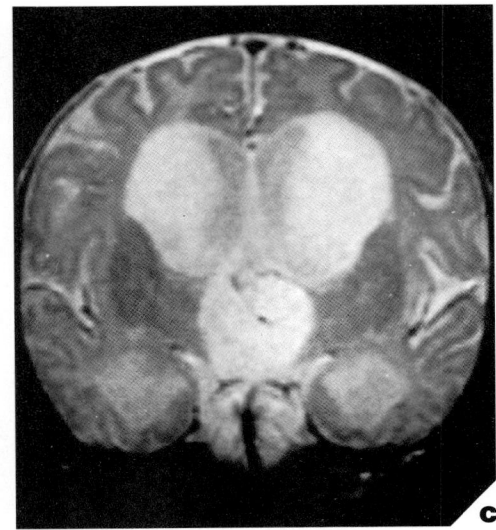

Figure 4.40

Intraventricular meningioma. Axial CT scans ***a*** *before and* ***b*** *after intravenous injection of contrast material show a high density, uniformly enhancing mass in the atrium of the left lateral ventricle. There is obstruction to CSF flow at this level causing the so-called "trapped" left temporal horn.*

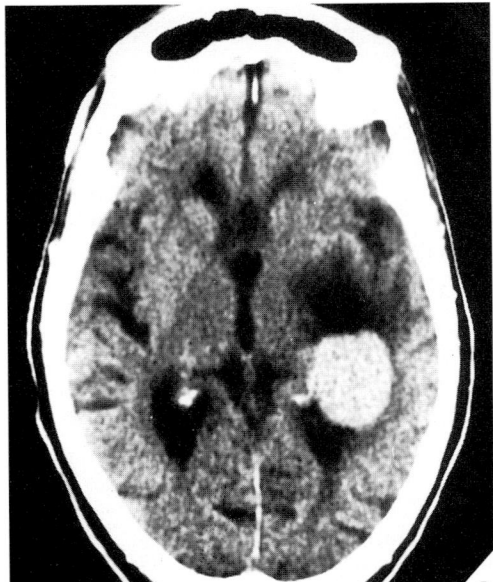

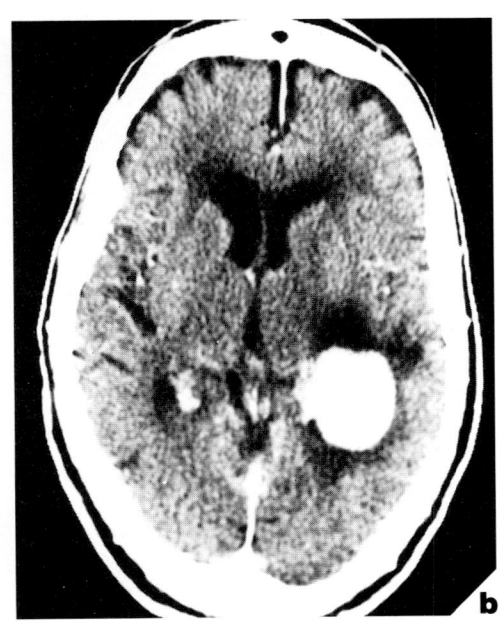

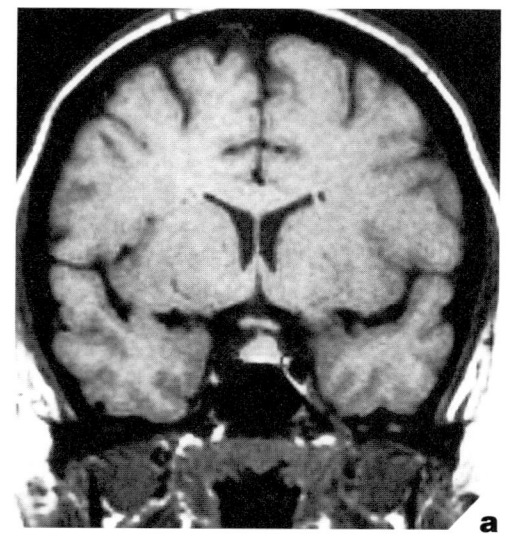 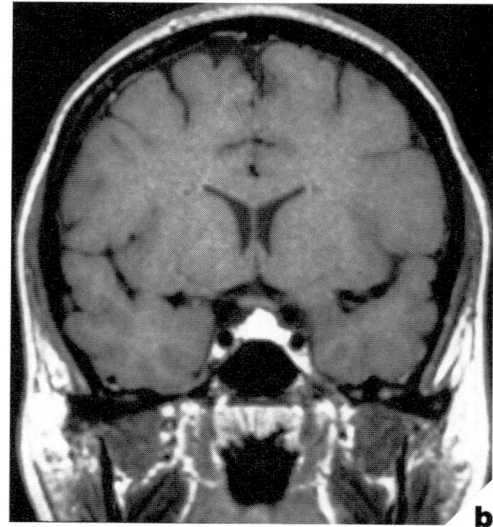 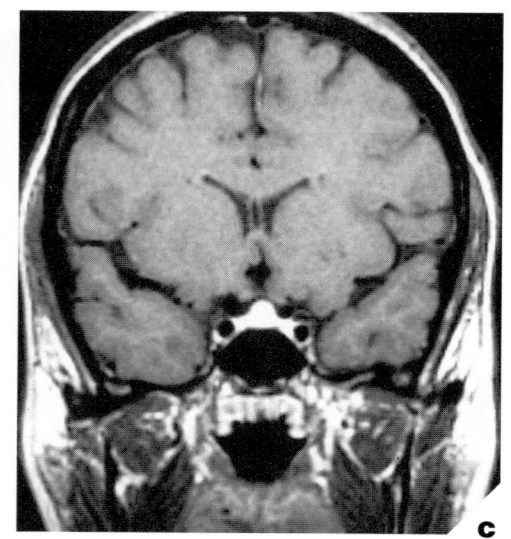

Figure 4.41

*ACTH-secreting pituitary adenoma. **a** Unenhanced and **b,c** Gadolinium-enhanced T1-weighted coronal MR images demonstrate a mass expanding the left side of the pituitary gland and extending into the suprasellar cistern. The mass demonstrates uniform contrast enhancement.*

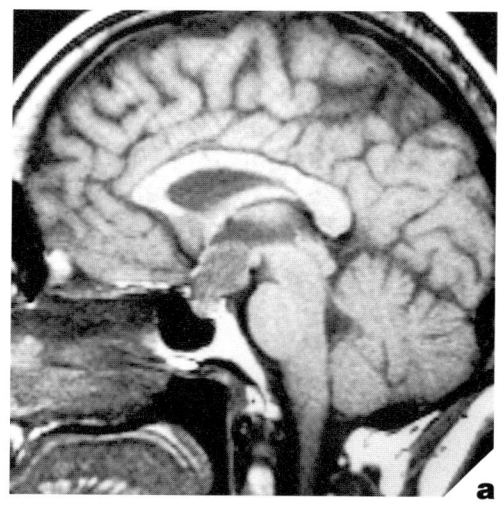 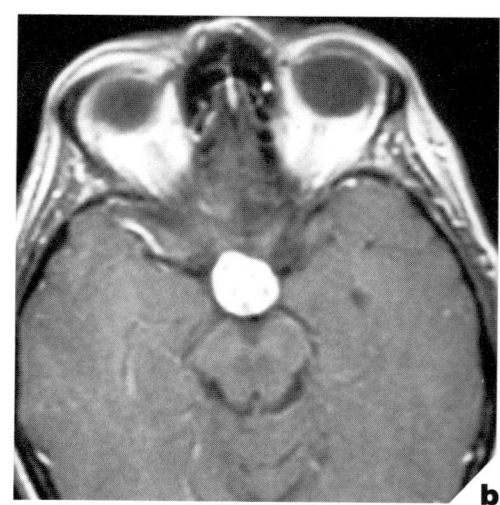 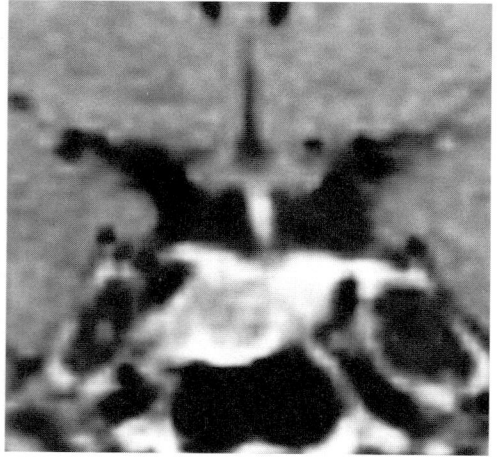

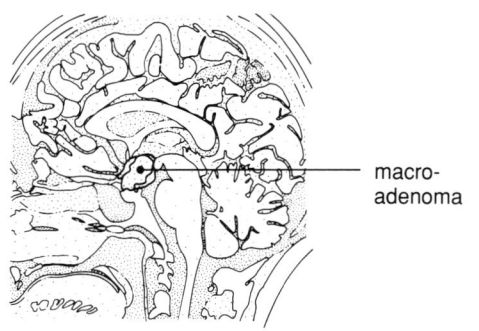

macro-
adenoma

macro-
adenoma

micro-
adenoma

Figure 4.42

*Growth hormone-secreting pituitary adenoma. **a** Unenhanced sagittal and **b** contrast-enhanced axial T1-weighted images demonstrate a large mass in the suprasellar cistern with intense contrast enhancement and small, central areas of decreased enhancement.*

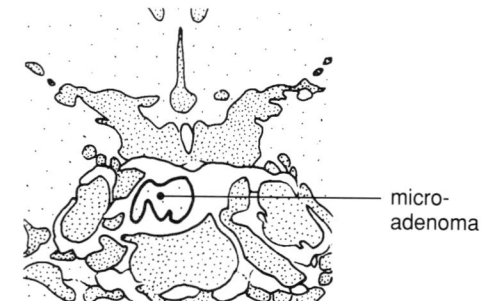

Figure 4.43

Pituitary microadenoma. Direct coronal contrast-enhanced T1-weighted MR image through the pituitary gland demonstrates an area of decreased enhancement in the right side of the pituitary gland. The mass results in convex inferior bowing of the floor of the sella turcica.

SELLAR AND PARASELLAR NEOPLASMS

Pituitary Adenoma

Pituitary adenomas comprise approximately 15% of all intracranial tumors in adults and are the most common tumors of the sellar and parasellar regions. These lesions are currently classified according to whether or not they are endocrinologically active. Hormone-secreting tumors are, in turn, categorized according to the particular hormone which they secrete: Cushing's disease is caused by a pituitary adenoma that secretes adrenocorticotropic hormone (ACTH) (Fig. 4.41); acromegaly is associated with growth hormone-secreting tumors (Fig. 4.42); the syndrome of amenorrhea, galactorrhea, and hyperprolactinemia are caused by prolactin-secreting tumors (Fig. 4.43). Because endocrinologically active tumors are symptomatic, they tend to present clinically at a much smaller size than nonsecreting tumors (formerly called *chromophobe adenomas*) (Fig. 4.44). The latter may attain great size and cause symptoms by causing compression of adjacent cranial nerves.

Pituitary tumors may be identified by CT or MRI because of the resultant enlargement of the pituitary gland, areas of abnormal signal/density, or areas of increased or decreased enhancement. The normal pituitary gland should not exceed 1 cm in height.

Figure 4.44

*Nonsecreting pituitary adenoma. **a** Coronal and **b** sagittal contrast enhanced T1-weighted MR images show a mass arising at the base of the pituitary stalk and extending superiorly and laterally into the suprasellar cistern. It compresses and displaces the optic chiasm superiorly.*

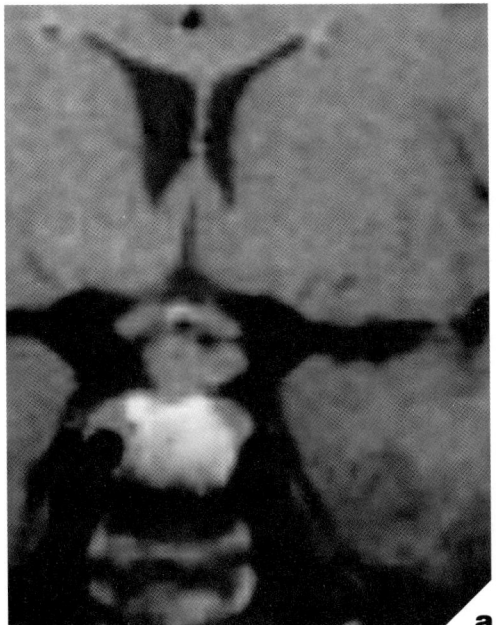
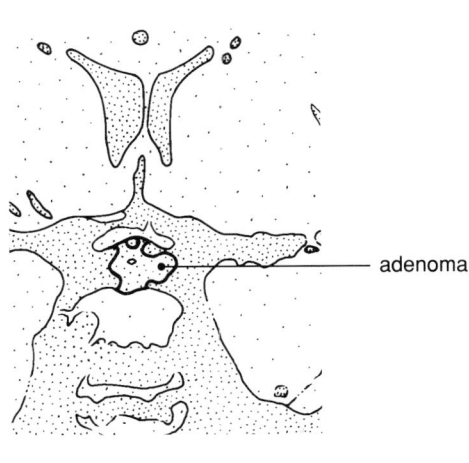

adenoma

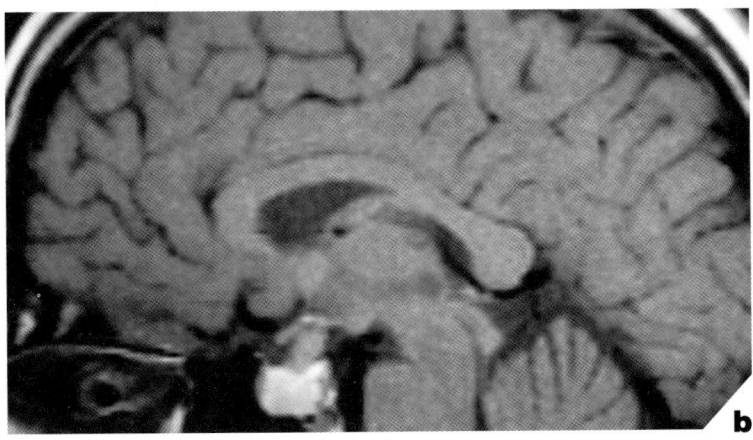
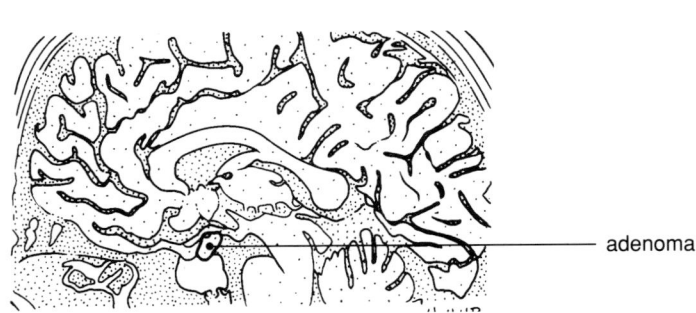

adenoma

Moreover, except in the case of young females of childbearing potential, the roof of the pituitary gland should be flat or slightly depressed centrally. Tumors smaller than 1 cm are termed *microadenomas* (Fig. 4.45) and show decreased enhancement on both CT and MRI compared to the rest of the gland. Lesions greater than 1 cm are called *macroadenomas*. They often extend into the suprasellar cistern and compress the optic chiasm (Fig. 4.46). This results in bitemporal hemianopsia. Pituitary tumors may encase the adjacent carotid arteries (Fig. 4.47) and extend into the cavernous sinuses.

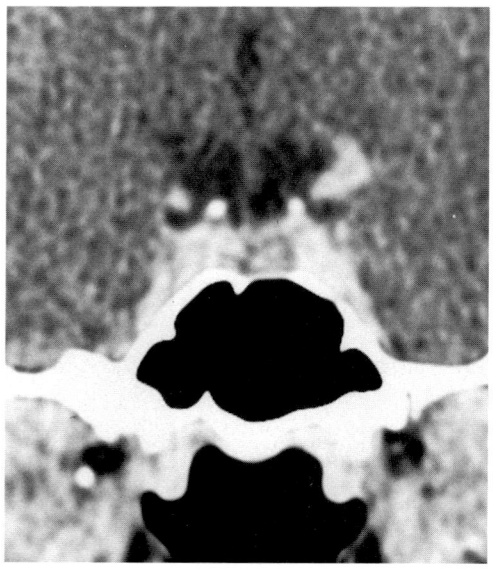

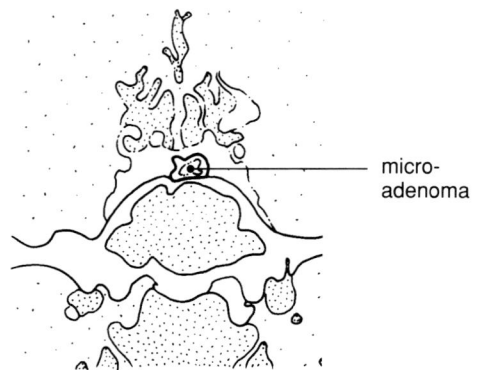

Figure 4.45
Pituitary microadenoma. Contrast-enhanced direct coronal CT scan through the pituitary gland shows a left paracentral area of decreased enhancement. Pituitary microadenomas typically show less enhancement than the normal, surrounding pituitary gland. The roof of the pituitary gland maintains a normal, flat shape; the gland as a whole is not enlarged.

micro-adenoma

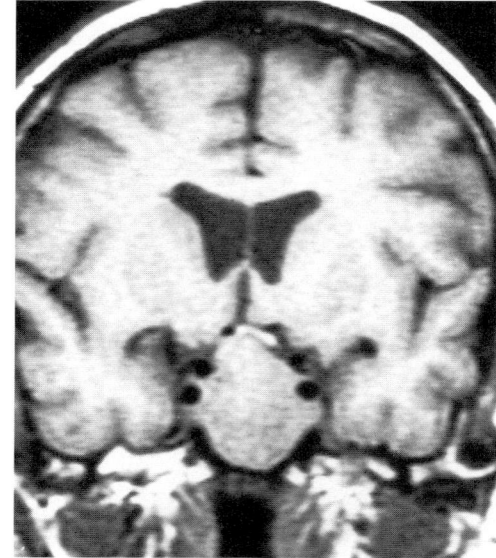

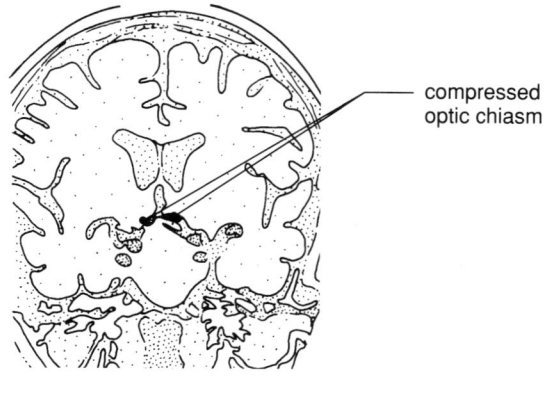

Figure 4.46
Pituitary macroadenoma. This unenhanced coronal T1 image shows a large pituitary mass extending into the suprasellar cistern and causing compression and displacement of the optic chiasm.

compressed optic chiasm

Figure 4.47
Prolactinoma. The main direction of growth of this pituitary mass is laterally. Contrast-enhanced T1-weighted image shows encasement of both distal internal carotid arteries by tumor extension into the right cavernous sinus.

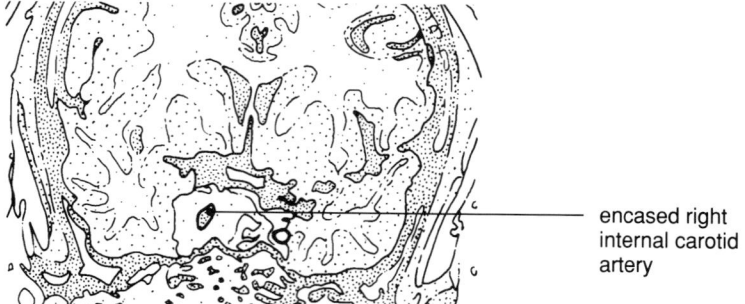

encased right internal carotid artery

Craniopharyngioma

Craniopharyngiomas are neoplasms which arise from remnants of Rathke's cleft. They are composed of elements of stratified and columnar epithelium, containing cholesterol, keratin, and necrotic debris. Calcification is present in approximately 80% of these tumors (Fig. 4.48). They have bimodal incidence peaks in the first and sixth decades. They most commonly arise in the suprasellar region. Craniopharyngiomas may present clinically with bitemporal hemi-anopsia due to compression of the optic chiasm, diabetes insipidus, hydrocephalus secondary to third ventricular obstruction, and/or growth retardation. CT and MRI usually reveal a lobulated, partially cystic or solid mass lesion centered in the suprasellar region. Craniopharyngiomas usually enhance on CT and MRI. Sometimes there is only a small, nodular area of enhancement. Craniopharyngiomas may contain thick mucoid material ("crank case oil") which produces a bright signal on T1-weighted images.

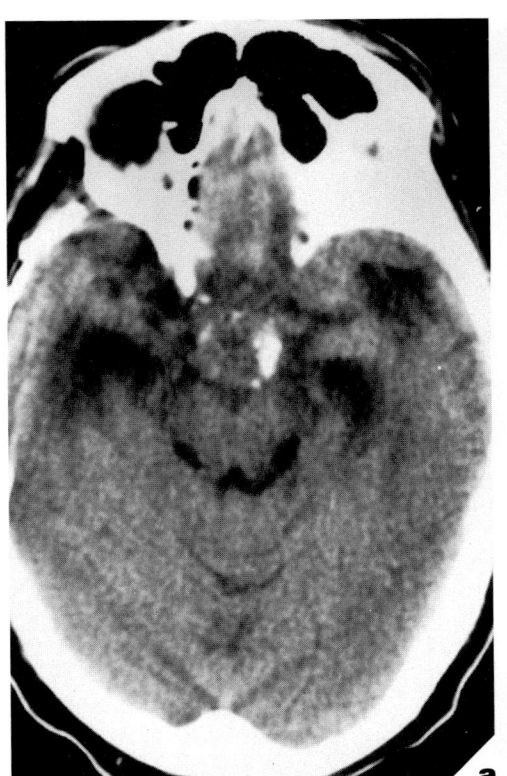 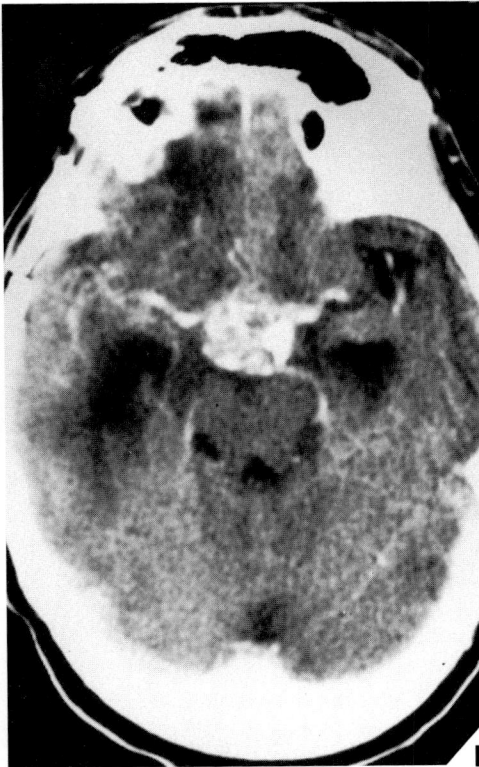 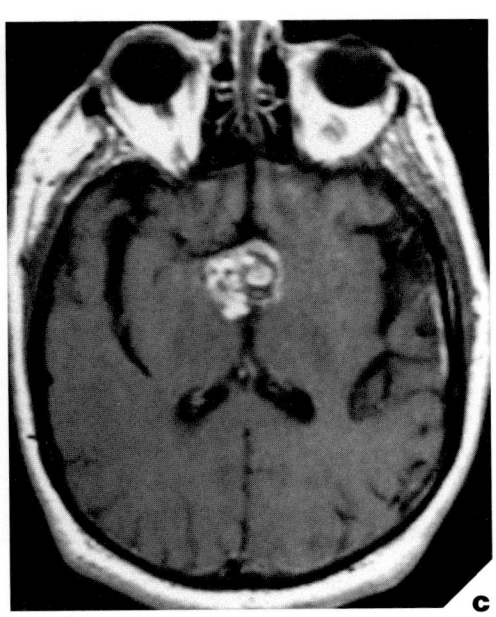

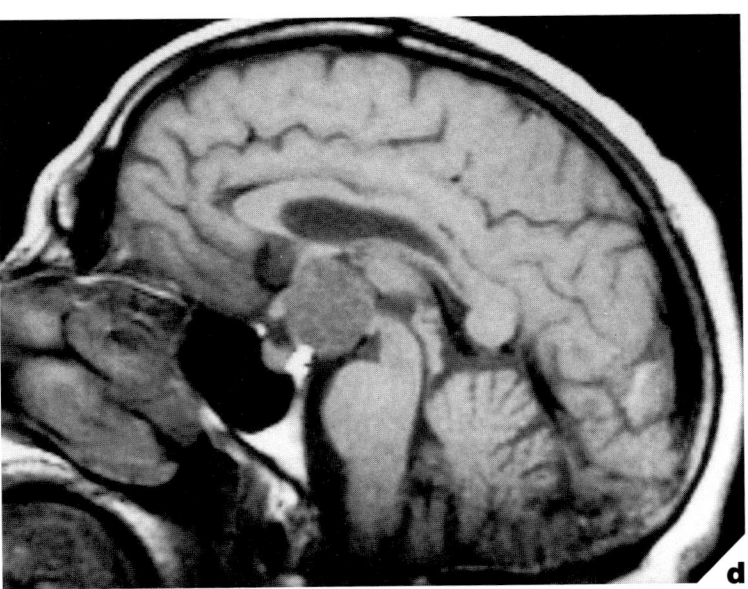

Figure 4.48

*Craniopharyngioma. **a** Unenhanced CT scan shows characteristic calcification which is present in 80% of craniopharyngiomas. Irregular enhancement is demonstrated on **b** CT and **c** MR images. **d** Sagittal T1 image shows the suprasellar location of this lesion to best advantage.*

Optic Glioma

These tumors arise from the optic chiasm in the suprasellar cistern or nearby portions of the optic nerves, tracts, or radiations (Fig. 4.49). Most present in the first decade of life with visual disturbance, hydrocephalus, or hypothalamic dysfunction. Optic and hypothalamic gliomas are quite common in patients with neurofibromatosis. There may be enlargement of one or both optic foramina. Optic gliomas frequently show contrast enhancement (Fig. 4.50).

DEVELOPMENTAL AND PINEAL REGION TUMORS

Neoplasms of developmental origin include epidermoids, dermoids, and teratomas. Some other devel-

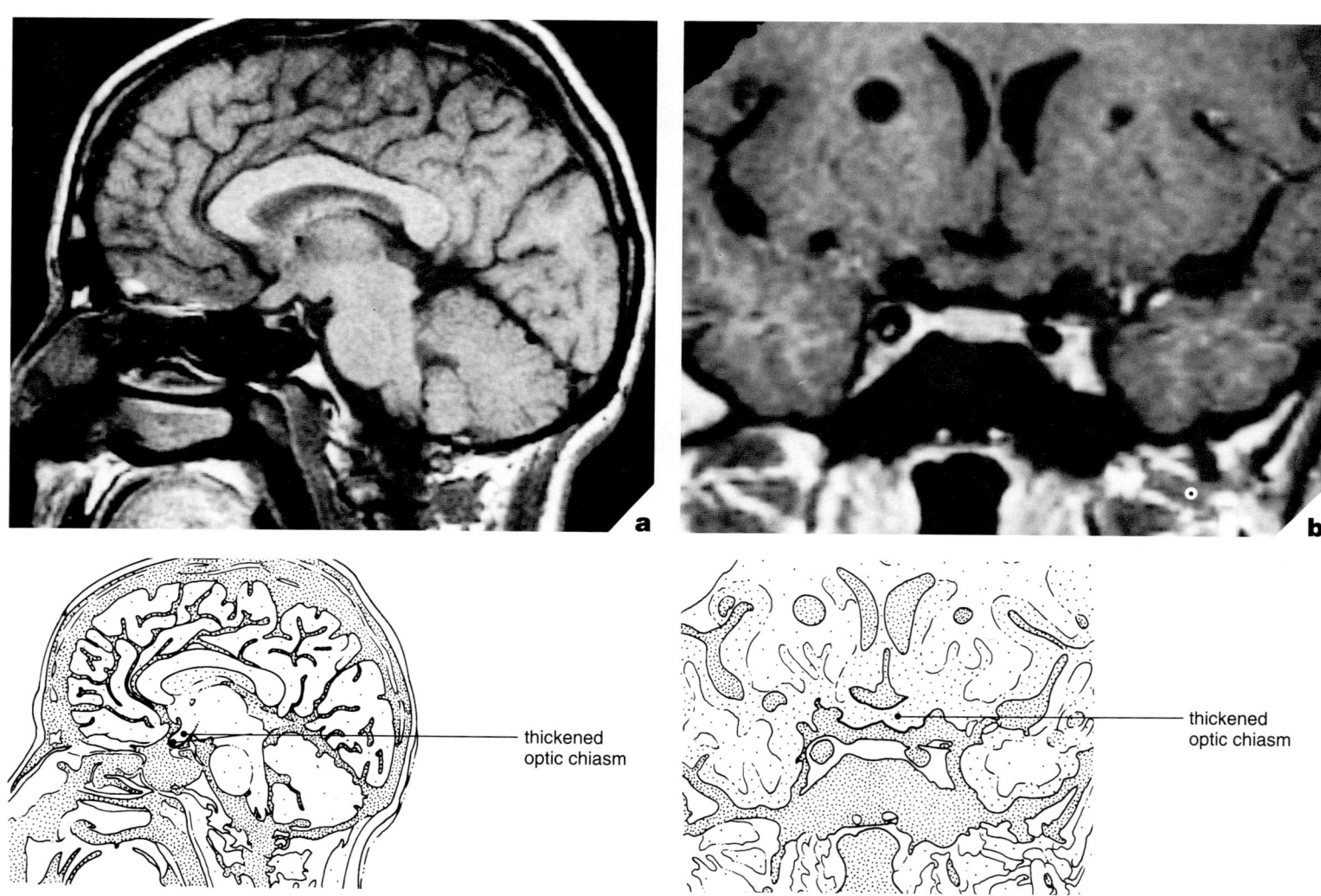

thickened
optic chiasm

thickened
optic chiasm

Figure 4.49

*Optic nerve and optic chiasm glioma. **a** Sagittal and **b** coronal T1-weighted MR images demonstrate thickening of the optic nerves and optic chiasm, a typical feature of optic gliomas.*

opmental tumors such as craniopharyngiomas, colloid cysts, and lipomas of the corpus callosum, have already been discussed.

Epidermoid

These congenital neoplasms generally occur in para-midline, extra-axial locations. They most likely occur secondary to incomplete separation of the neural and cutaneous ectoderm early in gestation with inclusion of ectodermal tissue into the neural groove. Epidermoids are often isodense to CSF on CT (Fig. 4.51), and thus, difficult to distinguish from arachnoid cysts. However, MRI usually is helpful in this regard since the lesions are mildly hypointense on T1 images but not of low enough signal intensity to be isointense to

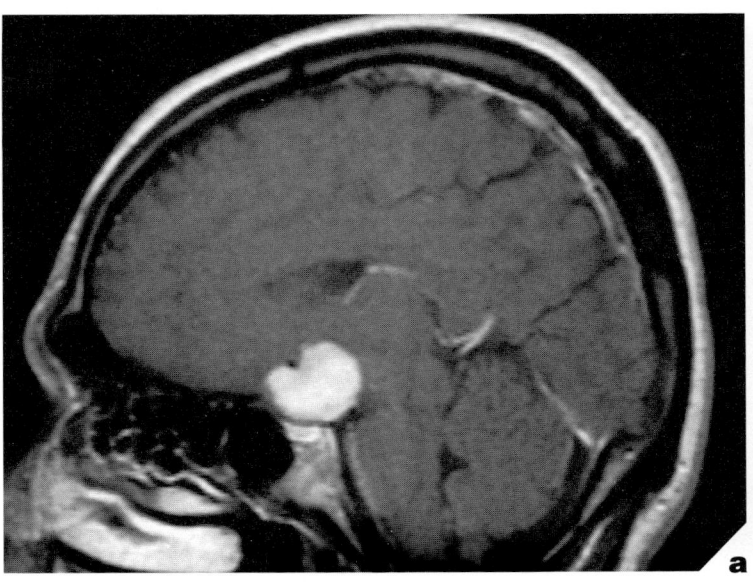

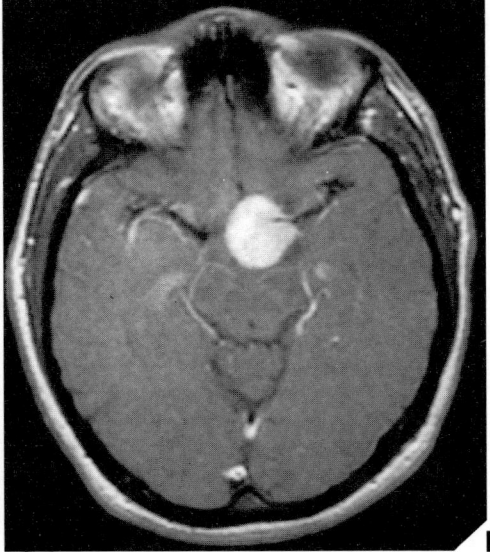

a   b

Figure 4.50
*Optic glioma. **a,b** Intense Gadolinium enhancement is demonstrated in this glioma of the optic chiasm and hypothalamus.*

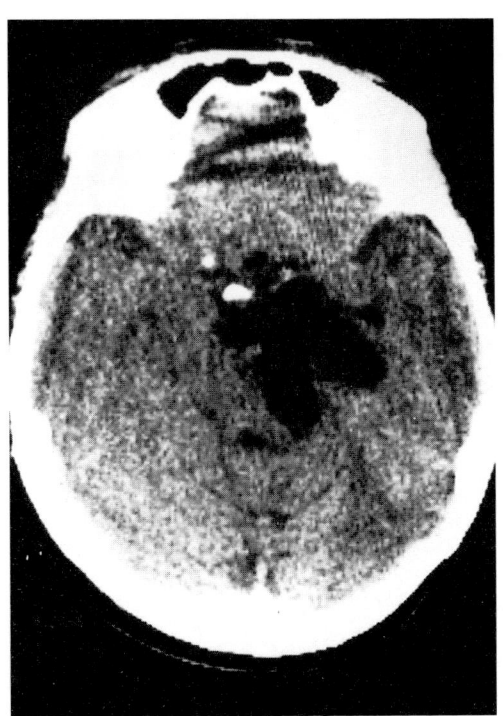

Figure 4.51
Epidermoid. Axial CT image demonstrates a large, irregularly shaped area of decreased attenuation which is isodense to CSF. Its para-midline location is typical of an epidermoid.

CSF (Fig. 4.52). Since epidermoids have an irregular, frond-like surface, nonionic contrast administered into the CSF via lumbar puncture and made to layer around the mass may distinguish an epidermoid from the smooth surface of an arachnoid cyst.

Teratoma

Teratomas are tumors composed of all three germ cell layers and tend to occur at or close to the mid-line. The presence of calcification, fat, and soft tissue is a characteristic feature of these tumors (Fig. 4.53). They may rupture into the ventricles and cause a chemical meningitis.

Pineal Region Tumors

Pineal cysts (Fig. 4.54) are the most common lesions in the pineal region. When they are smaller than 1 cm, they are usually considered to be clinically insignificant.

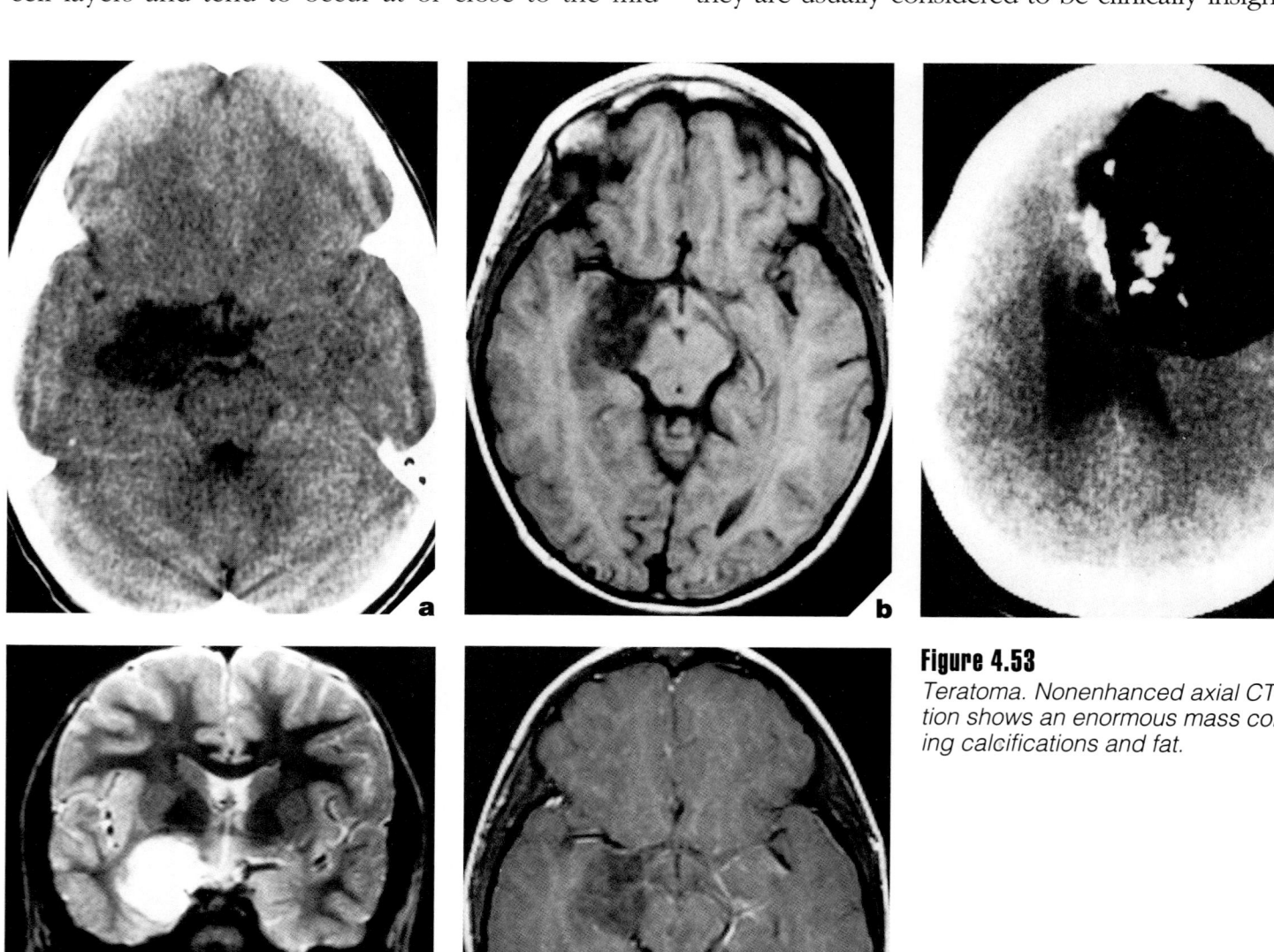

Figure 4.53
Teratoma. Nonenhanced axial CT section shows an enormous mass containing calcifications and fat.

Figure 4.52
*Epidermoid. **a** CT, **b** T1, **c** T2, and **d** Gadolinium-enhanced T1-weighted images show a nonenhancing mass which is isodense to CSF and of dark-T1, bright-T2 signal characteristics. Since the T1 images show that the mass is not isointense to CSF, the diagnosis favors an epidermoid rather than an arachnoid cyst.*

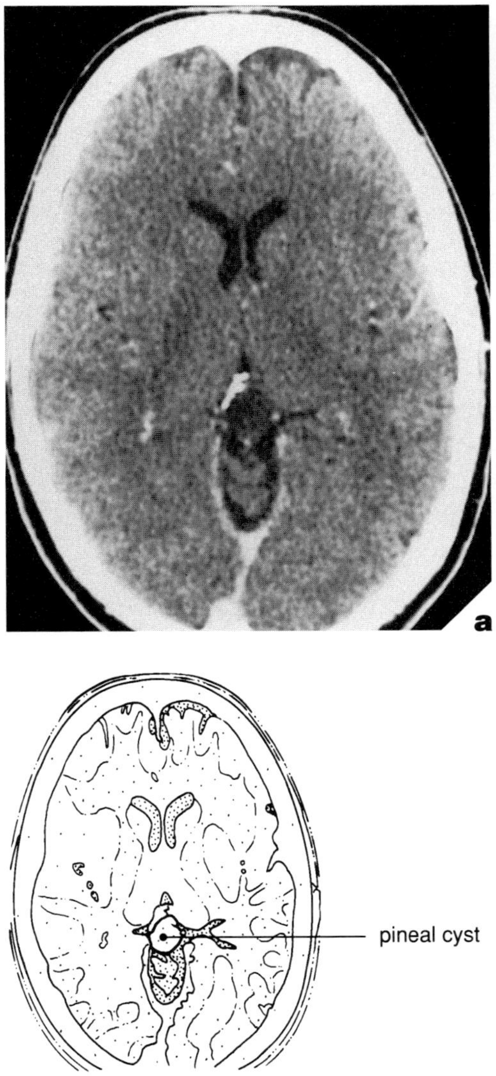

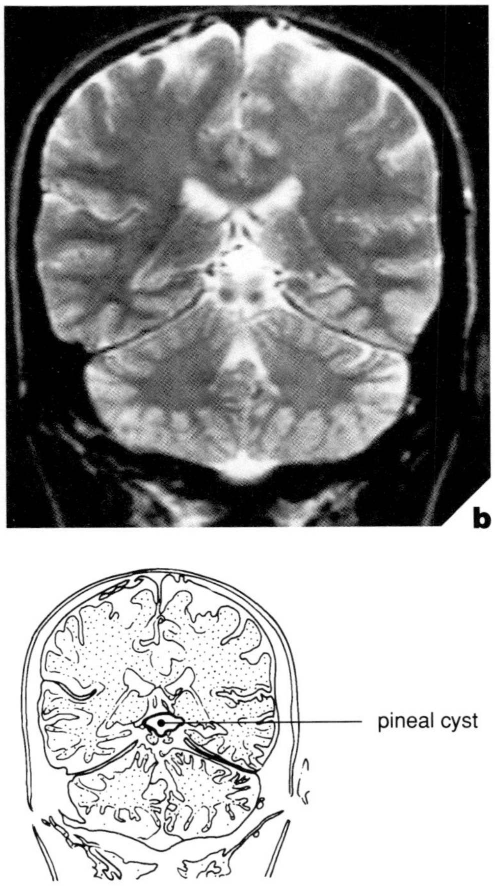

Figure 4.54
Pineal cyst. **a** CT, **b** T2-weighted coronal MR, and **c** sagittal, contrast-enhanced T1-weighted MRI scans demonstrate a 1-cm cyst in the pineal gland.

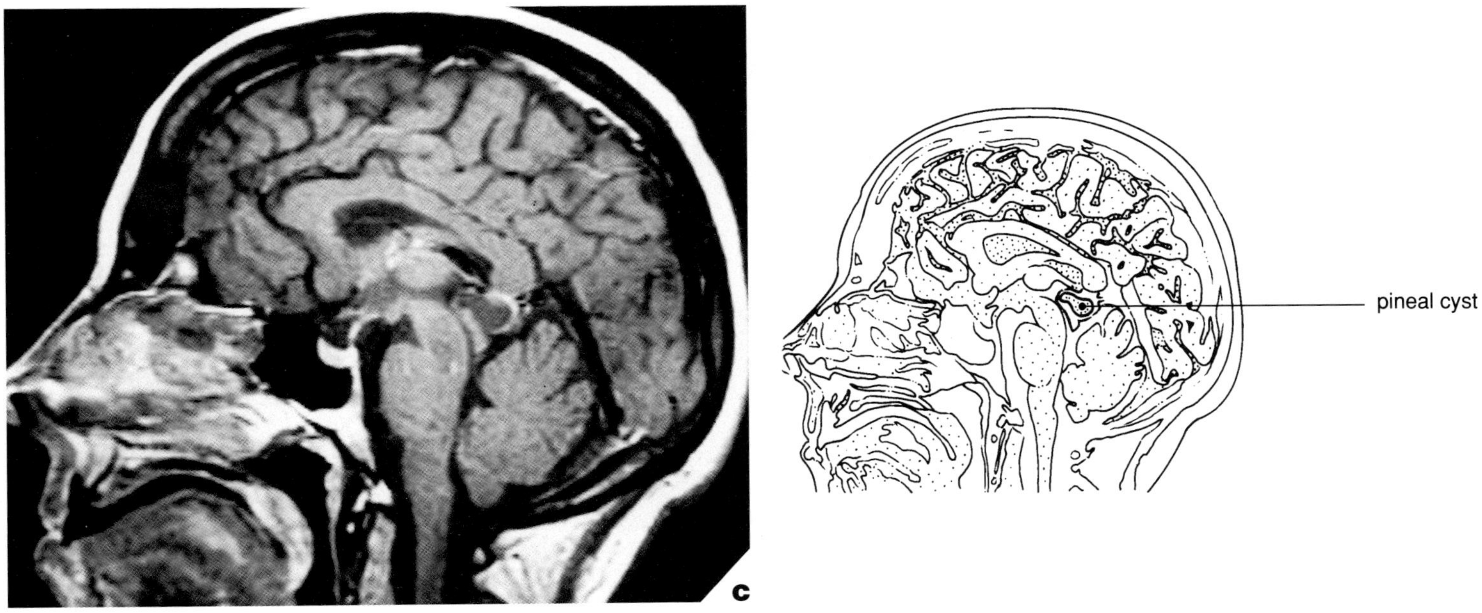

pineal cyst

pineal cyst

pineal cyst

When pineal lesions are large, they may compress the colliculi of the midbrain and produce paralysis of upward gaze (Pirinaud's syndrome). Solid pineal region tumors include developmental tumors (germinoma and teratoma), as well as true tumors of pineal cell origin (pineocytoma and pineoblastoma). Germinomas are the most common type of solid pineal tumor (Figure 4.55). When these lesions occur in the suprasellar region, they have been misnamed *ectopic pinealomas.*

POSTERIOR FOSSA TUMORS

While many of the tumors discussed thus far may also occur in the posterior fossa, certain neoplasms tend to occur with greater frequency in this region and are considered as a separate group. The age of the patient is a critical factor in evaluating the type of lesion; thus, astrocytomas are most common in children, hemangioblastomas are most common in young adults, and metastases are most common in elderly patients. Key criteria which must be regarded include location of the mass, its density and/or signal intensity, enhancement characteristics, calcifications and the presence of cysts. In certain circumstances, angiographic correlation is very helpful in making a specific diagnosis pos-

sible. Cerebellar masses can obstruct the fourth ventricle and patients occasionally present with signs of hydrocephalus. Brainstem masses usually do not cause hydrocephalus early in their course; they typically present with signs of cranial nerve dysfunction.

Cerebellar Astrocytoma

Cerebellar astrocytomas are the most common pediatric posterior fossa neoplasm. They typically contain cystic portions (Fig. 4.56) and frequently have a good prognosis. A particularly benign form is the pilocytic astrocytoma; this lesion is usually partially cystic and contains a mural nodule of enhancing solid tumor. It is difficult to distinguish on CT or MRI from other types of cerebellar astrocytomas.

Brainstem Glioma

Most brainstem gliomas occur during the first decade of life. Pontine astrocytomas are the most common lesions. They typically present with cranial nerve deficiencies rather than hydrocephalus. MRI is the best method for imaging these lesions (Fig. 4.57) since they are often infiltrative rather than compressive; also, the brainstem may be poorly seen on CT due to petrous bone-derived beam-hardening artifacts.

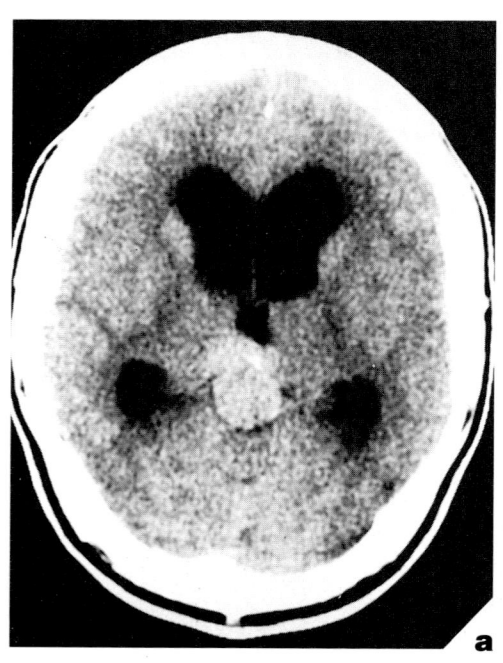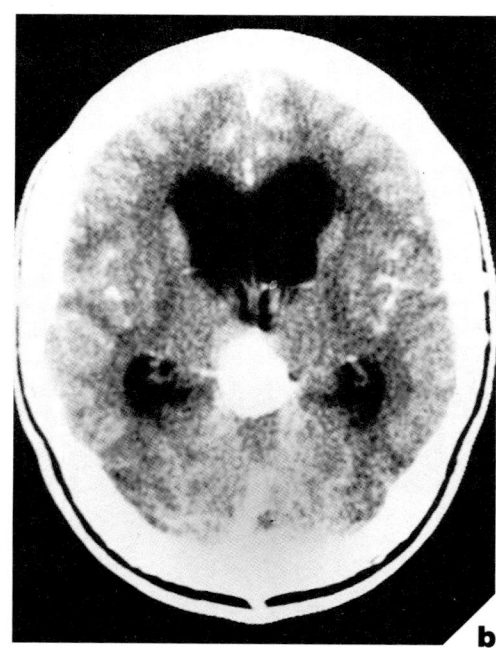

a   b

Figure 4.55

*Pineal region germinoma. Axial CT scans **a** before and **b** following intravenous injection of contrast material show a high-density, lobulated, intensely enhancing mass in the region of the pineal gland. There is hydrocephalus due to obstruction of the flow of CSF in the posterior third ventricle-aqueduct region.*

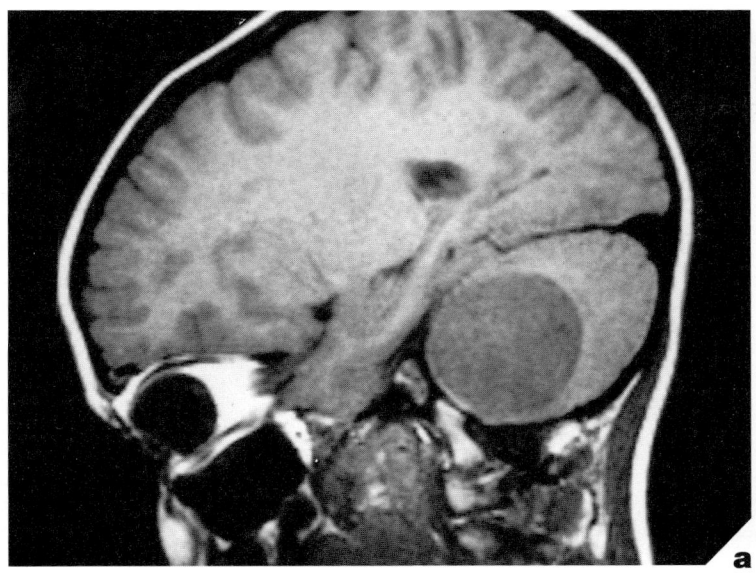

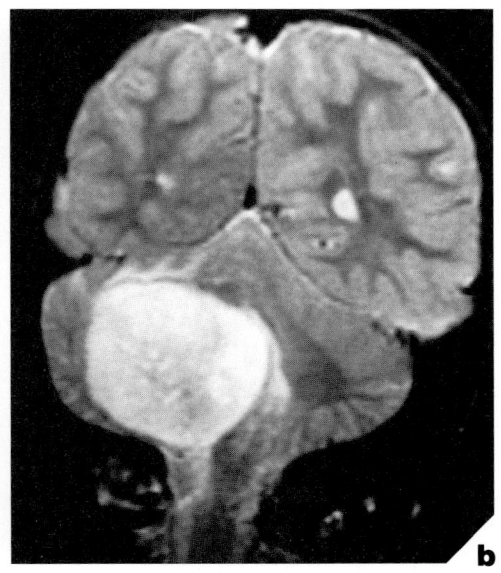

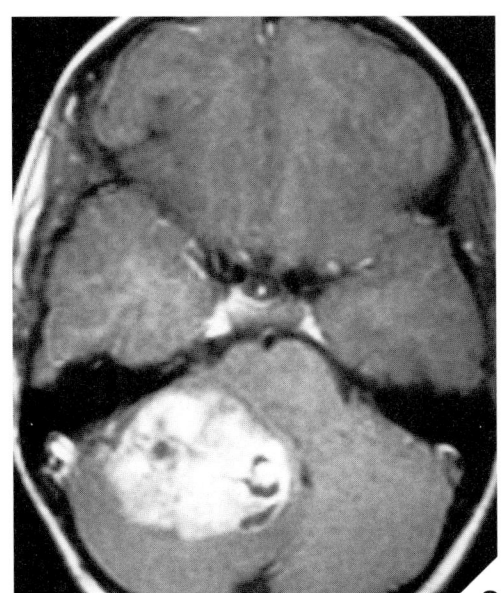

Figure 4.56

*Cerebellar astrocytoma. **a** Sagittal T1, **b** coronal T2, and **c** axial, Gadolinium-enhanced T1 images through the posterior fossa in this five-year-old demonstrate a well-demarcated, smooth, round, irregularly enhancing mass in the right cerebellar hemisphere which compresses the fourth ventricle and displaces it across the midline to the left.*

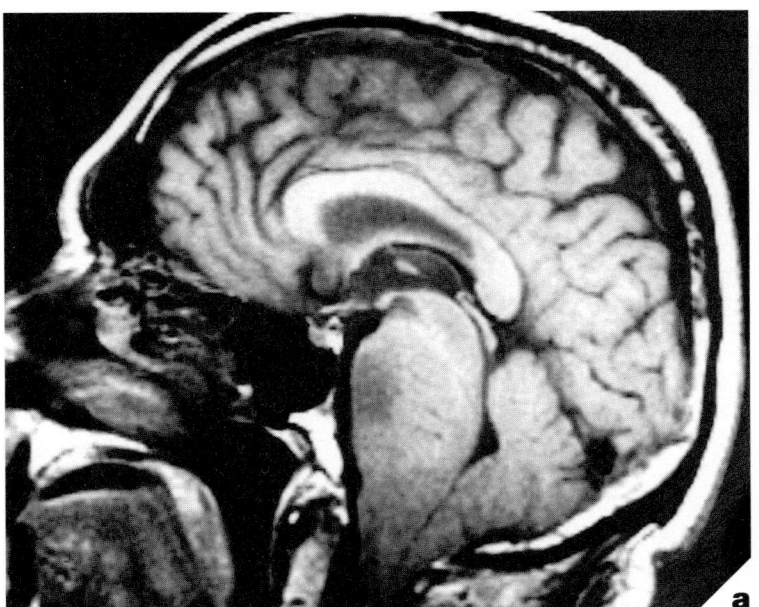

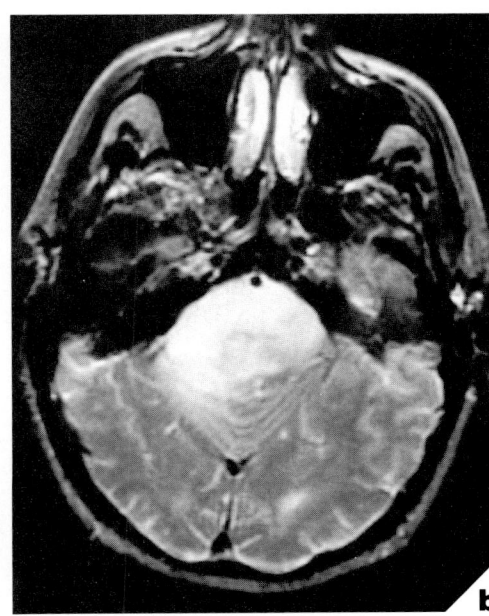

Figure 4.57

*Brainstem glioma. **a** Sagittal T1- and **b** axial T2-weighted images show diffuse enlargement and dark-T1, bright-T2 signal abnormality in the basis pontis. Brainstem gliomas such as this are usually slowly growing, infiltrative lesions.*

Intracranial Neoplasms

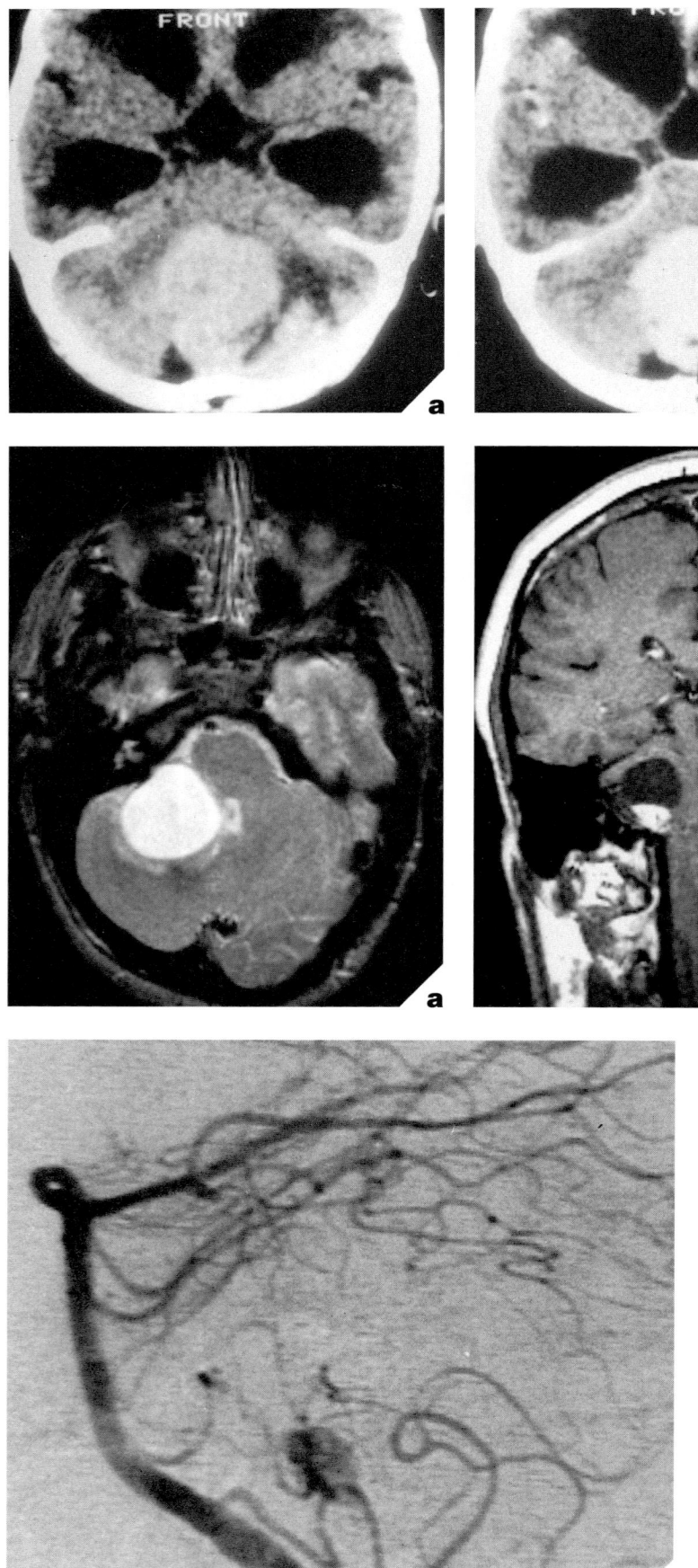

Figure 4.58

Medulloblastoma. **a** *Unenhanced and* **b** *contrast-enhanced CT sections show a hyperdense, homogeneously enhancing mass in the cerebellar vermis compressing and filling the fourth ventricle. There is obstructive hydrocephalus.*

pial surface enhancement

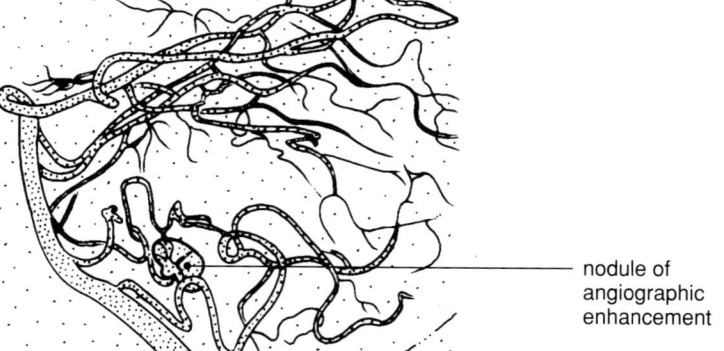

nodule of angiographic enhancement

Figure 4.59

Cerebellar hemangioblastoma. **a** *T2-weighted axial image shows a mass in the right cerebellar hemisphere compressing the fourth ventricle.* **b** *Following Gadolinium administration, there is a pial-based, mural nodule of enhancement. This nodule is well seen during* **c** *posterior fossa angiography and is virtually pathognomonic of a cerebellar hemangioblastoma.*

Medulloblastoma

Medulloblastomas are childhood tumors that are generally classified as *primitive neuroectodermal tumors.* They are characteristically located in the cerebellar vermis and frequently protrude into the fourth ventricle. Medulloblastomas are extremely cellular and therefore often appear more dense than surrounding brain on noncontrast CT scans. Calcification is unusual. The tumor is frequently homogeneous; it often enhances uniformly (Fig. 4.58). Low-density zones may be present, indicating central necrosis.

Hemangioblastoma

Hemangioblastomas are the most common cerebellar tumors of young adults (Fig. 4.59). There is a higher incidence of hemangioblastoma in patients with von Hippel-Lindau syndrome than the general population. Since hemangioblastomas are frequently multiple (particularly in patients with von Hippel-Lindau syndrome), the cervical spinal cord should be carefully studied for other lesions.

Hemangioblastomas are usually cystic and typically contain a nodule of solid tumor which occurs along the most superficial portion of the mass. This mural nodule enhances intensely on CT, MRI, and angiography, and is a specific feature of hemangioblastomas. The solid nidus must be completely removed at surgery or the lesion is likely to recur.

Ependymoma

Ependymomas arise from the ependymal lining of the ventricular system or from periventricular ependymal cell rests within the white matter. Ependymomas most frequently arise from the ependymal lining of the fourth ventricle and are usually classified with posterior fossa tumors. Calcification is common. The tumor has a propensity to grow through the foramina of Luschka (Fig. 4.60).

Schwannoma

Schwannomas are tumors which arise in the sheath of cranial nerves. The acoustic schwannoma (frequently called *acoustic neuroma*) arises in the vestibular portion of the eight cranial nerve. The tumor may be quite large and cause obstruction of the fourth ventricle, or it may be quite small and exclusively intracanalicular. Since these lesions are centered in the cerebellopontine angle, they are usually easy to identify (Fig. 4.61), but must be distinguished from menin-

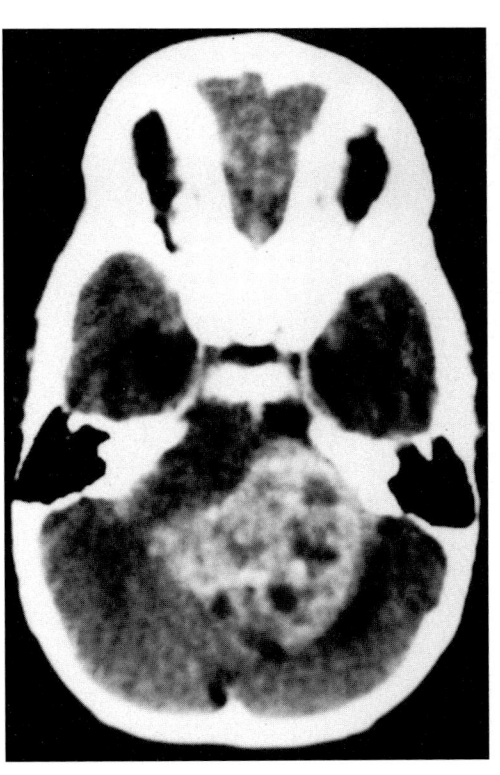

Figure 4.60
Ependymoma. Axial, contrast-enhanced CT images show a heterogeneous, enhancing mass in the fourth ventricle extending through the left foramen of Luschka. This is a characteristic growth pattern for fourth ventricular ependymomas. Tiny areas of calcification were demonstrated on the unenhanced scan. Calcification is statistically more common in ependymomas than in other posterior fossa tumors.

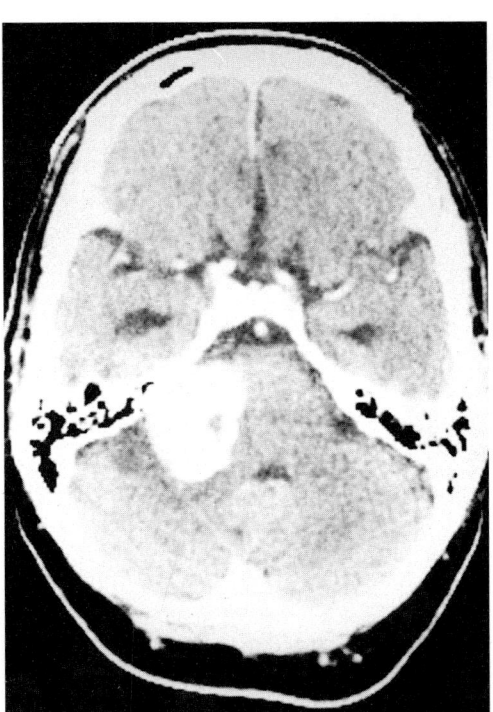

Figure 4.61
Acoustic schwannoma. Axial CT image obtained following intravenous administration of contrast material shows a lobulated, enhancing mass in the right cerebellopontine angle cistern.

giomas. Meningiomas are usually not centered at the porus acousticus. MRI (Fig. 4.62) is the best imaging modality in studying acoustic schwannomas since it demonstrates the seventh/eighth cranial nerve complex directly. With Gadolinium, schwannomas typically show intense enhancement. Bilateral acoustic schwan-

nomas occur in patients with neurofibromatosis II.

Schwannomas of the fifth and ninth (Fig. 4.63) cranial nerves are less common than those of the eighth nerve, but demonstrate similar features. Like most other extra-axial lesions, they exhibit intense contrast enhancement.

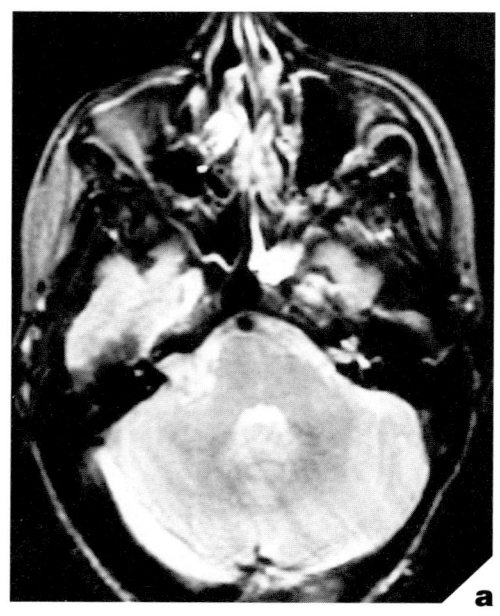

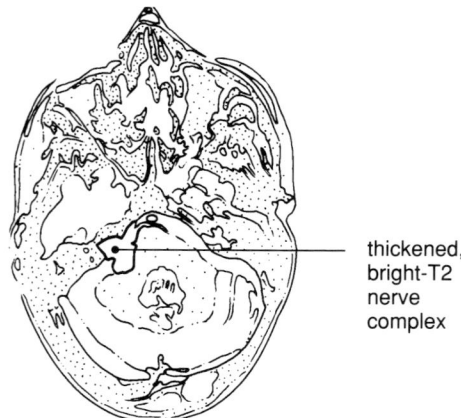

thickened, bright-T2 nerve complex

Figure 4.62

*Acoustic schwannoma. **a** T2-weighted axial MR scan shows marked widening of the right seventh/eighth cranial nerve complex when compared to the left. There is bright-T2 signal in this widened nerve complex. **b** Axial and **c** coronal Gadolinium-enhanced T1 images show the mass most clearly. There is intense, uniform enhancement, as is typically seen in acoustic schwannomas.*

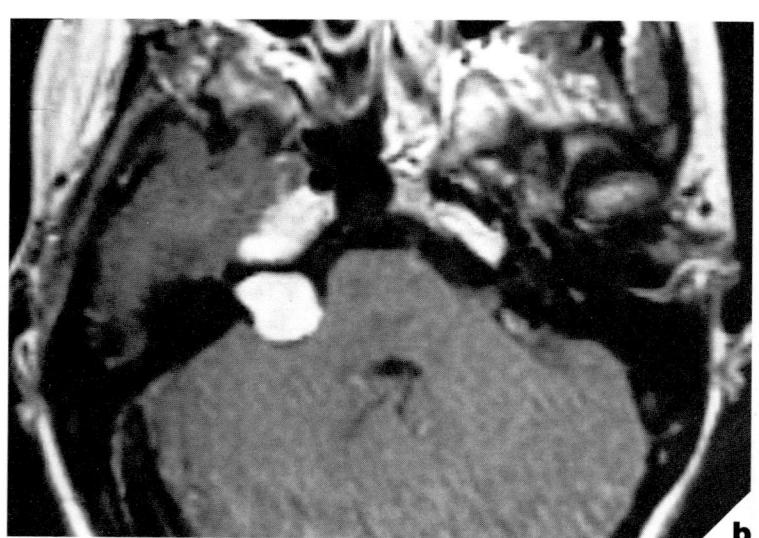

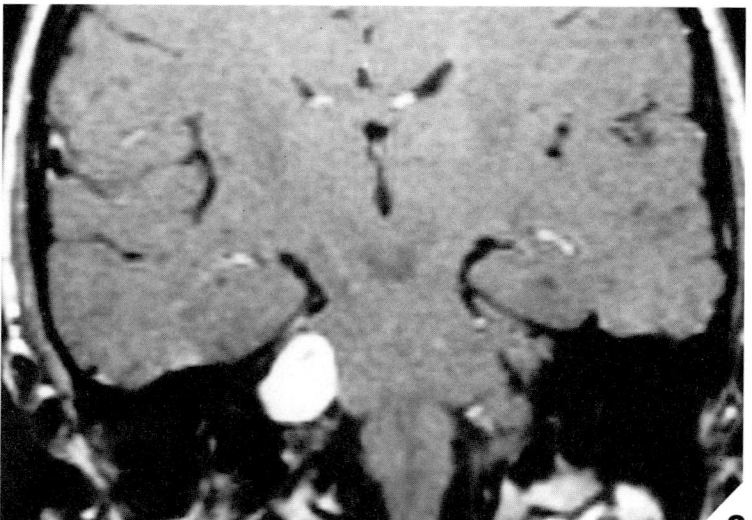

Brain

Xanthogranulomatosis

Xanthogranulomatosis is an extremely rare, idiopathic disorder which results in multiple calcified and hemorrhagic granulomatous posterior fossa lesions. These are typically manifested as extra-axial masses of dark-T2 signal intensity (Fig. 4.64) on magnetic resonance images.

Neuroenteric Cysts

Neuroenteric cysts are developmental/congenital cystic lesions that result from incorporation of endoderm into the neural tube. Lesions are typically present in the cervical spine (see Chapter 10) but may extend into the posterior fossa (Fig. 4.65). These cysts tend to recur following surgical removal.

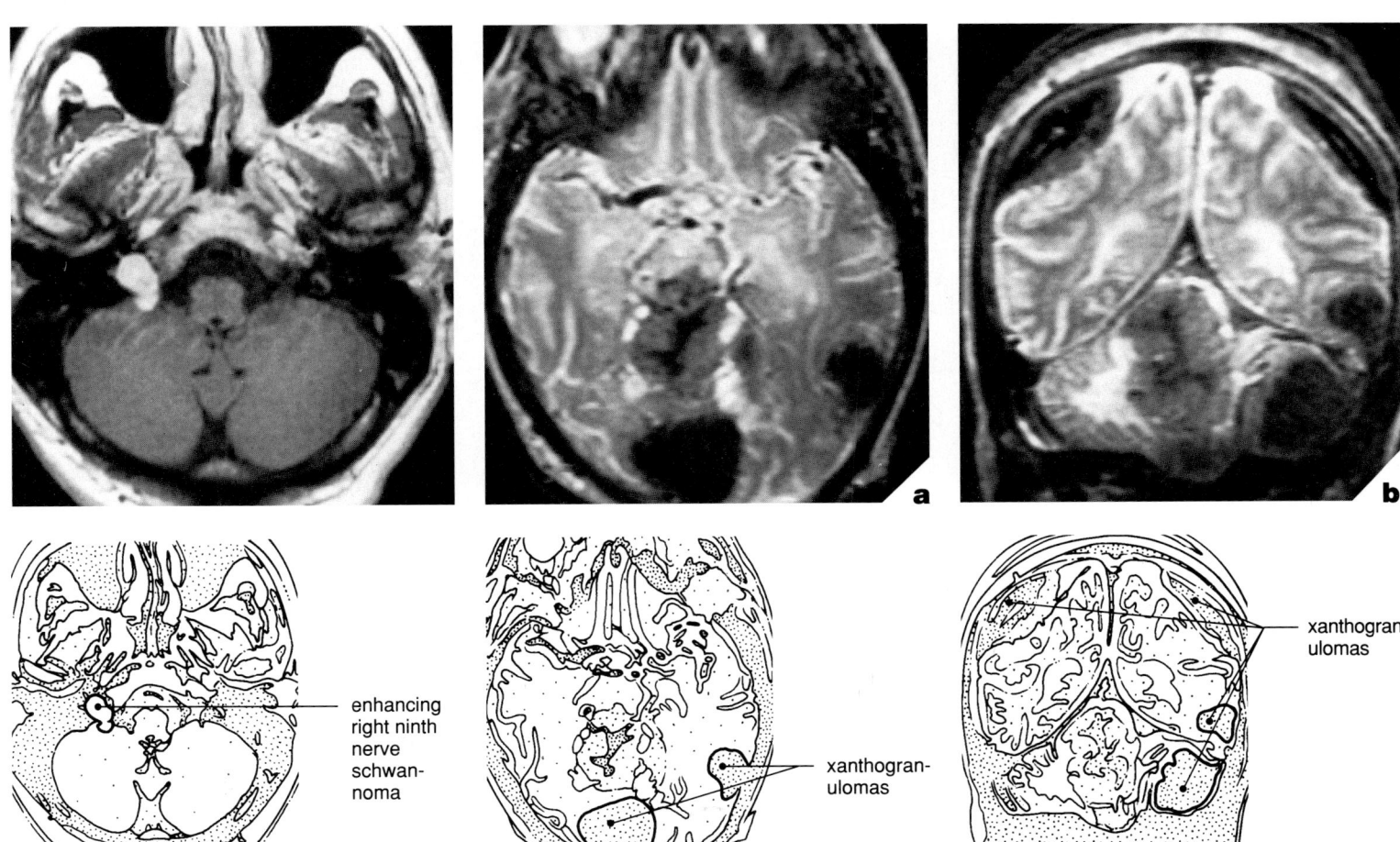

Figure 4.63

Ninth cranial nerve schwannoma. Contrast-enhanced T1-weighted MR image shows intense enhancement of an enlarged right ninth nerve sheath (compare with the normal left side).

Figure 4.64

*Xanthogranulomatosis. **a** Axial and **b** coronal T2-weighted MR images show multiple extra-axial masses in the posterior fossa which compress the adjacent* *cerebellum. The lesions are partly hemorrhagic and partly calcified, accounting for their dark-T2 signal.*

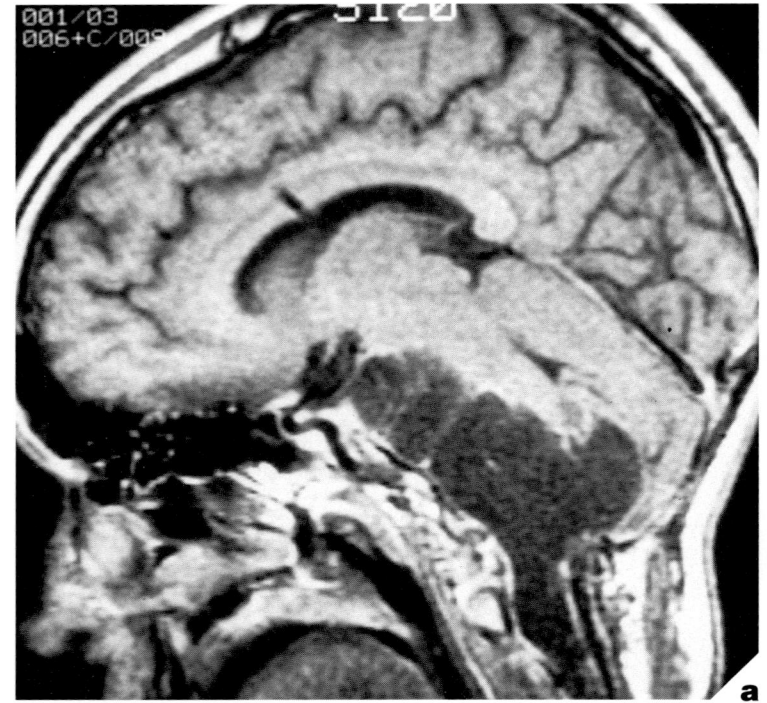

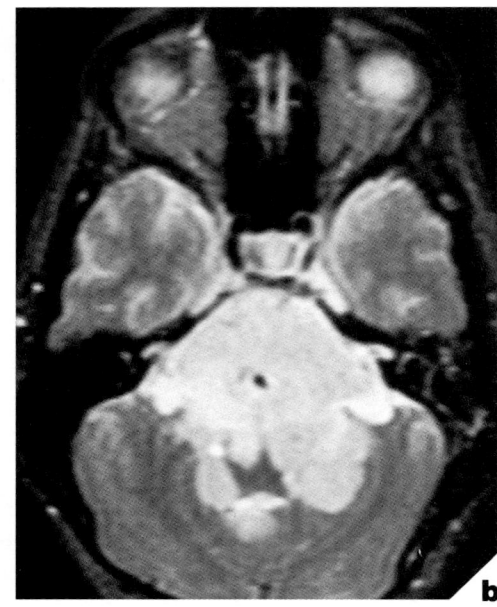

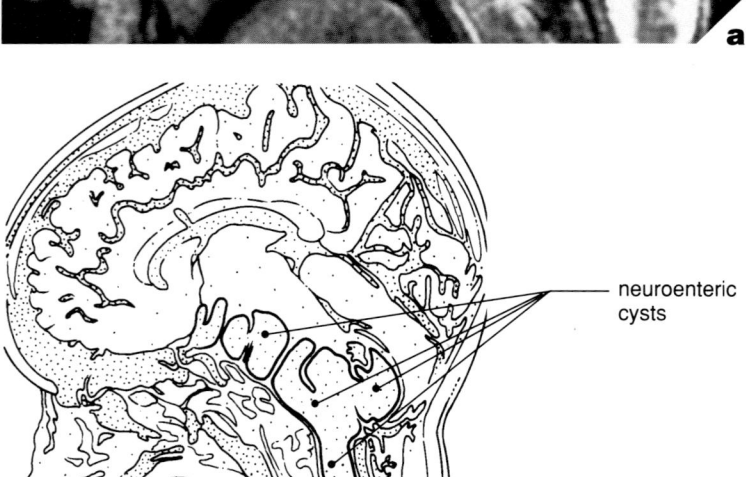

neuroenteric
cysts

Figure 4.65
Neuroenteric cysts. Numerous large,
confluent cysts arising from the cervical
spine have extended cephalad to compress the brainstem and cerebellum.
These cysts contain CSF and have
a dark-T1, **b** bright-T2 signal characteristics.

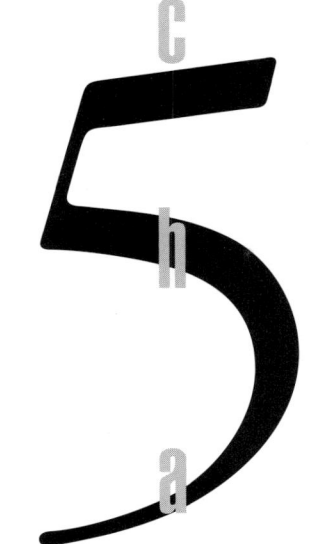

5

chapter

Cerebrovascular Diseases

Stroke is the third leading cause of death in the United States, after heart disease and cancer. The term *stroke* means a sudden, focal neurological deficit that is not due to a seizure disorder. Strokes range in severity from a trivial malady, with a deficit so mild that the patient is not prompted to seek medical attention, to gross hemiplegia or other major neurological deficit; the most severe lesions result in coma or death. A synonym for stroke is *cerebrovascular accident* (CVA). The term *cerebrovascular disease* broadly designates any abnormality of the brain due to pathology of the arteries or veins. A simplified classification of the common cerebrovascular diseases is presented in Fig. 5.1.

Cerebral infarction may be caused by a variety of mechanisms including thrombosis, embolic phenomena, and hemorrhage.

CEREBRAL INFARCTION

Most cerebrovascular accidents are clinically apparent simply from the history and neurological examination. The primary role of CT and MRI in these patients is (1) to distinguish a bland or ischemic infarct from a hemorrhagic infarct; and (2) to exclude the rare neoplasm or other lesion which presents with stroke symptoms.

There are no definite MRI or CT findings associated with a *transient ischemic attack* (TIA), defined as an ischemic deficit that resolves within 24 hours

(most resolve within minutes). Even when infarction is extensive, CT is frequently negative in the early stages. Twenty-four hours after the onset of the clinical deficit, the CT scan is still negative in up to 30% of patients with acute infarcts. MRI is usually positive after approximately 8 to 12 hours. The earliest CT finding in ischemic infarction is low density in the involved vascular territory. The low density can usually be appreciated 12 to 24 hours after the onset of the deficit. In the earlier stages, the low density may be due to oligemia in the infarcted territory; later, tissue necrosis and the resultant edema contribute to the low density.

The initial low-density (lucent) stage is followed by the development of a mass effect due to tissue necrosis and cerebral edema. At this stage, effacement of the cortical sulci and compression of nearby portions of the ventricular system can be demonstrated. The degree of mass effect can be enormous, resulting in brain herniation and death (Fig. 5.2). Hemorrhage into a zone of recent infarction occurs in a minority of patients (Fig. 5.3) and is seen most frequently in cases of embolic infarction. The following sequence of events has been postulated to explain hemorrhagic infarcts: (1) occlusion of a vessel by embolic material results in infarction and tissue necrosis; (2) subsequent fragmentation and distal migration of the embolus allows blood flow to be restored to the infarcted, necrotic zone; (3) seepage of blood through damaged or necrotic vessels results in focal hemorrhage.

The use of intravenous contrast material is usually unnecessary in the diagnosis of cerebral infarction ex-

Classification of Cerebrovascular Diseases

I. Cerebral infarction
II. Primary intracerebral hemorrhage
III. Subarachnoid hemorrhage/cerebral aneurysm
IV. Vascular malformations

Figure 5.1
Classification of cerebrovascular diseases.

cept to rule out other entities such as a neoplasm. A characteristic pattern of gyriform enhancement is often demonstrated in subacute infarcts, usually between 3 and 6 weeks old (Figs. 5.4, 5.5). Rare cases of enhancement persisting up 6 months following an infarct have been reported. As in neoplastic and inflammatory diseases, the mechanism of contrast enhancement in infarcts is leakage of contrast material into the brain substance through an incompetent blood–brain barrier. Luxury perfusion, due to regional loss of autoregulation of the cerebral circulation, may result in local dilatation of blood vessels within an infarct; however, the increased density in the blood pool in the infarcted zone contributes little to the enhancement seen on MRI or CT.

Late changes consist of findings due to loss of brain tissue, or encephalomalacia. The density/signal intensity of an old infarct can approach that of cerebrospinal fluid (CSF) (Fig. 5.6). Often there is displacement of normal structures toward the infarcted zone—a "negative" mass effect, that is associated with porencephalic dilatation of the adjacent ventricle.

The radiographic patterns of cerebral infarction reflect the vascular distribution affected. Because the middle cerebral territory is the largest, and because the middle cerebral artery is anatomically a direct continuation of the internal carotid artery, it is the vessel most frequently affected by thrombotic and embolic events. Anterior cerebral territory infarcts are recognizable as low-attenuation zones in the frontal

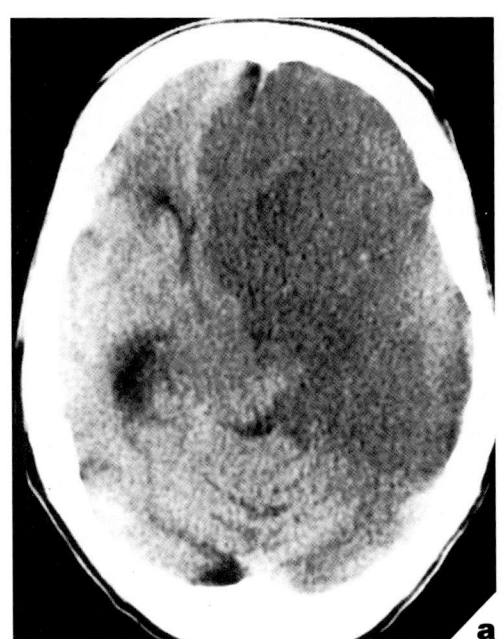 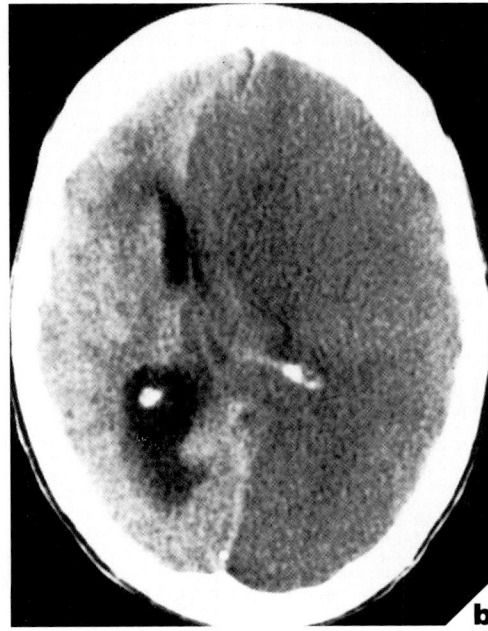 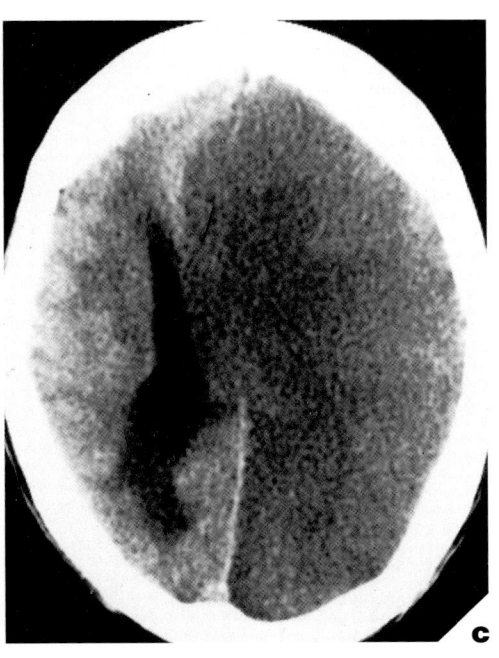

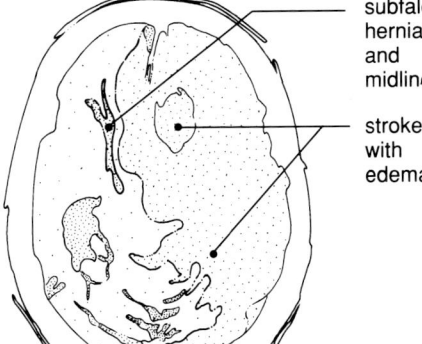

subfalcine herniation and midline shift

stroke with edema

Figure 5.2

*Acute cerebral infarction. **a,b,c** Axial unenhanced CT images show an acute infarct involving the entire left cerebral hemisphere. The associated swelling and edema produce extensive mass effect, midline shift, subfalcine and transtentorial herniation.*

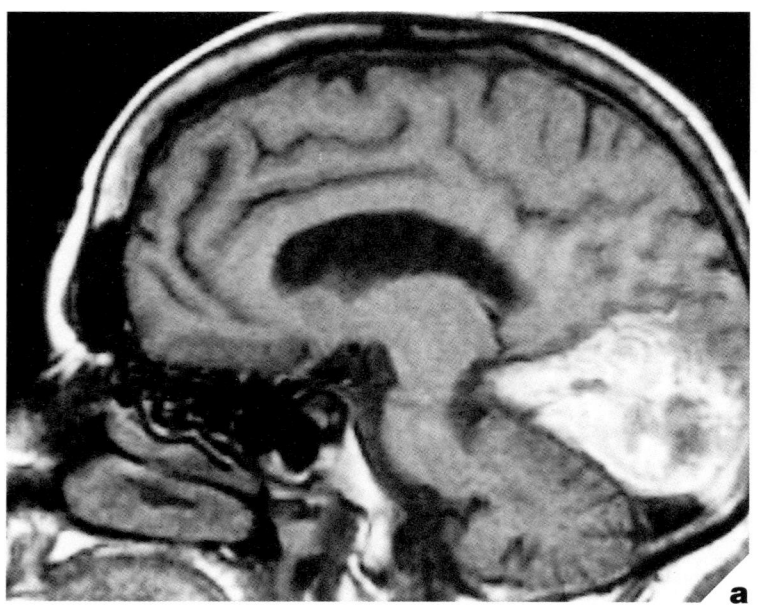
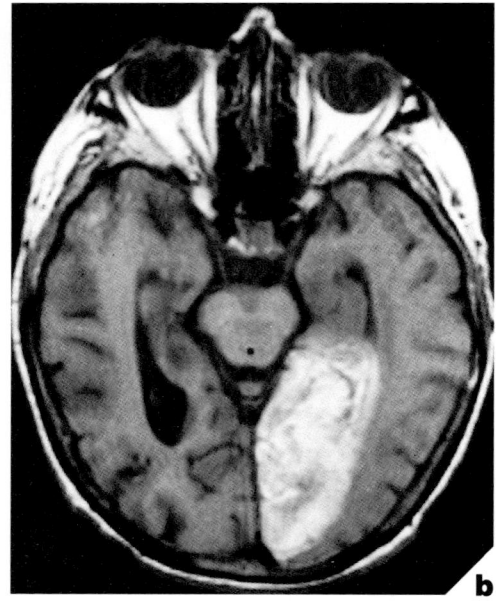

Figure 5.3
*Hemorrhagic cerebral infarction in the distribution of the left posterior cerebral artery. Unenhanced **a** sagittal and **b** axial T1 images show bright signal abnormality conforming to the distribution of the left posterior cerebral artery. **c** T2-weighted axial image shows mixed bright and dark signal abnormalities.*

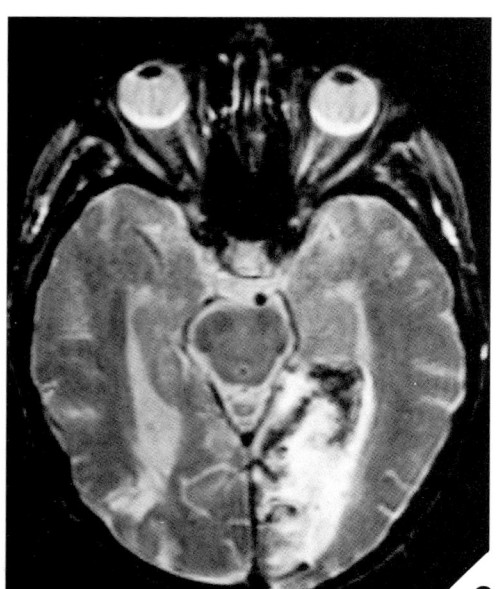

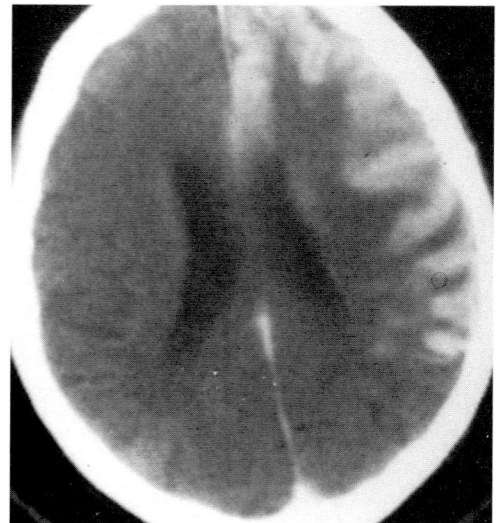

Figure 5.4
Enhancement in a subacute infarct. There is gyriform pattern of enhancement in the left frontal and parietal lobes in this patient who had an infarct in the distributions of the left anterior and middle cerebral arteries 4 weeks earlier.

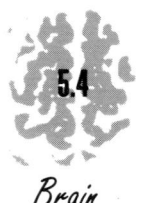

5.4

Brain

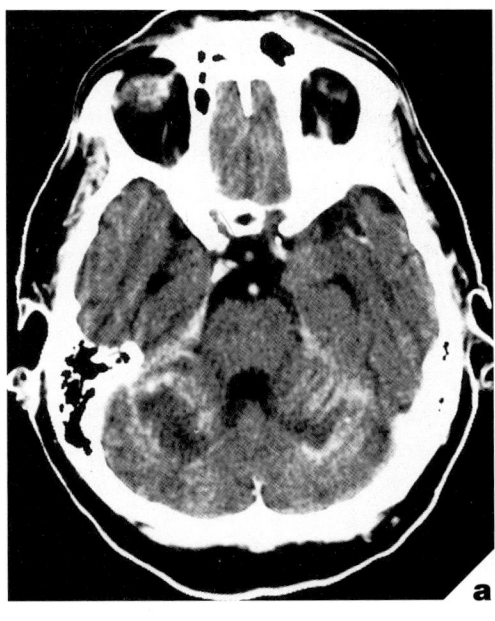

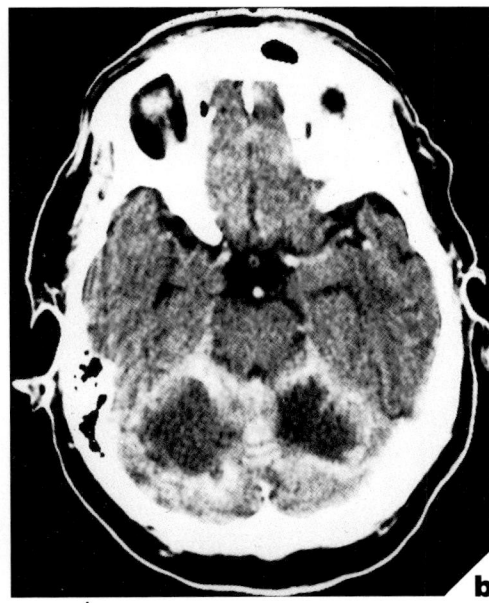

Figure 5.5

*Enhancing cerebellar infarcts. **a,b** Contrast-enhanced CT sections through the cerebellum demonstrate enhancement of the cerebellar cortical grey matter bilaterally, characteristic for subacute infarction.*

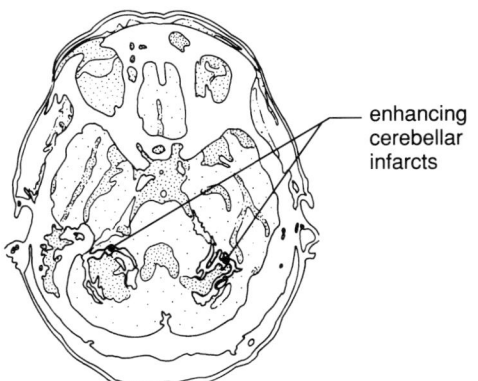

enhancing
cerebellar
infarcts

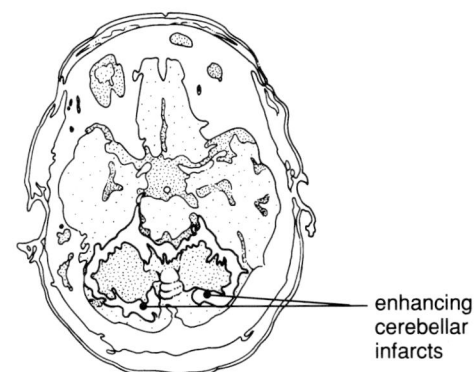

enhancing
cerebellar
infarcts

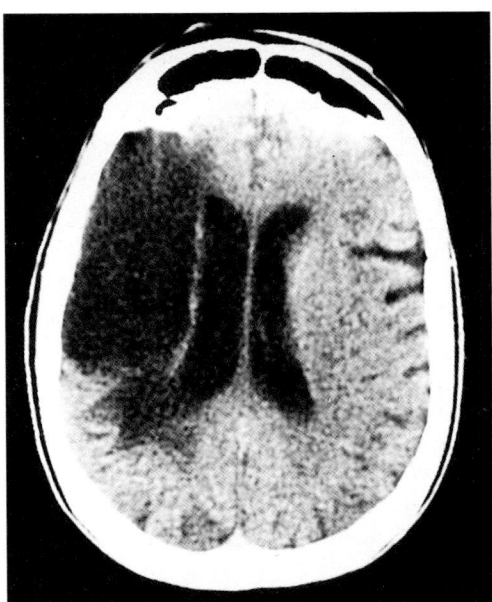

Figure 5.6

Old right middle cerebral artery distribution infarct. Axial CT section without contrast shows a sharply defined low-attenuation zone in the right cerebral hemisphere, in the distribution of the right middle cerebral artery. The density of the infarct is nearly as low as that of CSF in the ventricular system. There is compensatory dilatation (porencephalic dilatation) of the right lateral ventricle.

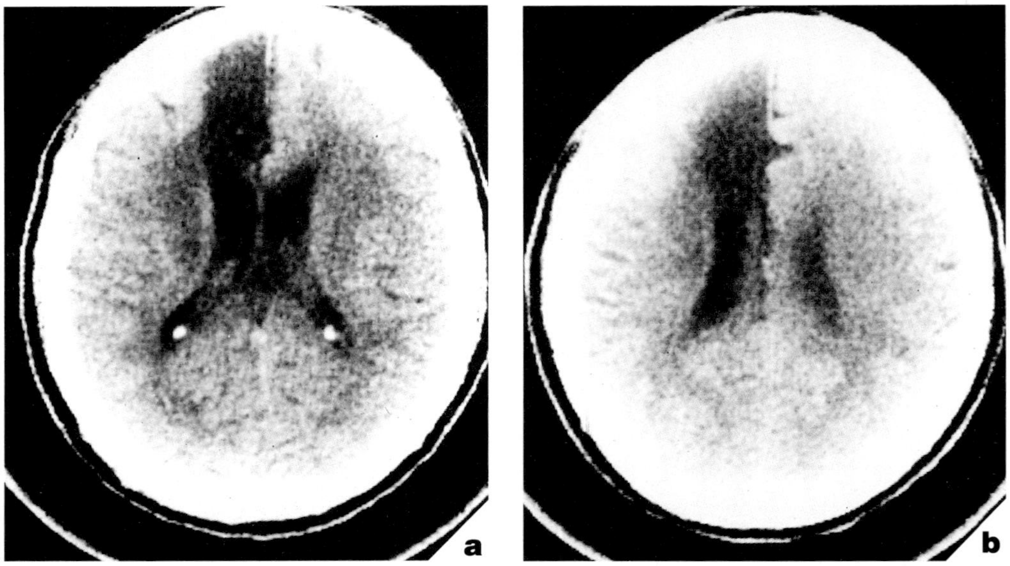

Figure 5.7

Old right anterior cerebral artery distribution infarct. **a,b** Axial CT sections show a sharply defined low attenuation zone in the right frontal parasagittal region typical of an old anterior cerebral artery distribution infarct.

bilateral occipital lobe infarcts

enhancing cerebral infarcts

enhancing cerebral infarcts

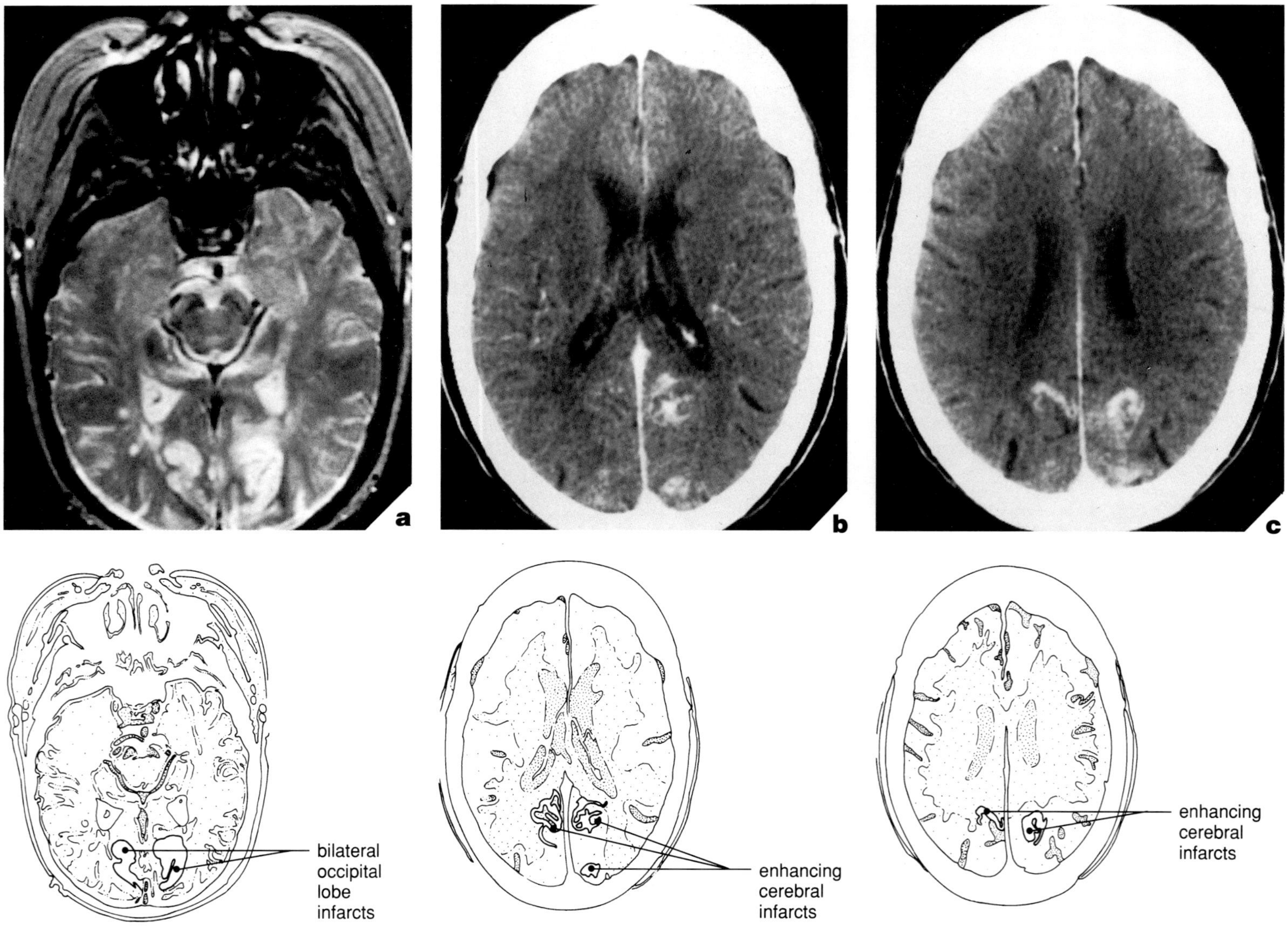

Figure 5.8

Enhancing posterior cerebral artery distribution infarcts. **a** Unenhanced T2-weighted axial MR image shows increased signal intensity in both occipital lobes. **b,c** Contrast-enhanced CT sections show gyriform enhancement in the same locations.

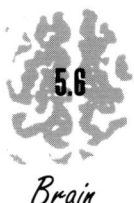

5.6

Brain

parasagittal region (Fig. 5.7). Infarcts involving the posterior cerebral artery distribution occur in the thalami, posterior temporal, and occipital lobes (Fig. 5.8). Infarction of the brainstem (Fig. 5.9) or cerebellum results from vertebro-basilar system disease.

When the brain substance in two adjacent vascular territories is infarcted, the cause is usually an internal carotid occlusion; in such cases the pattern of blood flow at the circle of Willis can be deduced.

Cerebral infarction can also occur in the boundary zone between adjacent vascular territories (Fig. 5.10). Such watershed infarcts are most commonly due to hypotensive episodes.

Lacunar infarcts are small, deep infarcts resulting

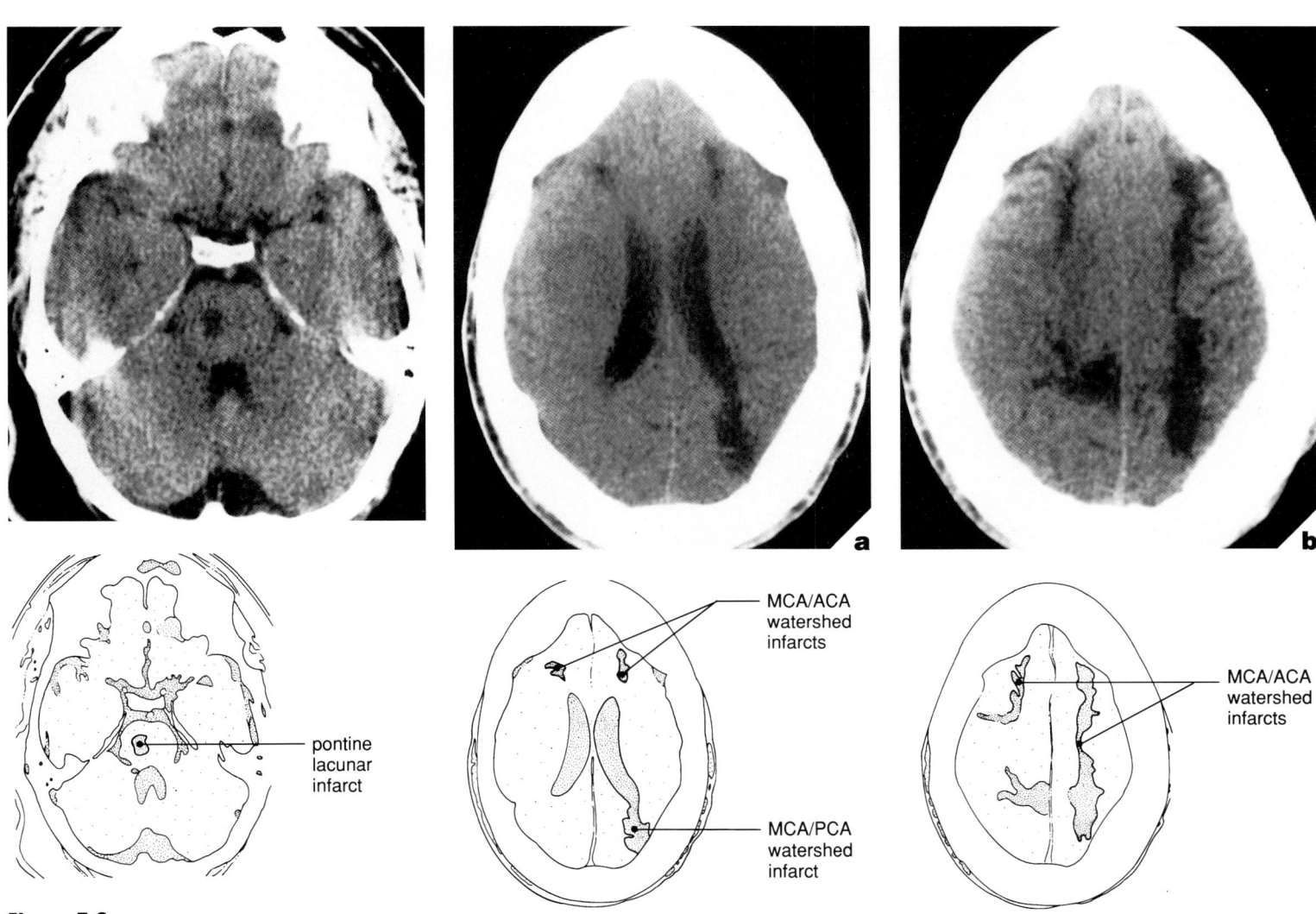

Figure 5.9
Pontine lacunar infarct. Unenhanced CT scan shows a focal area of decreased attenuation in the right side of the pons.

Figure 5.10
*Watershed infarcts. **a,b** Unenhanced axial CT images show decreased attenuation in the brain tissue between the middle cerebral artery distribution and the anterior and posterior cerebral artery distributions.*

from occlusion of the small penetrating branches of the cerebral arteries (Figs. 5.11, 5.12). The underlying lesion is infiltration of the arterial wall by fatty, fibrous material, a pathological process called *lipohyalinosis*. The presence of lacunes is strongly correlated with hypertension and athersclerosis, and to a lesser extent with diabetes mellitus. Extensive destruction of the white matter due to occlusive disease of the lenticulostriate and thalamoperforating arteries is associated with a type of dementia called *subcortical arteriosclerotic encephalopathy* or Binswanger's disease; CT and MRI show diffuse or multifocal abnormalities in the hemispheric white matter. MRI is more sensitive than CT to the white matter changes associated with vascular disease or aging (see Fig. 5.11).

Venous infarcts are less common than infarction due to arterial occlusion. The major causes are cerebral thrombophlebitis due to infection of the paranasal sinuses or mastoids, sickle cell anemia, hypercoagulative states, Behçet's disease, the puerperium, and polycythemia. Magnetic resonance imaging has the advantage of being able to depict thrombosis of the major dural venous sinuses as well as infarction in the territories of their tributaries (Fig. 5.13). Superior sagittal sinus thrombosis occurs in neonates, particularly in the setting of dehydration and meningitis (see Chapter 3).

Cerebral infarction may be caused by carotid artery dissection (Fig. 5.14) with subsequent distal vascular insufficiency. Vasculitis may result in large

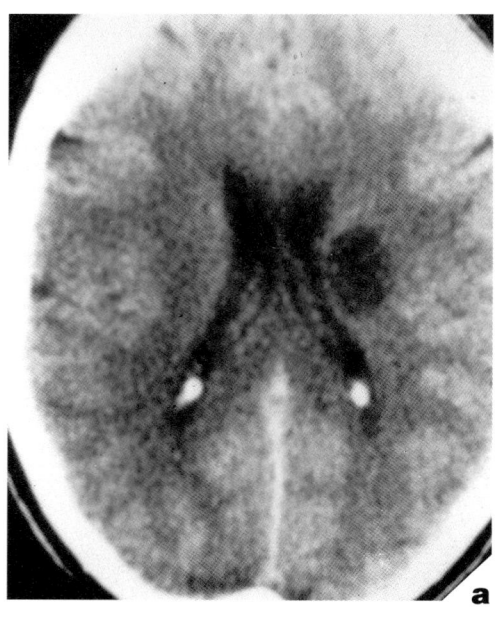
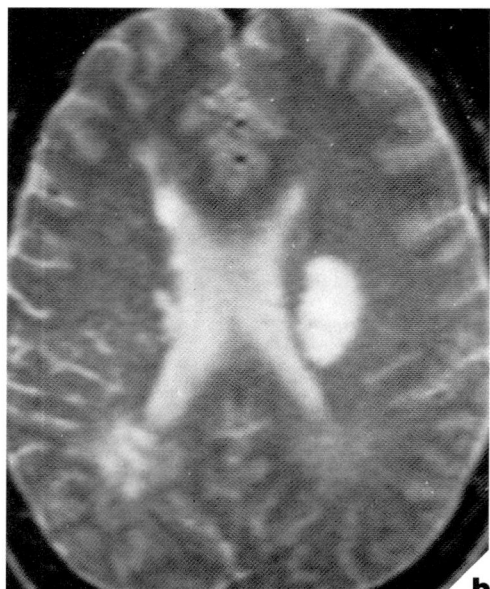

Figure 5.11
*Lacunar infarction. **a** CT scan without contrast shows an oval-shaped area of decreased attenuation in the left centrum semiovale which represents a lacunar infarction. **b** This is well seen on a T2 MR image as bright signal abnormality conforming to the same location. MRI also shows signal abnormalities in the right peri-atrial region and periventricular white matter not demonstrated on the CT image.*

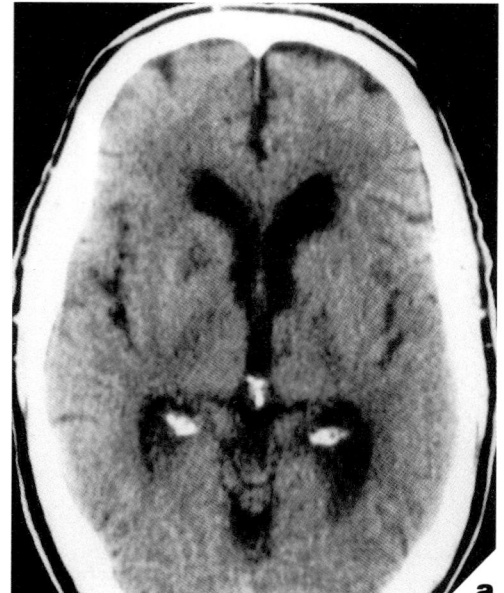
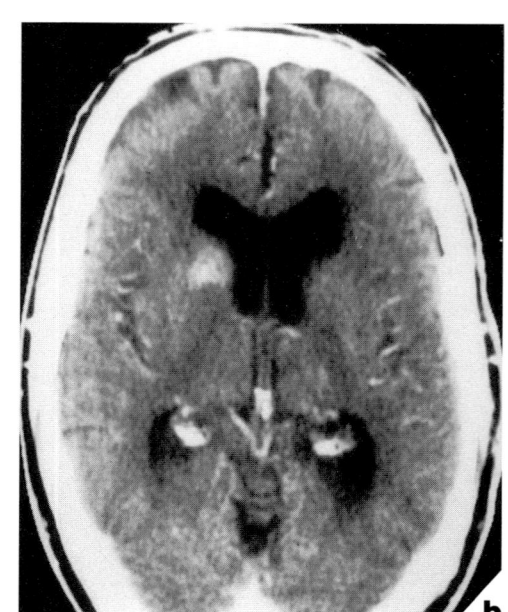

Figure 5.12
*Lacunar infarction. There is a wedge-shaped area of decreased attenuation **a** in the head of the right caudate nucleus and anterior limb of the right internal capsule, which homogeneously enhances **b** following intravenous administration of contrast material.*

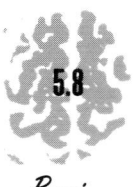

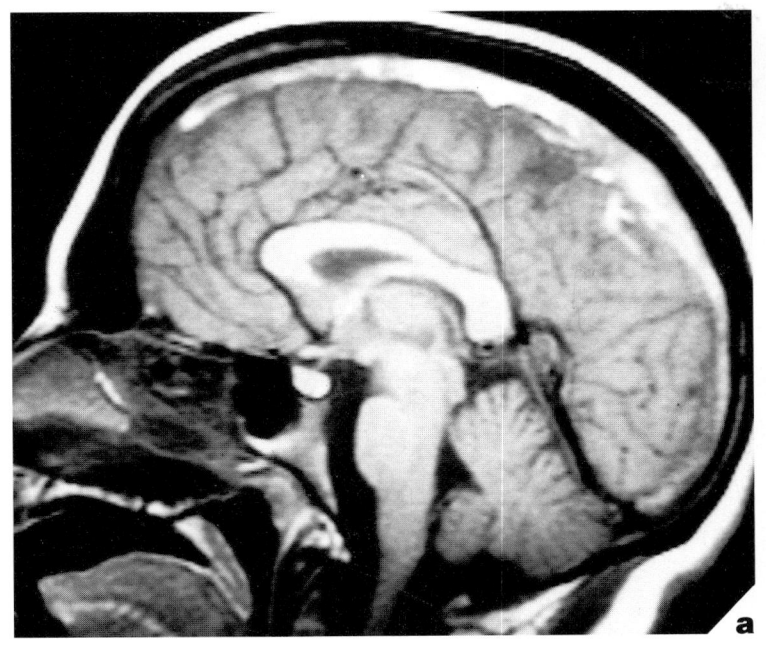

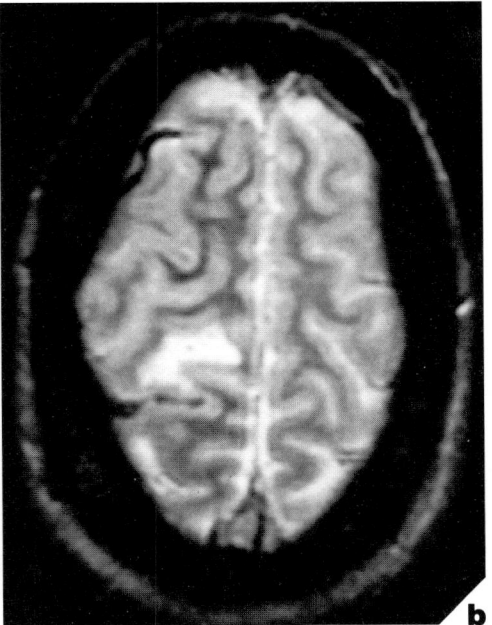

Figure 5.13

*Superior sagittal sinus thrombosis and venous infarct. **a** Sagittal T1 MR image shows abnormal bright-T1 signal in the superior sagittal sinus indicating thrombosis. **b** An associated venous infarct is demonstrated in the right parietal lobe on the T2-weighted axial image.*

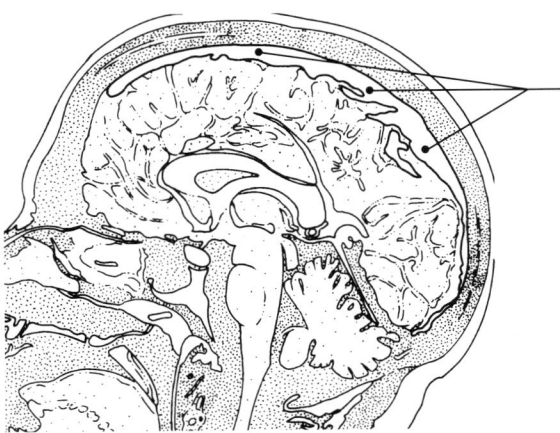

thrombosed superior sagittal sinus

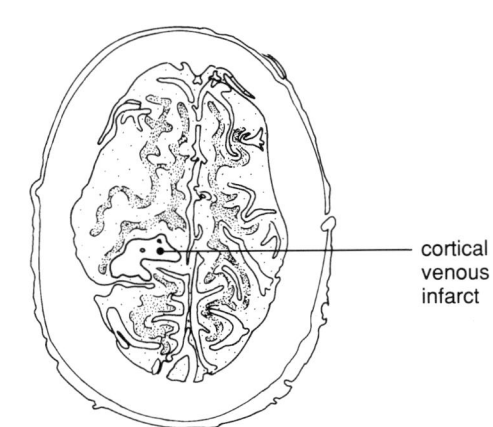

cortical venous infarct

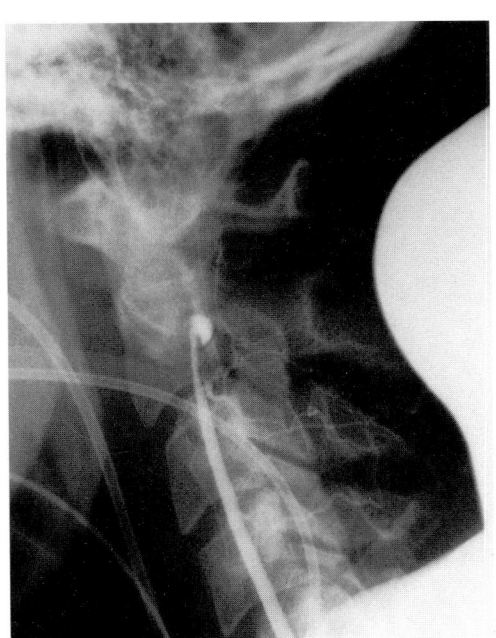

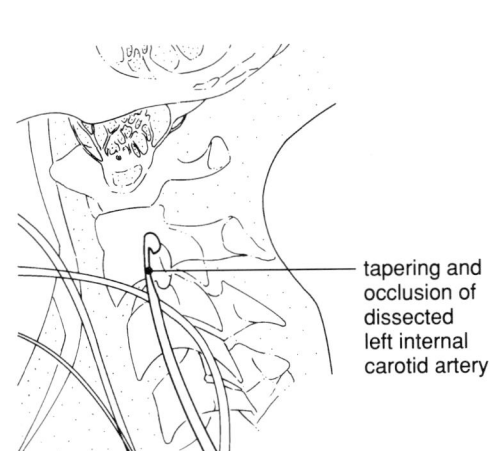

tapering and occlusion of dissected left internal carotid artery

Figure 5.14

Left internal carotid artery dissection. Left carotid artery injection shows tapering of the cervical portion of the left internal carotid artery with occlusion and slight dilatation of this vessel at the level of C2. This 22-year-old male presented with right-sided hemiparesis and severe headache.

or small vessel disease (Fig. 5.15). The vessels may have a beaded or cork-screw appearance, or there may be large or small vessel occlusions. Cerebral vasculitis may be idiopathic or due to systemic lupus erythematosis, Takayasu's arteritis (Fig. 5.16), giant cell arteritis, and other disorders.

Atherosclerotic disease of the carotid arteries and great vessels produces significant morbidity and mortality in the United States. When the carotid arteries are involved, there is typically stenosis involving the carotid artery bifurcation and proximal portions of the internal (Fig. 5.17) and/or external carotid arteries. There are often hemodynamic shifts of blood flow within the cerebral arteries associated with

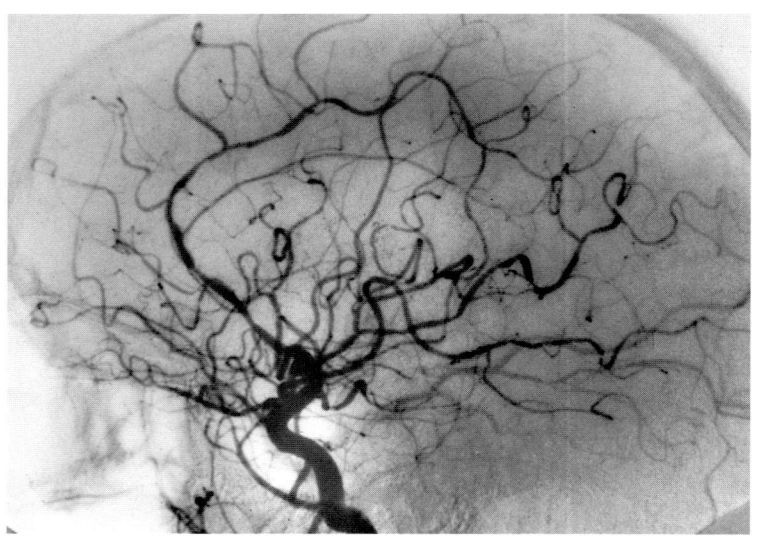

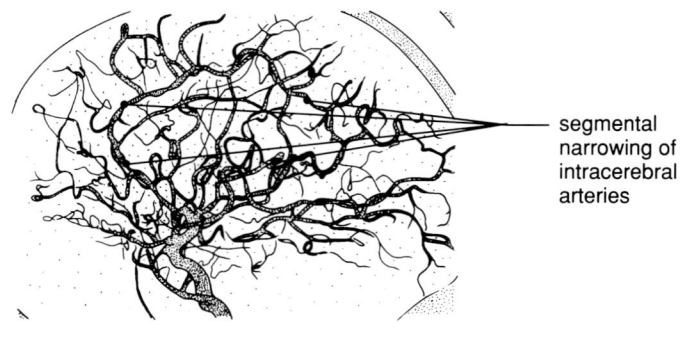

segmental narrowing of intracerebral arteries

Figure 5.15
Cerebral vasculitis. There are numerous segmental areas of narrowing in the branches of the anterior and middle cerebral arteries in this patient with systemic lupus erythematosis.

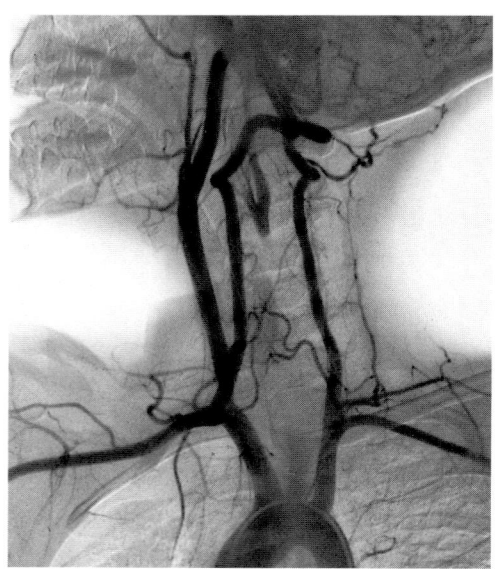

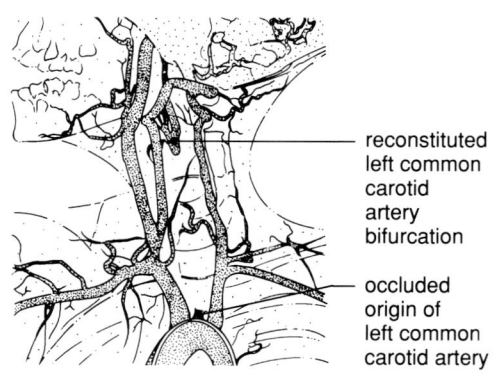

reconstituted left common carotid artery bifurcation

occluded origin of left common carotid artery

Figure 5.16
Takayasu's arteritis. Aortic arch angiogram demonstrates occlusion at the origin of the left common carotid artery with reconstitution of the left common carotid bifurcation via retrograde filling from branches of the left external carotid artery and vertebral arteries.

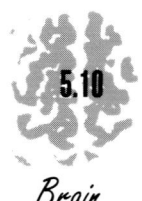

carotid artery stenosis. For example, unilateral internal carotid artery stenosis (less than 2.5 mm residual lumen) will result in cross-flow of blood through a patent anterior communicating artery from the opposite, normal side (Fig. 5.18). Intracranial occlusions may cause lepto-meningeal collateral blood flow with resultant retrograde filling of cerebral arteries distal to the site of the occlusion. Collateral pathways frequently include the ophthalmic artery, ethmoidal arteries, and the anterior and posterior callosal arteries.

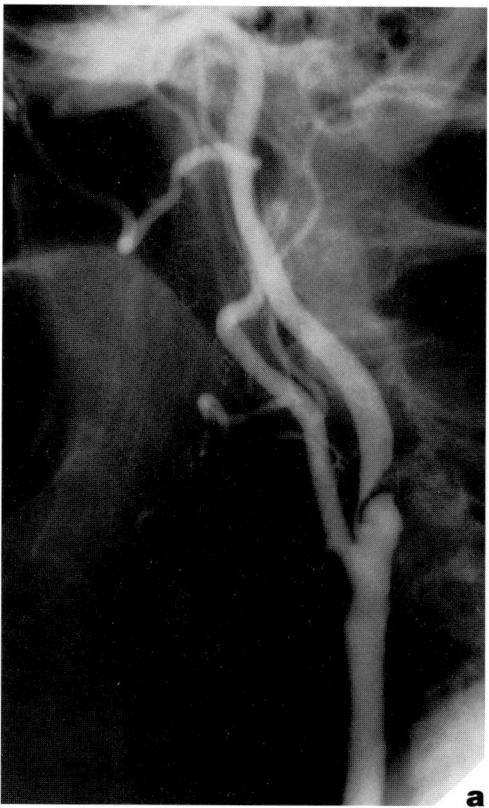

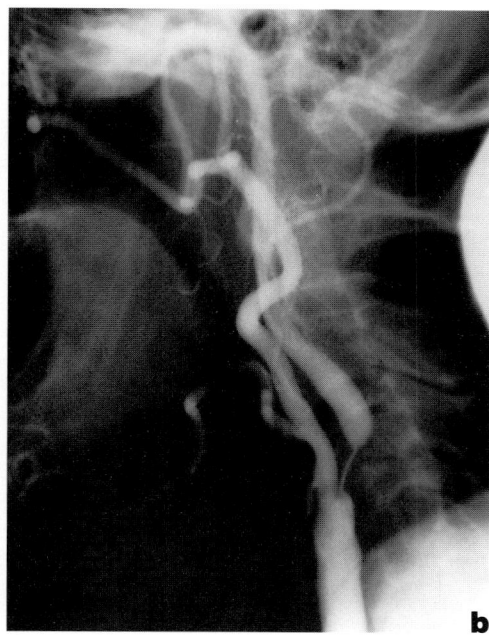

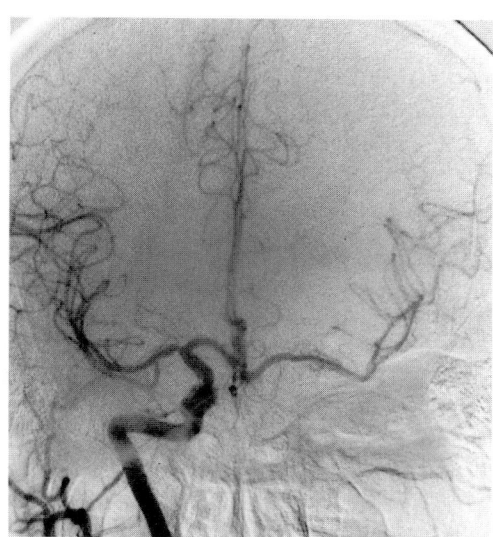

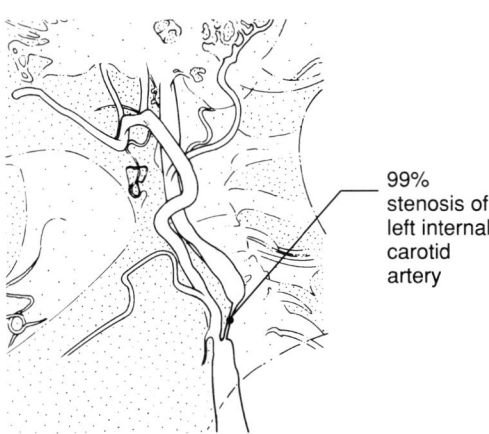

99% stenosis of right internal carotid artery

ulcerated plaque

99% stenosis of left internal carotid artery

cross filling of left anterior and middle cerebral vasculature during right carotid injection

Figure 5.17

Bilateral carotid stenosis. *a,b* Bilateral carotid angiography shows 99% stenosis at the origins of both internal carotid arteries. There is an outpouching of contrast at the origin of the right internal carotid artery which was due to an ulcerating plaque.

Figure 5.18

Hemodynamic shift. This patient has severe stenosis of the left internal carotid artery. A right common carotid artery injection demonstrates contrast media flowing from right to left across the anterior communicating artery to fill the branches of the left anterior and middle cerebral arteries.

Occlusion or severe stenosis of the left subclavian artery proximal to the origin of the left vertebral artery may result in retrograde flow down the left vertebral artery to supply blood to the left upper extremity (subclavian "steal" syndrome) (Fig. 5.19). This deprives the posterior fossa circulation of some of its blood; symptoms such as syncope or vertigo may arise when the left arm is exerted. This may be treated by percutaneous angioplasty (Fig. 5.20).

Degenerative Microangiopathy

As discussed in Chapter 2, there are a multitude of different pathological causes for the small bright foci seen on T2-weighted MR images in many patients.

The majority of these lesions (facetiously called "UBOs" for "unidentified bright objects") are due to demyelination or vascular disorders including lacunar infarctions. However, pathological inspection of many of these vascular-induced lesions shows that they are not due to frank cerebral infarction but rather to less severe ischemic injury. Pathologically there is gliosis, demyelination and myelin pallor, which is called *degenerative microangiopathy* (Fig. 5.21). These lesions typically occur in the deep and/or subcortical white matter and the basal ganglia (Fig. 5.22). This is unlike the periventricular white matter predominance of multiple sclerosis plaques.

One pitfall in the diagnosis of bright-T2 lesions on MRI is the occurrence of perivascular (Virchow-

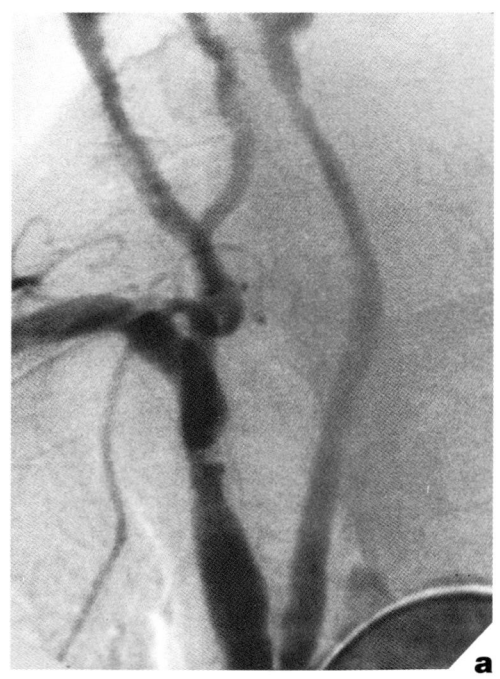

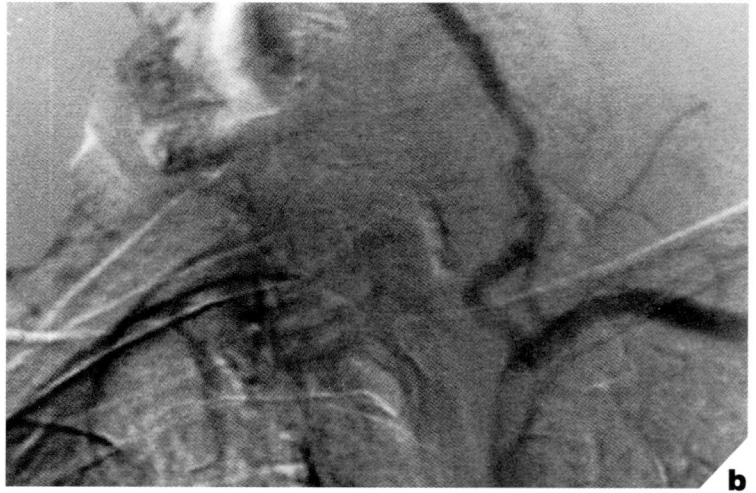

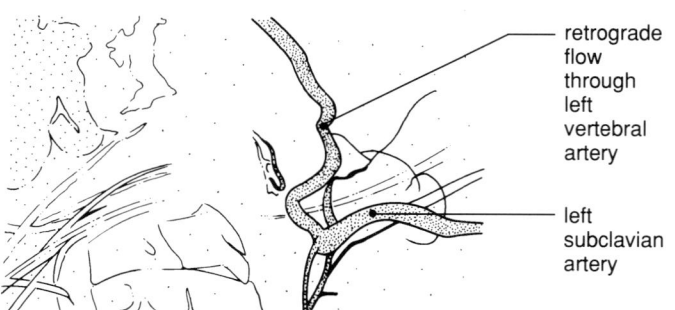

retrograde flow through left vertebral artery

left subclavian artery

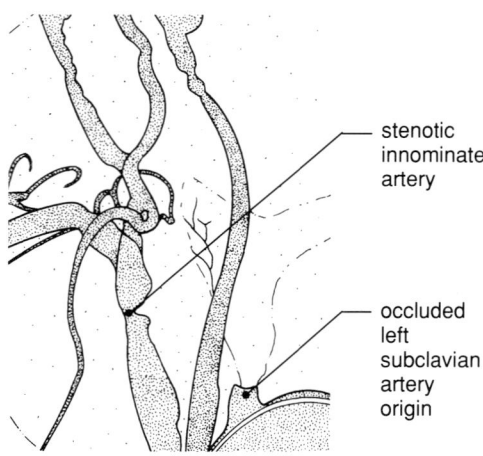

stenotic innominate artery

occluded left subclavian artery origin

Figure 5.19
Subclavian "steal" syndrome. **a** *Digital subtraction film during the early arterial phase of an aortic arch injection shows occlusion of the proximal left subclavian artery. Also demonstrated is stenosis involving the distal inominate artery and left carotid artery bifurcation.* **b** *Several seconds later, retrograde flow down the left vertebral artery is demonstrated with subsequent filling of the left subclavian artery distal to its occlusion site.*

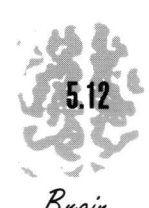

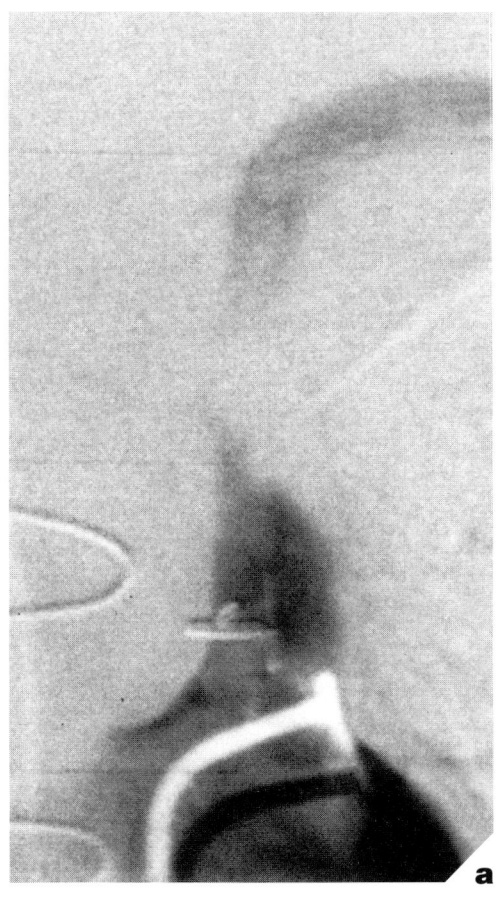

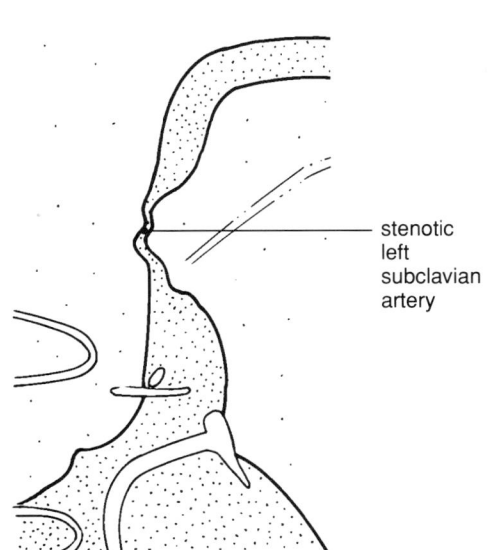

stenotic
left
subclavian
artery

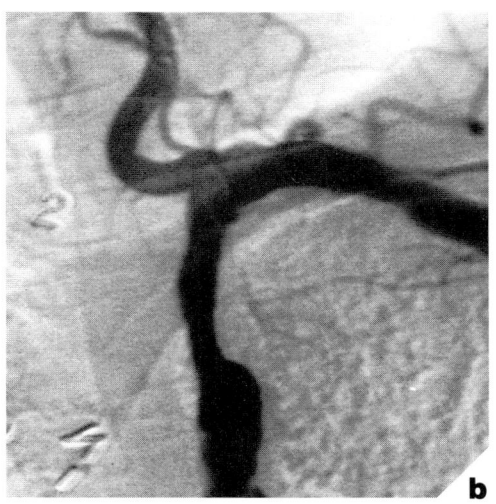

Figure 5.20

*Percutaneous transluminal angioplasty of a subclavian artery stenosis. **a** Left subclavian artery injection demonstrates a severe, irregular stenosis of the left subclavian artery proximal to the origin of the left vertebral artery (which fills in a retrograde fashion). **b** Following balloon angioplasty, there is marked improvement in the caliber of the proximal left subclavian artery and anterograde filling of the left vertebral artery.*

Figure 5.21

Degenerative microangiopathy. There are numerous small bright foci of T2 signal abnormality in the deep and subcortical white matter of both cerebral hemispheres. Upon pathological examination these are found to represent focal areas of gliosis, demyelination, myelin pallor, and etat criblet.

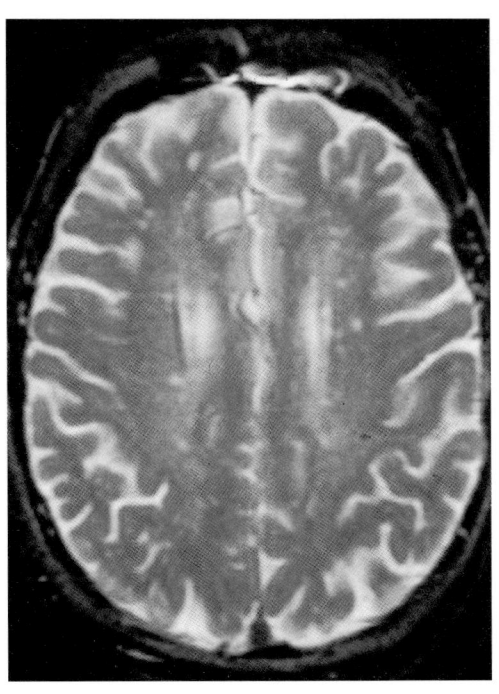

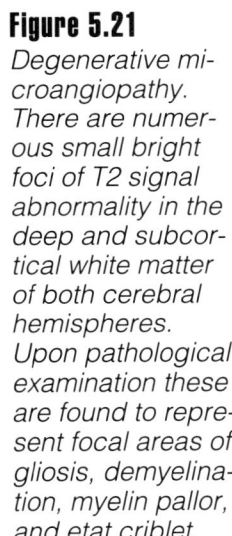

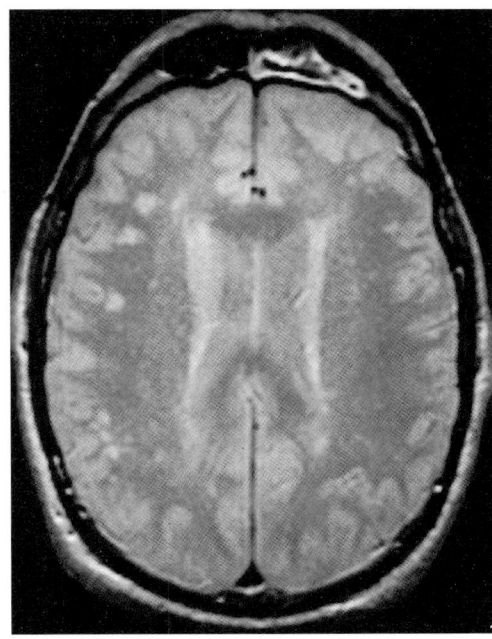

Figure 5.22

Degenerative microangiopathy. Proton density MR images show numerous subcortical hyperintensities. These are the typical location for lesions caused by degenerative microangiopathy and represent one of the most common abnormalities demonstrated by MRI.

Robin) spaces which may be normal. These look like pathological processes on T2-weighted images but occur in typical locations (deep white matter near the vertex or inferior one third of the basal ganglia) and are unusually sharply demarcated on both T1- and T2-weighted sequences (Fig. 5.23). Since these perivascular spaces contain CSF, and since CSF is isointense to cerebral white matter on proton density images, no signal abnormality is seen on this pulse sequence. There is an increase in prevalence of these perivascular spaces with aging due to tortuosity and kinking of small blood vessels. This results in a "sieve-like" appearance to the brain upon pathological inspection and is termed *etat criblet* (Fig. 5.24).

Intracerebral hemorrhage occurs in a wide variety of disorders including hypertension, trauma, aneurysms, and vascular malformations. Neoplasms and infection are relatively less frequent causes of intracerebral hemorrhage. The terms *primary* or *spontaneous* brain hemorrhage, as currently used, are virtually synonymous with hypertensive hemorrhage and thus refer to hemorrhage in the absence of an underlying aneurysm, vascular malformation, neoplasm, or traumatic injury. CT and MRI are very sensitive to the presence of intracerebral hematomas. The high attenuation on CT of an intracerebral hematoma is due to the presence of proteins in the plasma and red blood

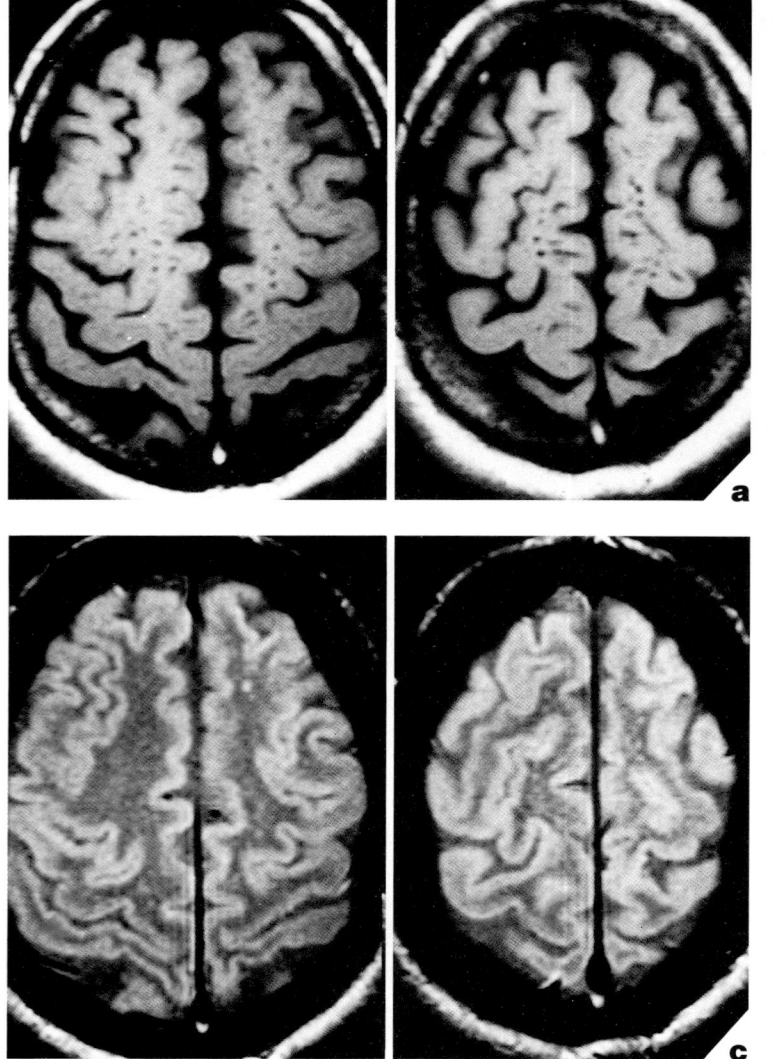

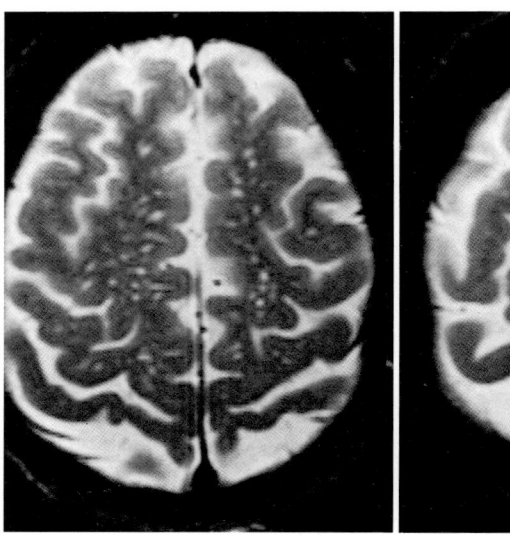
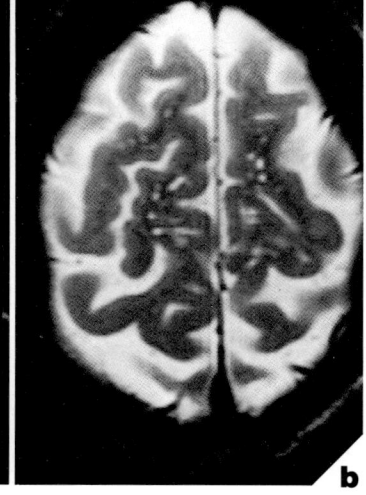

Figure 5.23

*Prominent Virchow-Robin spaces. Axial **a** T1 and **b** T2 images near the cranial vertex show extremely well circumscribed, sharply outlined punctate, symmetrical foci of dark-T1, bright-T2 signal abnormality. These signal abnormalities are absent on the **c** proton density images and represent prominent CSF spaces around penetrating vessels. Since CSF is isointense to the adjacent cerebral white matter on proton density images, Virchow-Robin spaces cannot be identified on proton density sequences.*

cells. Thus, in severe anemia or a clotting disorder, intracerebral hemorrhage may be hypodense or iso-dense with respect to the surrounding brain. The most common sites for hypertensive hemorrhage are the lenticular nucleus and adjacent portions of the internal capsule (Fig. 5.25), thalamus, pons (Fig. 5.26), cerebral white matter (Fig. 5.27), cerebral cortex (Fig. 5.28), and the cerebellar hemispheres. There may be associated subarachnoid or intraventricular rupture (Fig. 5.29). The blood vessel involved is usually a perforating artery. While the exact nature of the vascular lesion is not known, serial sections in some cases have shown the hemorrhage apparently

arising from an artery altered by the effects of hypertension (lipohyalinosis). Tiny (Charcot-Bouchard) aneurysms at the origin of penetrating arteries from major vascular trunks have been observed in some hypertensive patients and may represent another possible mechanism for hypertensive intracerebral hemorrhage.

Amyloidosis of the cerebral arterial walls, observed in elderly, sometimes demented patients, may give rise to solitary or multiple intracerebral hemorrhages (Fig. 5.30). These hemorrhages are often large and are usually located in or near the cerebral cortex. This disorder is termed *amyloid angiopathy.*

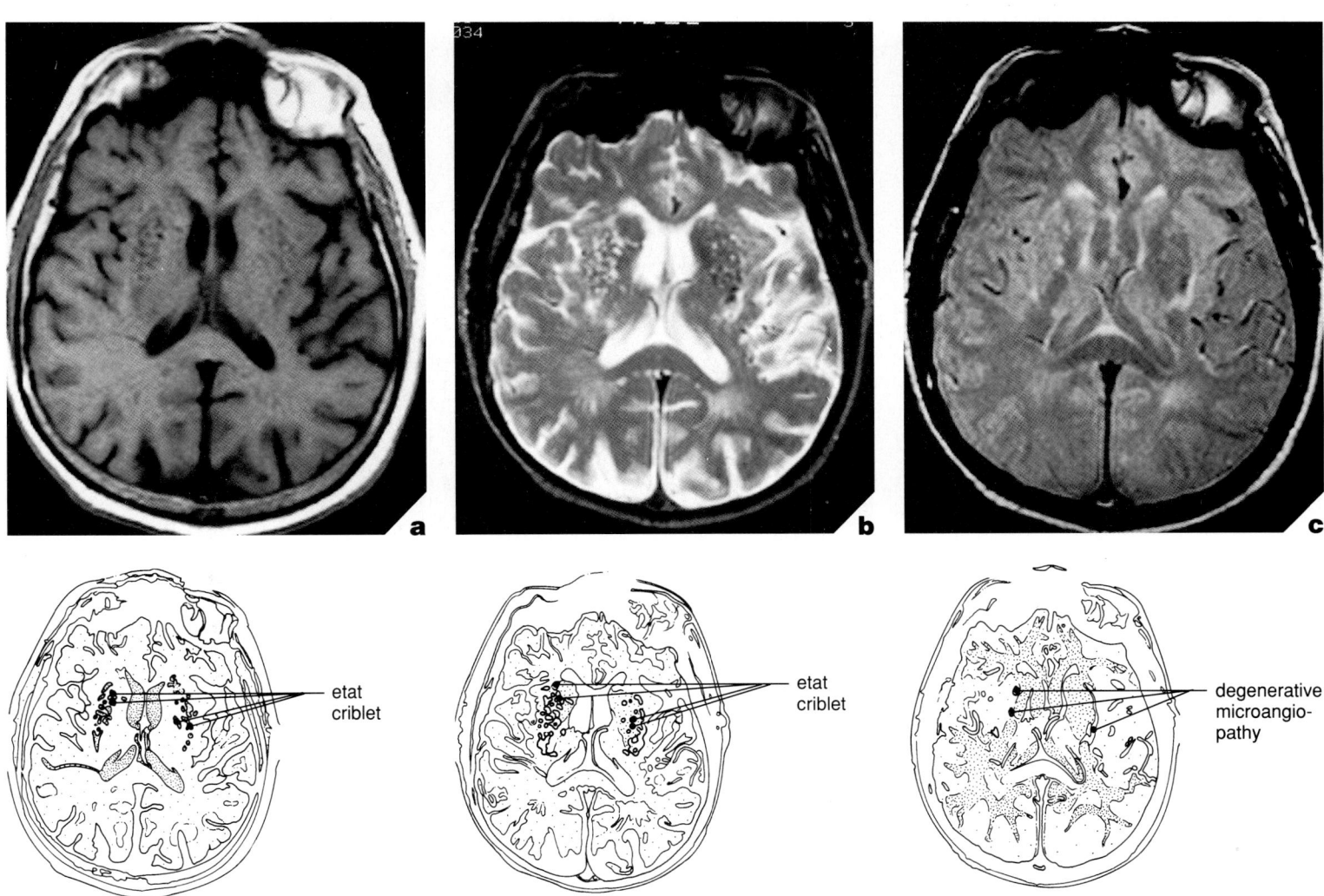

Figure 5.24
*Etat criblet. **a** Dark-T1, **b** bright-T2 lesions, which are invisible on a corresponding **c** proton density image represent dilated perivascular spaces. Lesions visible on the proton density image represent degenerative microangiopathy.*

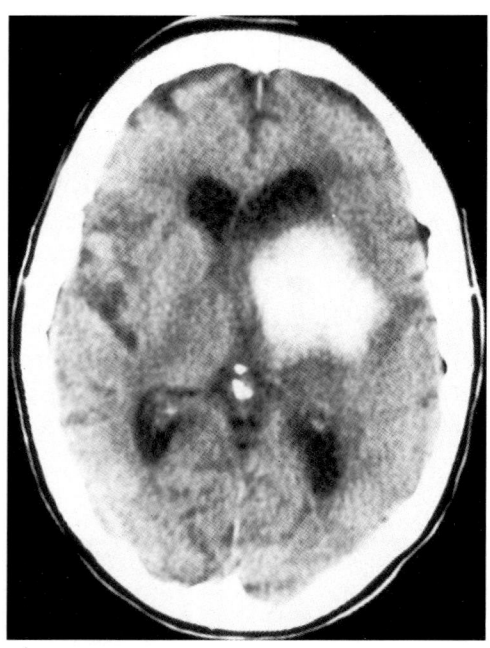

Figure 5.25
Basal ganglia and internal capsule hemorrhage. Un-enhanced axial CT scan shows a large, solitary acute hemorrhage in the left basal ganglia and internal capsule in this hypertensive patient. There is mass effect on the adjacent third and left lateral ventricles.

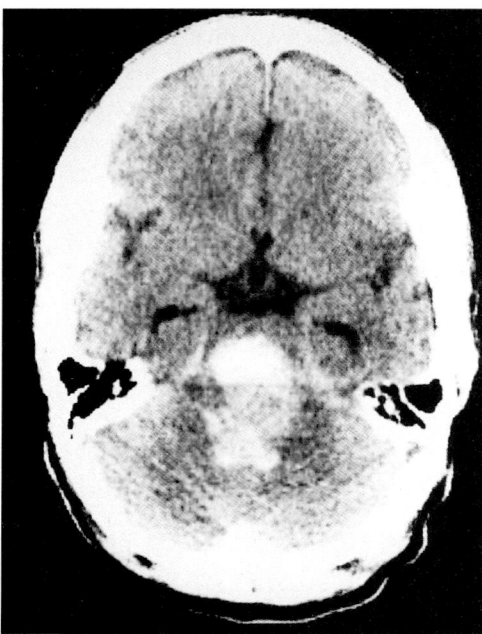

Figure 5.26
Brainstem hemorrhage. A noncontrast axial CT section demonstrates an area of hemorrhage in the pons with extension posteriorly into the fourth ventricle.

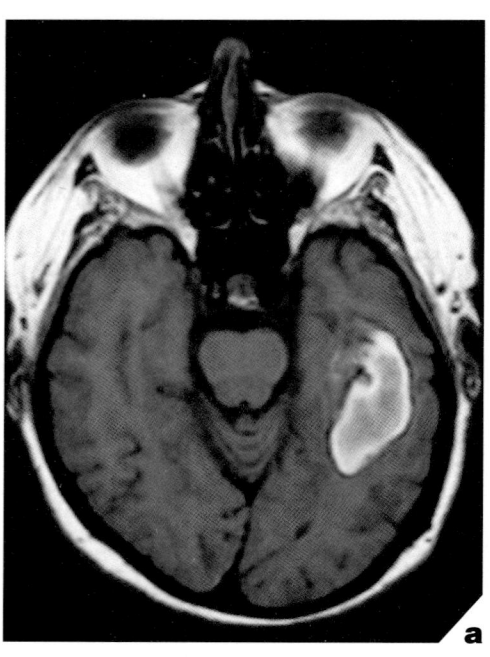

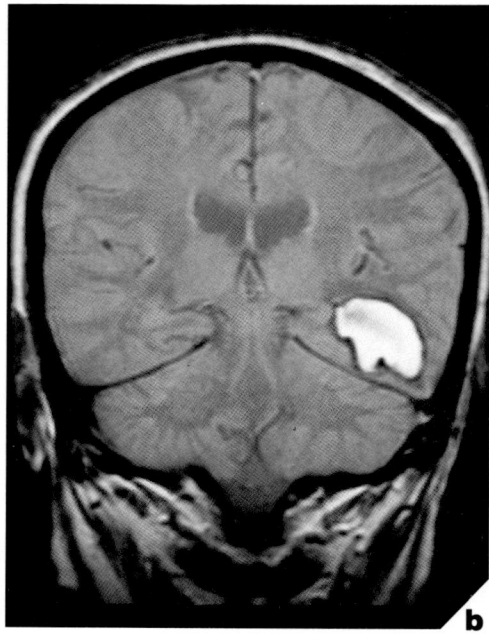

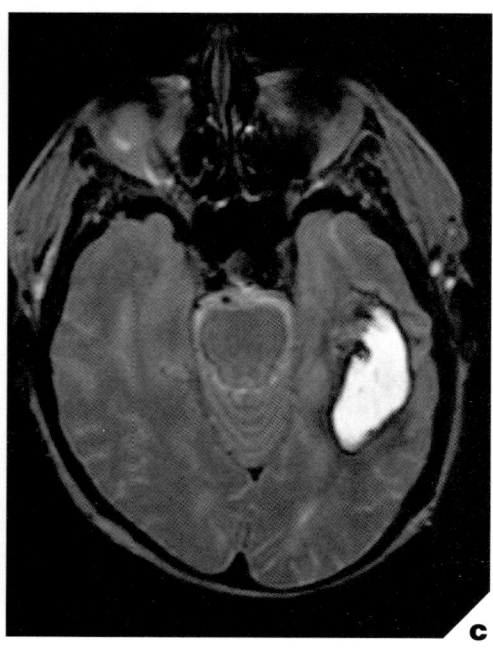

Figure 5.27
*White matter hemorrhage. **a** T1-weighted, **b** proton density, and **c** T2-weighted images show areas of mixed signal inten-* *sity on all pulse sequences in the white matter of the left temporal lobe.*

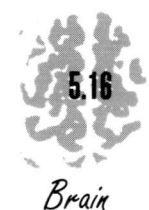

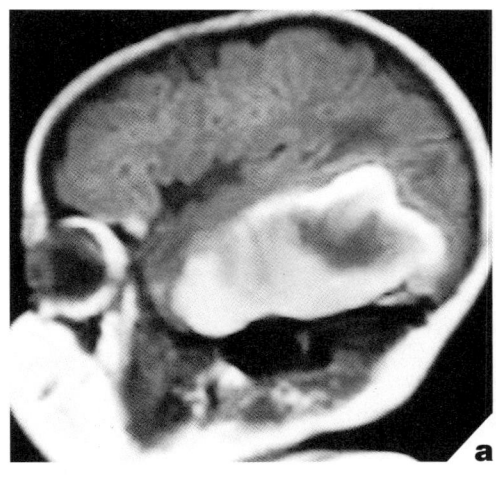

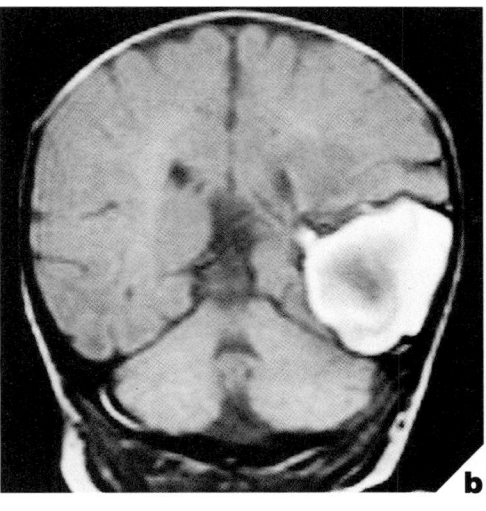

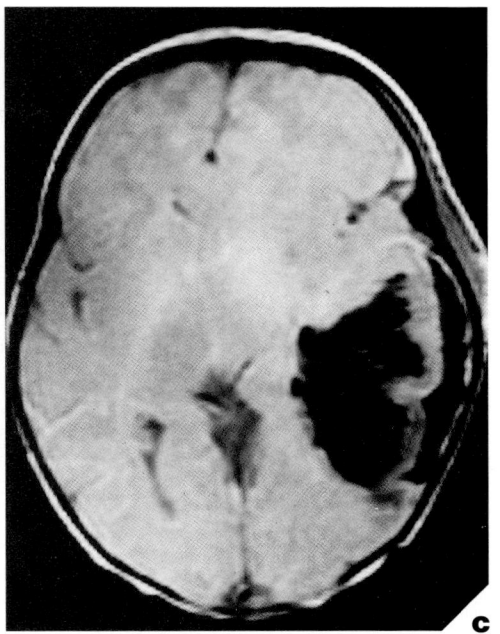

Figure 5.28

*Cerebral hemorrhage. **a,b** T1-weighted and **c** proton density images show hemor-rhage in the grey and white matter of the left temporal lobe.*

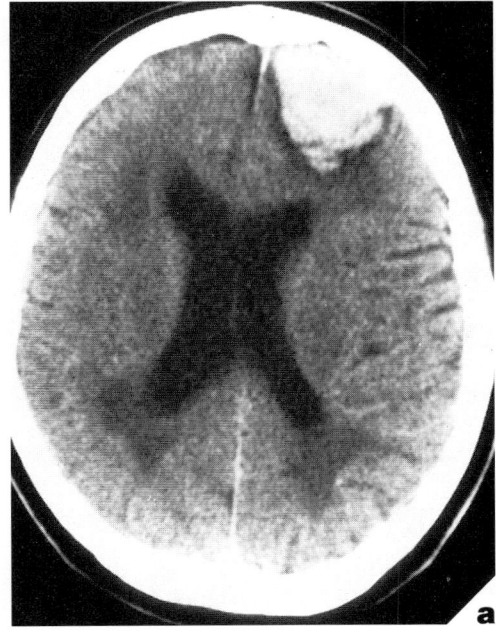

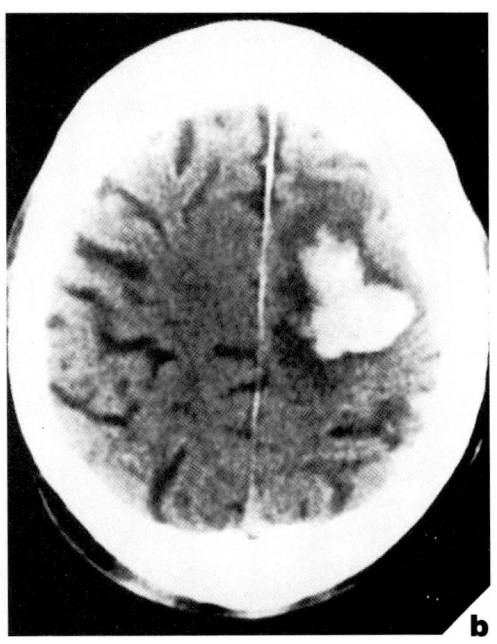

Figure 5.29

Cerebral hemorrhage with associated intraventricular extension. Unenhanced axial CT shows a large parenchymal hemorrhage in the inferior right parietal lobe and acute blood in the right frontal horn and third ventricle.

Figure 5.30

*Amyloid angiopathy. **a,b** This elderly patient presented on different occasions with large, cortical cerebral hemor-rhages.*

At the opposite end of the age spectrum are premature infants. They frequently develop hemorrhage within the lateral ventricles and in the germinal matrix (Fig. 5.31).

Cranial CT is usually able to depict the presence of blood in the subarachnoid space (Fig. 5.32). Occasionally, a small volume of subarachnoid hemorrhage

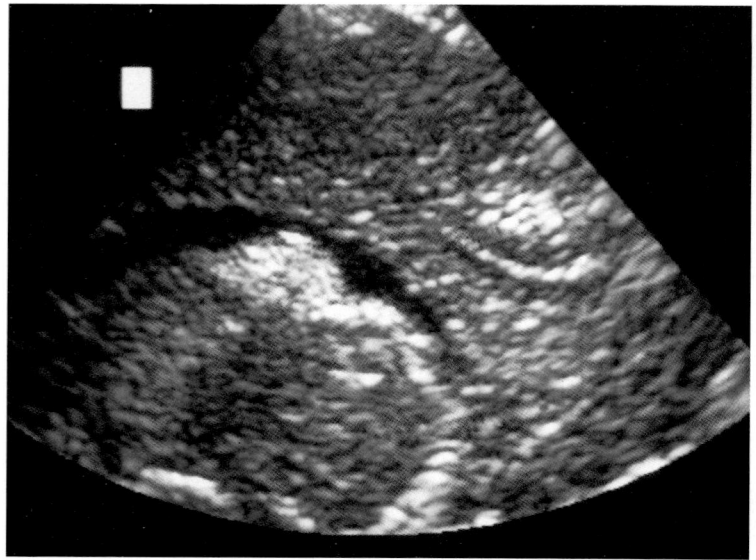

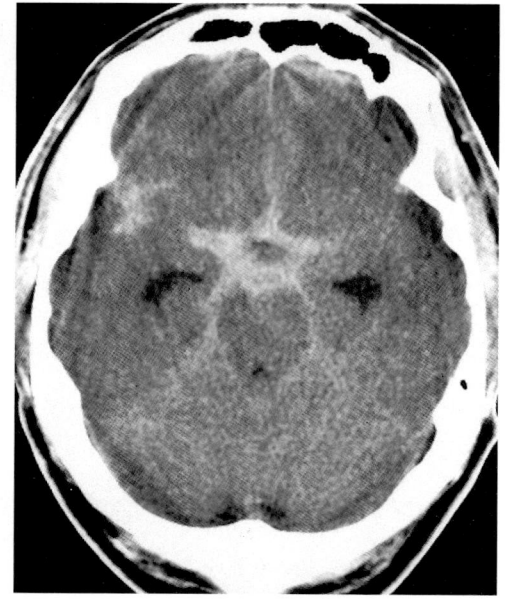

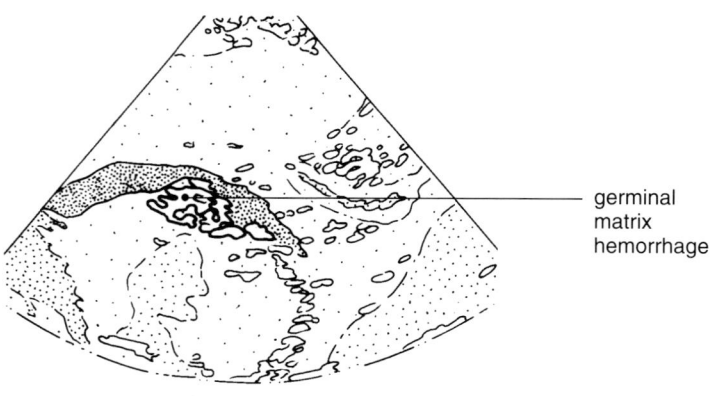

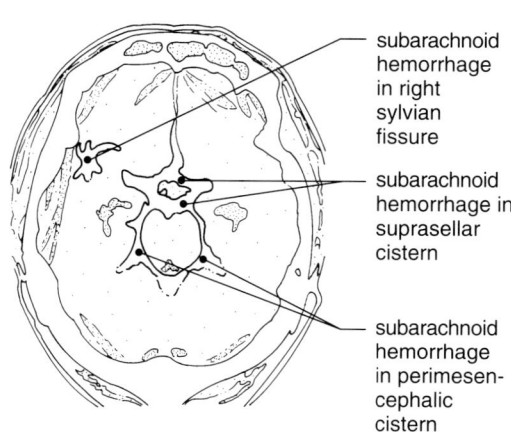

Figure 5.31

Germinal matrix hemorrhage. Sagittal image from a head ultrasound in a premature neonate shows an area of increased echogenicity in the right caudo-thalamic groove. This is the location of the germinal matrix, a common location for intracranial hemorrhage in premature infants.

Figure 5.32

Subarachnoid hemorrhage. There are symmetrical areas of increased density throughout the subarachnoid spaces representing hemorrhage. In this particular case, the hemorrhage is demonstrated in the suprasellar cistern, the right sylvian fissure, the perimesencephalic cisterns, and the anterior interhemispheric fissure. Normally, low density CSF occupies these locations. Note the dilatation of the temporal horns, indicating hydrocephalus.

is undetectable and a lumbar puncture is required to confirm the diagnosis. While subarachnoid hemorrhage may result from trauma or extension into the subarachnoid space from other areas of hemorrhage, the source of primary subarachnoid hemorrhage is usually a ruptured saccular ("berry") aneurysm. Hemorrhage from an arteriovenous malformation is the second leading cause of primary subarachnoid hemorrhage. Since subarachnoid hemorrhage from a ruptured aneurysm is potentially both lethal and treatable, its early detection is of paramount importance. When CT shows diffuse subarachnoid hemorrhage, exact localization of the aneurysm is difficult. However, it is usually possible to suggest the location of a ruptured aneurysm from the pattern of blood distribution within the cisternal spaces.

In subarachnoid hemorrhage due to rupture of an aneurysm arising from the anterior communicating complex, blood tends to accumulate in the anterior portion of the interhemispheric fissure (Fig. 5.33); if the dome of the aneurysm is adherent to the brain substance, blood may extend into the parenchyma of the medial frontal lobes (Fig. 5.34). Following rupture of an aneurysm at the junction of the internal carotid and posterior communicating arteries, there may be a blood clot within only the ipsilateral, lateral aspect of the suprasellar cistern. A preponderance of blood in the sylvian fissure often indicates rupture of a middle cerebral artery aneurysm.

Giant aneurysms (≥2.5 cm in diameter) can often be visualized by using contrast-enhanced CT scans

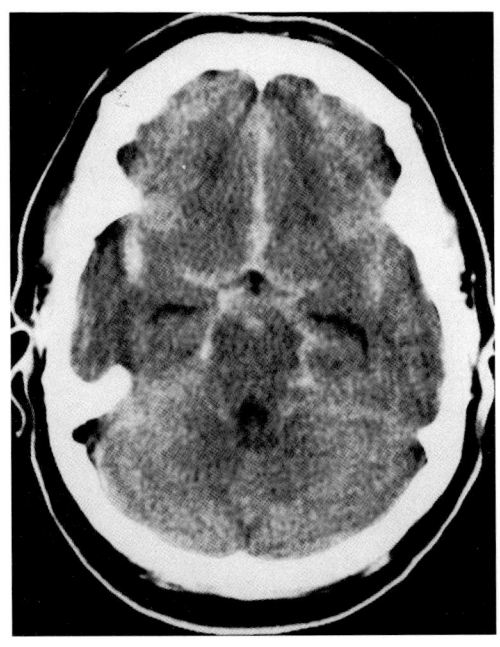 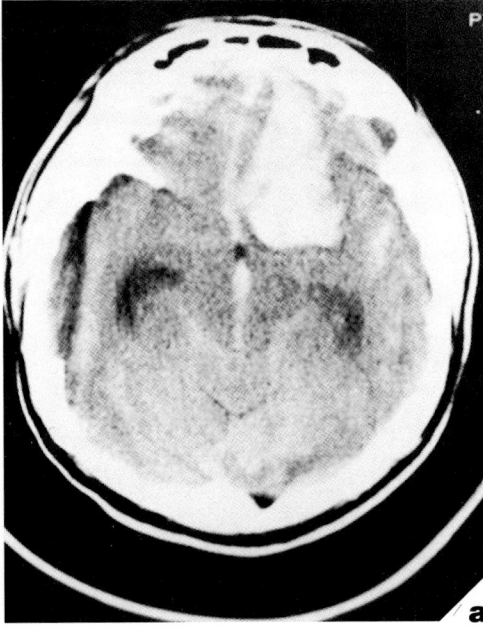 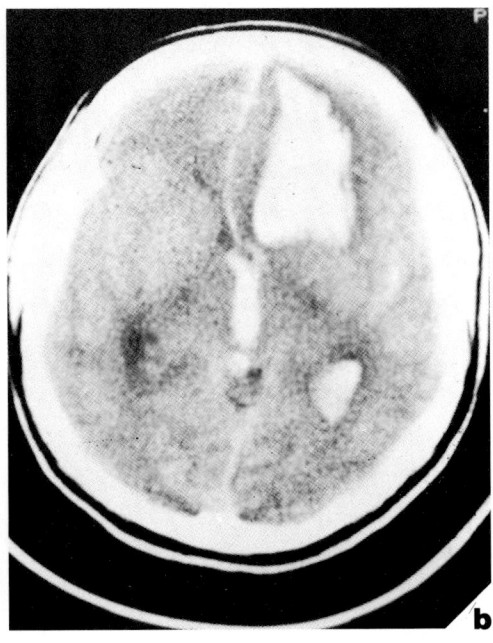

Figure 5.33

Subarachnoid hemorrhage from a ruptured anterior communicating artery aneurysm. Unenhanced CT shows blood in the suprasellar and perimesencephalic cisterns, sylvian fissures, and anterior interhemispheric fissure.

Figure 5.34

*Intraparenchymal hemorrhage due to rupture of an anterior communicating artery aneurysm. **a,b** Noncontrast axial CT sections demonstrate a large area of intraparenchymal hemorrhage in the left frontal lobe. There is also blood in*

the interhemispheric fissure anteriorly, the sylvian fissure on the left side, the left lateral ventricle, and the third ventricle. Note the enlarged temporal horns of the lateral ventricles, indicating acute hydrocephalus.

(Fig. 5.35). While a giant aneurysm is also usually demonstrable on an unenhanced MR or CT scan (Fig. 5.36), the contrast enhancement usually helps to separate thrombosed portions of the aneurysm from patent regions. Patients with giant aneurysms may present with signs and symptoms related to mass effect rather than subarachnoid hemorrhage. Fusiform aneurysms of the cerebral arteries secondary to atherosclerosis and hypertension also may present with neurological signs related to compression of the brain substance (Fig. 5.37).

Intracranial aneurysms occur in many different, but typical, locations. Supraclinoid internal carotid artery aneurysms are common. Ophthalmic artery aneurysms (Fig. 5.38), like others, may be initially diagnosed by CT or MRI, but require angiography for detailed evaluation. Posterior communicating artery aneurysms (Fig. 5.39) are second only to anterior communicating artery aneurysms (Fig. 5.40) in incidence. Not only are anterior communicating artery aneurysms the most common type (30%) of "berry" aneurysm, they are also the type most likely to bleed. Aneurysms at the internal carotid artery bifurcation (Fig. 5.41) and middle cerebral artery bifurcation or trifurcation are also common. Basilar tip artery aneurysms (Fig. 5.42) represent 5% of intracranial

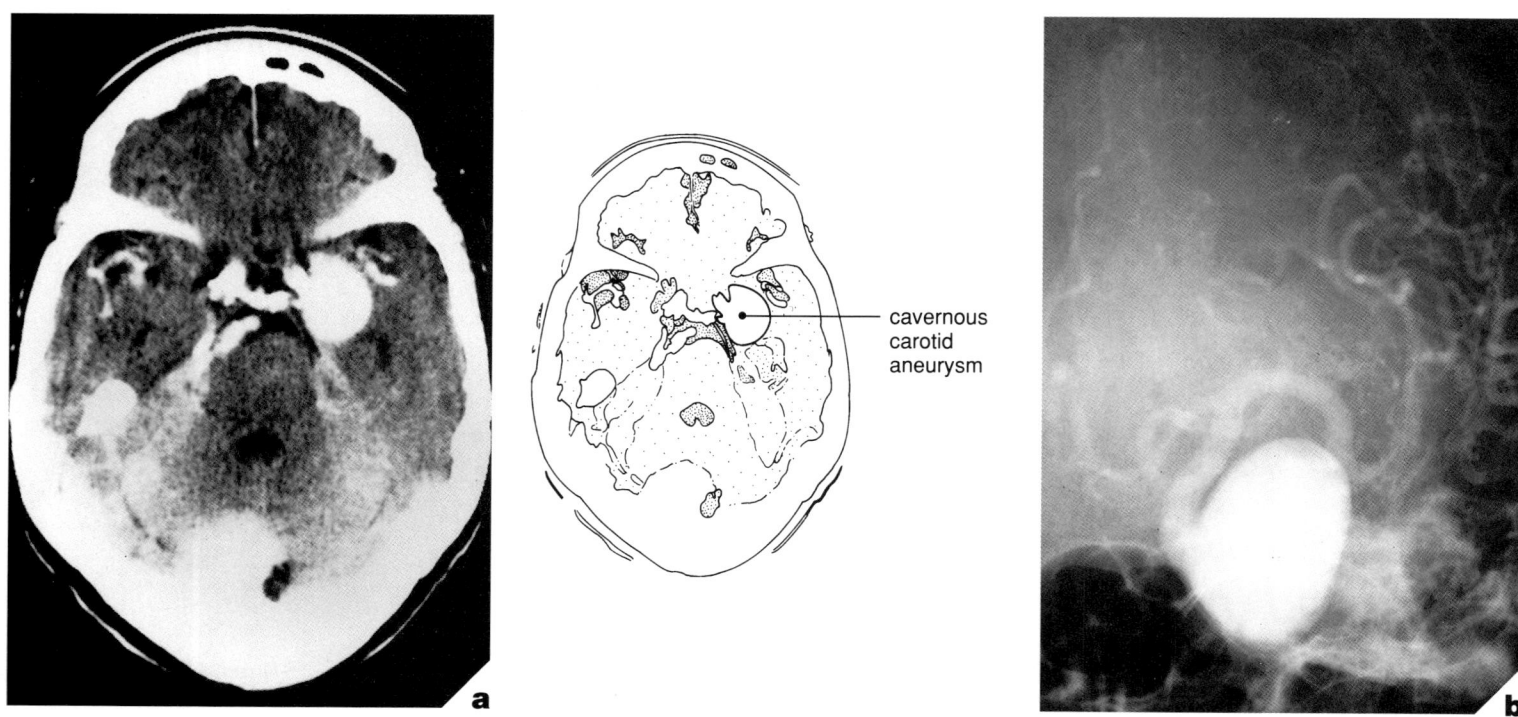

cavernous carotid aneurysm

Figure 5.35

*Giant aneurysm. **a** Contrast-enhanced CT shows a large enhancing mass in the left middle cranial fossa which was proven on **b** angiography to represent a giant cavernous carotid artery aneurysm.*

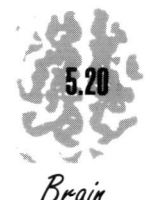

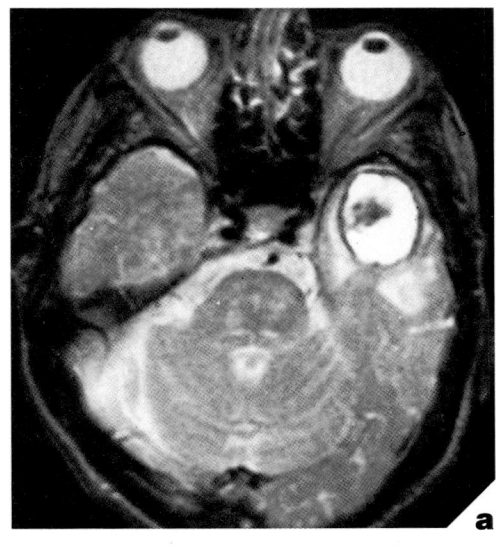

Figure 5.36

*Giant middle cerebral artery bifurcation aneurysm. **a** Unenhanced T2-weighted MRI and **b** CT scans show a mass in the left middle cranial fossa. **c** Contrast-enhanced CT shows rim enhancement more posterior to the hyperdensity seen on unenhanced CT. This rim outlines an area of isodense thrombus in the posterior portion of the aneurysm and explains why the aneurysm appeared larger on the MRI (which showed the entire aneurysm) than on unenhanced CT.*

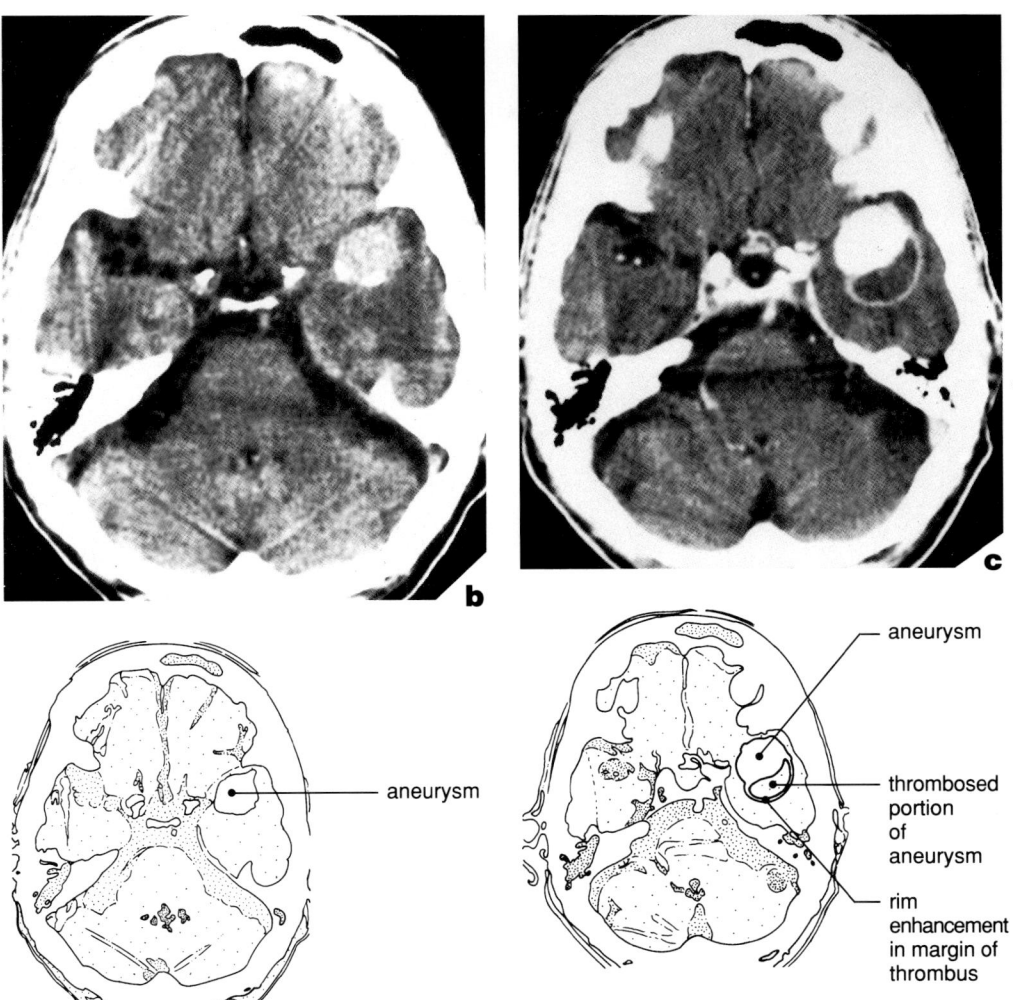

aneurysm

aneurysm

thrombosed portion of aneurysm

rim enhancement in margin of thrombus

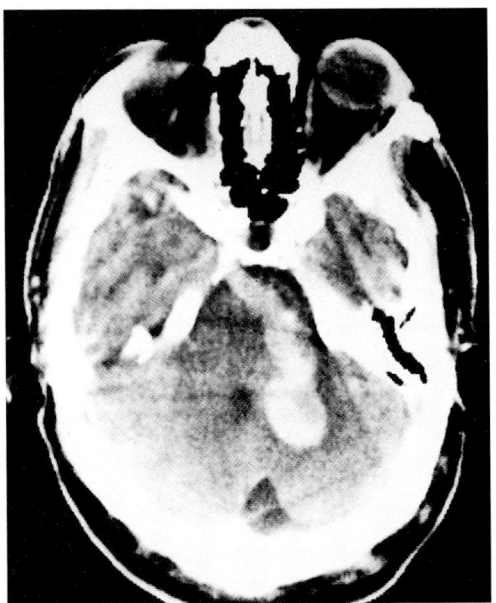

Figure 5.37

Dolichoectasia of the basilar artery. An axial CT section through the posterior fossa following intravenous injection of contrast material demonstrates a large tubular enhancing structure representing marked fusiform dilatation of the basilar artery.

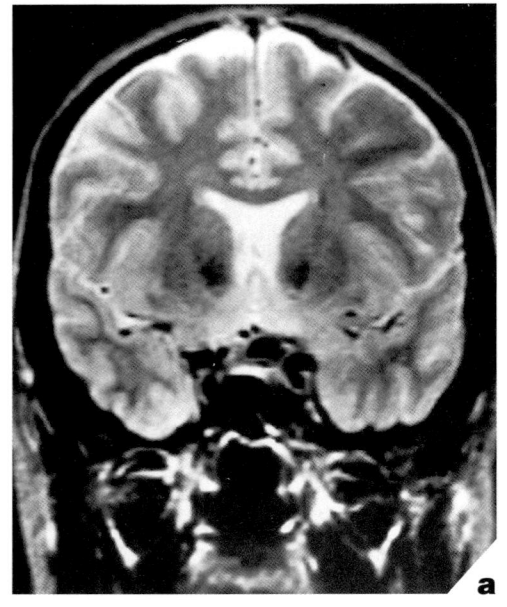

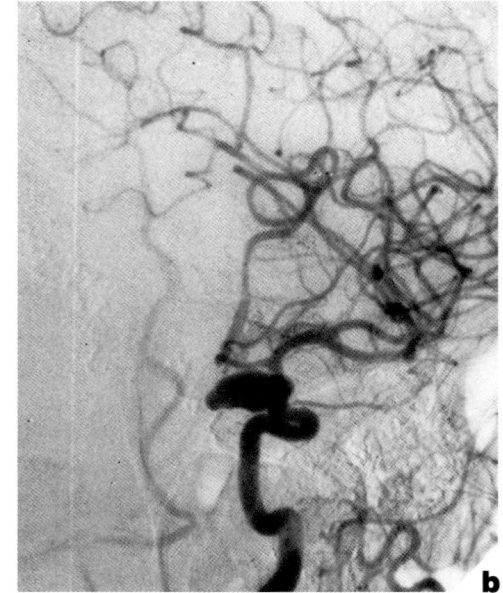

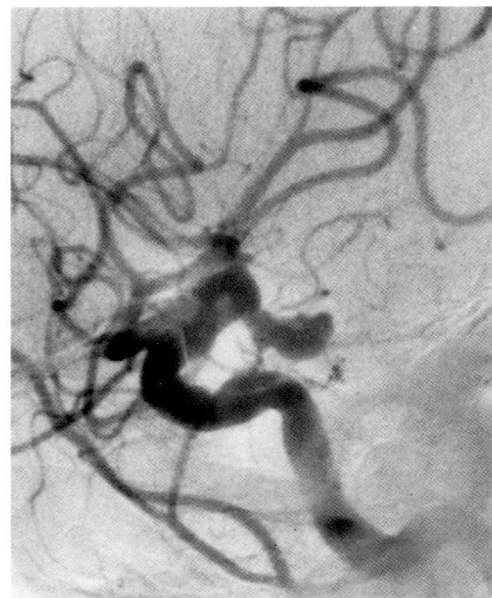

ophthalmic
artery
aneurysm

flow void
within
cavernous
portions of
internal
carotid
arteries

ophthalmic
artery
aneurysm

posterior
communicating
artery
aneurysm

Figure 5.38

*Ophthalmic artery aneurysm. **a** T2 coronal MRI shows a flow void signal abnormality medial to the cavernous portion of the left internal carotid artery. **b** Left in-*

ternal carotid arteriogram confirms the presence of an aneurysm at the junction of the left ophthalmic artery and the supraclinoid left internal carotid artery.

Figure 5.39

Posterior communicating artery aneurysm. Lateral view from a cerebral angiogram shows a large outpouching of contrast media from the wall of the supraclinoid internal carotid artery at the site of the origin of the posterior communicating artery.

Figure 5.40

Anterior communicating artery aneurysm. There is a lobulated outpouching at the site of the anterior communicating artery representing an aneurysm. Anterior communicating aneurysms are the most common type of "berry" aneurysm as well as the most likely type to rupture.

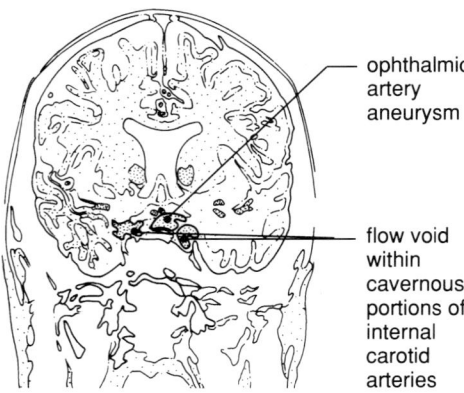

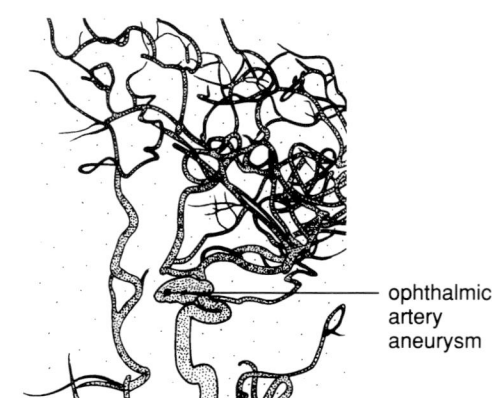

anterior
communicating
artery
aneurysm

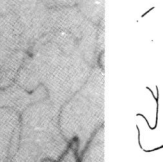

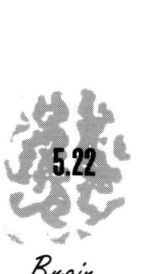

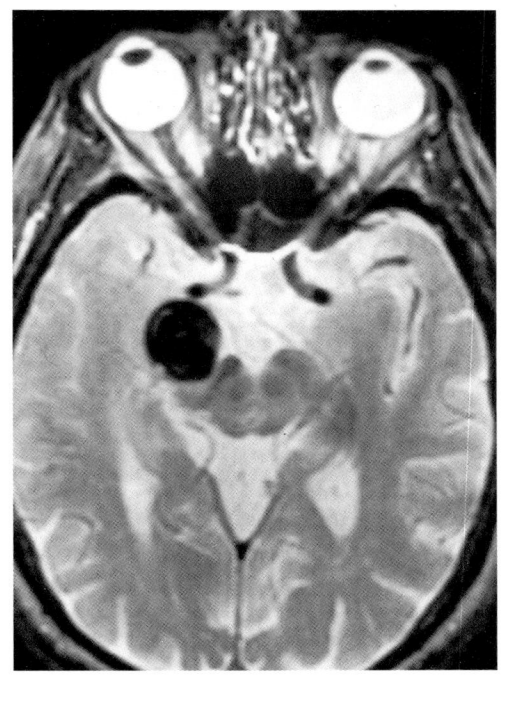
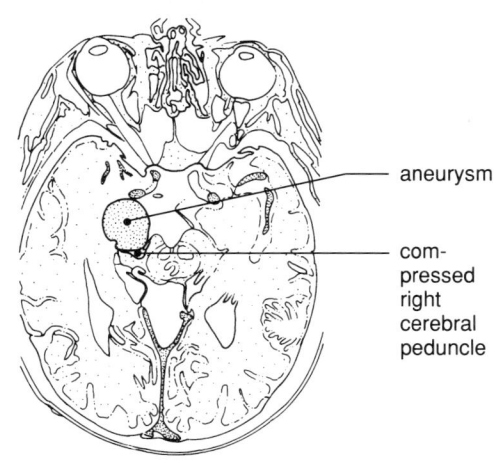

aneurysm

com-
pressed
right
cerebral
peduncle

Figure 5.41

Right internal carotid artery bifurcation aneurysm. Axial T2-weighted MR image shows a large area of dark signal abnormality at the site of the right internal carotid artery bifurcation. There is compression of the adjacent right cerebral peduncle. The aneurysm was found during a workup for Bell's palsy; there was no subarachnoid hemorrhage.

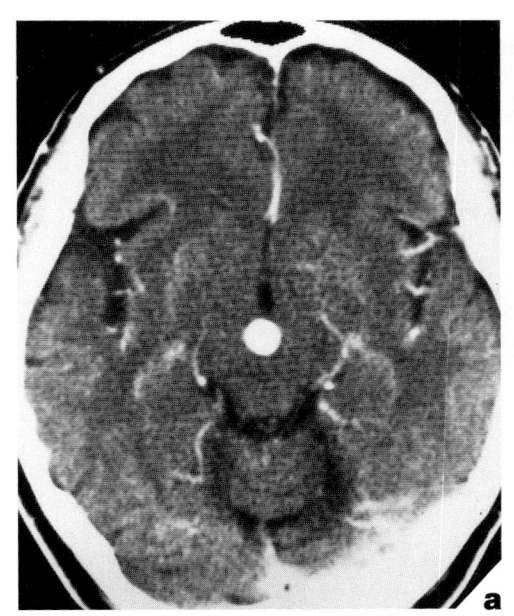
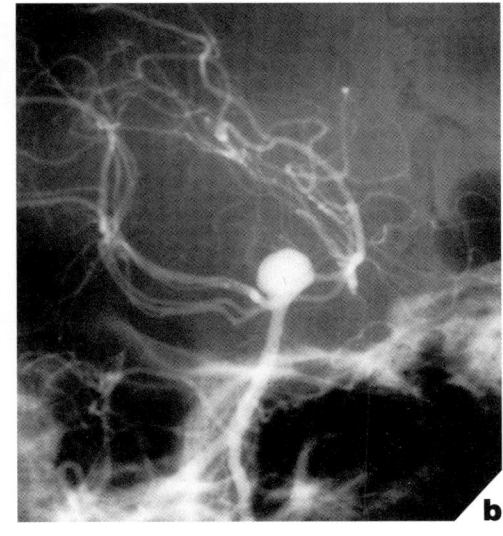
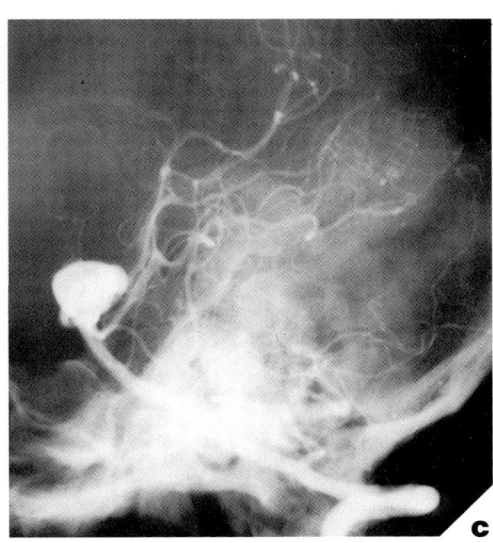

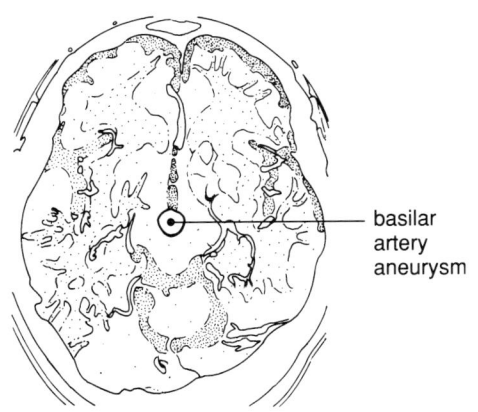
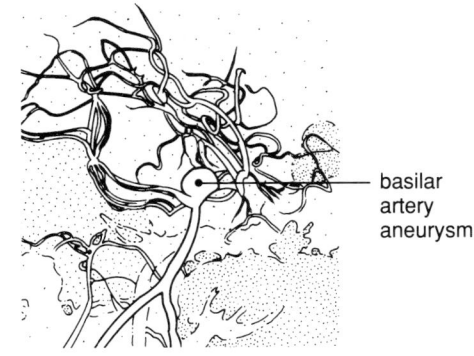

basilar
artery
aneurysm

basilar
artery
aneurysm

basilar
artery
aneurysm

Figure 5.42

*Basilar tip aneurysm. **a** Contrast-enhanced CT and **b,c** posterior fossa angiographic images show a rounded aneurysm of the basilar tip. Basilar tip aneurysms comprise 5% of intracranial aneurysms.*

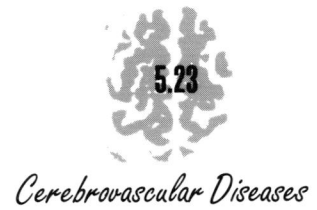

aneurysms. Posterior inferior cerebellar artery (PICA) aneurysms (Fig. 5.43) represent approximately 1% of intracranial aneurysms.

Twenty percent of patients with intracranial aneurysms have multiple aneurysms. Therefore, it is important to study the entire brain during angiography in order not to miss an additional lesion. When multiple aneurysms are demonstrated, it may be difficult to determine which aneurysm has bled. Generally, the aneurysm that bled may be determined by the distribution of blood on CT, but in equivocal cases, it is generally the largest and most lobulated aneurysm which has bled. Surrounding vasospasm and mass effect are also angiographic clues. Although the likelihood that an aneurysm will rupture is proportional to its size, giant aneurysms have a somewhat lower incidence of rupture than would be expected by size criteria alone.

A dreaded complication of subarachnoid hemorrhage is vasospasm. Although this may be treated medically with calcium channel blockers and other agents, the results are often unsatisfactory. Recently angioplasty has been reported to be remarkably suc-cessful in treating patients with intracranial vasospasm (Fig. 5.44).

VASCULAR MALFORMATIONS

Vascular malformations of the brain include arteriovenous malformation (AVM), venous angioma, cavernous angioma, and capillary telangectasia. AVMs are abnormal connections between arteries and veins without intervening capillaries. The feeding arteries and draining veins may be quite large.

An AVM in and around the vein of Galen (Fig. 5.45) is the most common type of intracranial vascular malformation in the neonatal period. AVMs usually come to medical attention later in life because of intracerebral or subarachnoid hemorrhage, because of cerebral infarction due to "steal" of blood flow from adjacent normal tissues, or as a result of a seizure. In a patient with a ruptured AVM, the CT and MRI findings are those of an intraparenchymal hematoma and/or subarachnoid hemorrhage and dilated feeding arteries or draining veins. In a patient

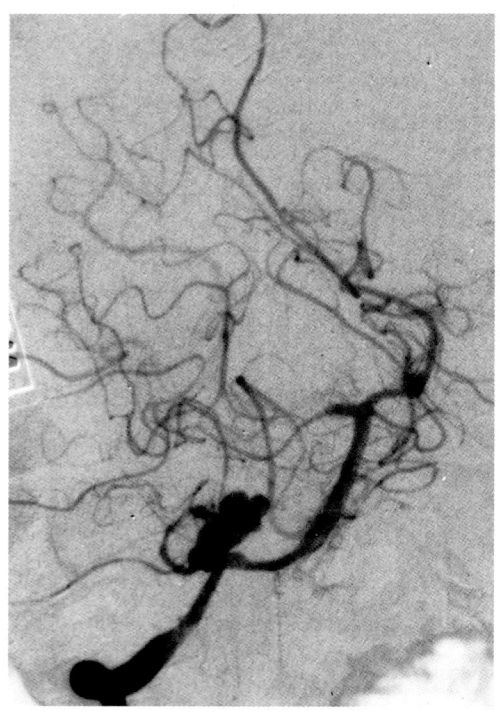

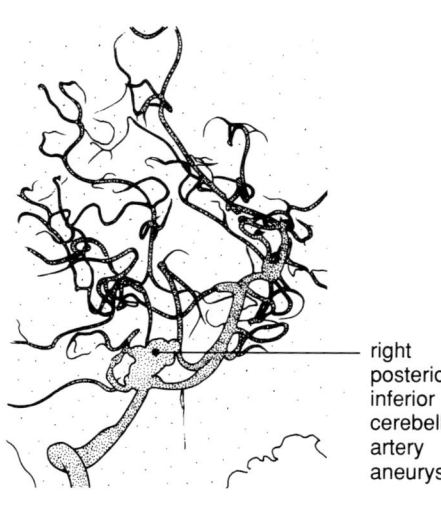

right posterior inferior cerebellar artery aneurysm

Figure 5.43

Posterior inferior cerebellar artery aneurysm. Right vertebral artery injection demonstrates a large, multilobulated aneurysm located at the origin of the right posterior inferior cerebellar artery (PICA). It is important to visualize both PICAs during angiography, either by reflux or direct anterograde filling.

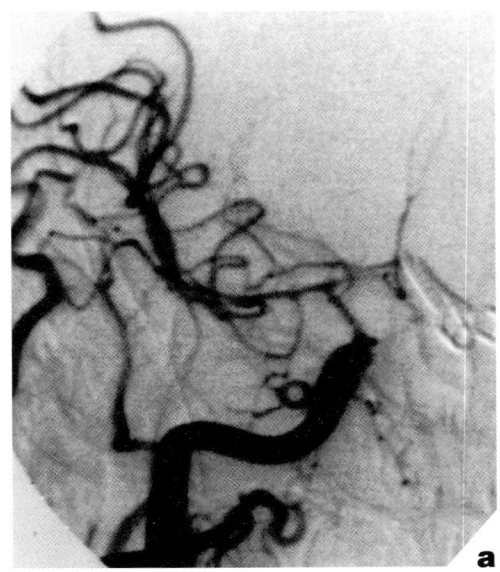
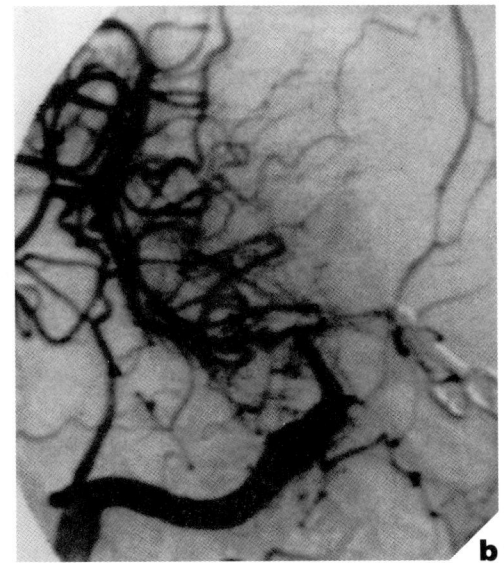

Figure 5.44

Postsubarachnoid hemorrhage vaso-spasm. One week following the rupture of a left-sided posterior communicating artery aneurysm, the patient's clinical condition rapidly deteriorated. **a** *The supraclinoid portion of the right internal carotid artery and proximal portions of the right anterior and middle cerebral arteries are severely narrowed, indicating vasospasm.* **b** *Following percutaneous balloon dilatation, there is considerable increase in diameter of the internal carotid artery and proximal right middle cerebral artery. Due to the severe nature of this vasospasm, the proximal right anterior cerebral artery could not be dilated.*

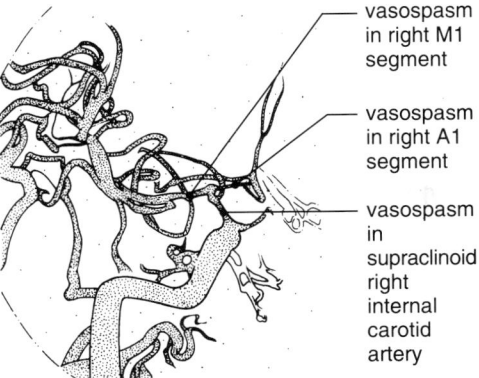

vasospasm in right M1 segment

vasospasm in right A1 segment

vasospasm in supraclinoid right internal carotid artery

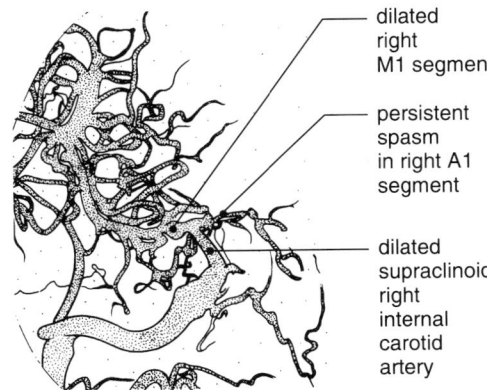

dilated right M1 segment

persistent spasm in right A1 segment

dilated supraclinoid right internal carotid artery

Figure 5.45

Vein of Galen AVM. CT scan with contrast of a neonate shows dilated tortuous vessels draining into an enlarged vein of Galen. This is the most common location for a neonatal AVM.

with an unruptured AVM, CT may show irregular areas of increased density representing the blood pool of the enlarged vascular channels . Following contrast administration, the intensely enhancing, serpiginous vessels are revealed (Fig. 5.46). Because of the rapidly flowing blood, the enlarged vessels appear as areas of signal void on MR images (Fig. 5.47).

AVMs frequently bleed (Fig. 5.48) and the hemorrhage may be difficult to distinguish from other causes of subarachnoid or intraparenchymal hemorrhage. AVMs may be treated by embolization; however, deep-seated lesions with many small arterial feeders (Fig. 5.49) may be impossible to embolize safely. Proton beam therapy or other specialized forms of radiation therapy may also be used to treat AVMs.

Cavernous angiomas consist of thin-walled, closely spaced sinusoidal vascular spaces. These vascular channels are frequently too small to be seen by angiography. The CT and MRI findings are characteristic but not specific. The most frequent appearance is a small, round, hyperdense or T1-hyperintense region that causes surprisingly little mass effect and exhibits little or no enhancement after intravenous injection of contrast material. MRI is more sensitive and specific than CT in detecting cavernous angiomas of the brainstem, a typical location (Fig. 5.50).

Venous angiomas are characterized by dilated venous channels and the absence of enlarged feeding arteries. MRI shows prominent, anomalous venous channels (Fig. 5.51), which often have a "spoke-wheel" or "caput-medusae" appearance. Venous angiomas are believed to be caused by abnormal development of the deep venous structures of the brain. The key point in differentiating venous angiomas from AVMs is their lack of early venous filling and the absence of dilated arterial feeders.

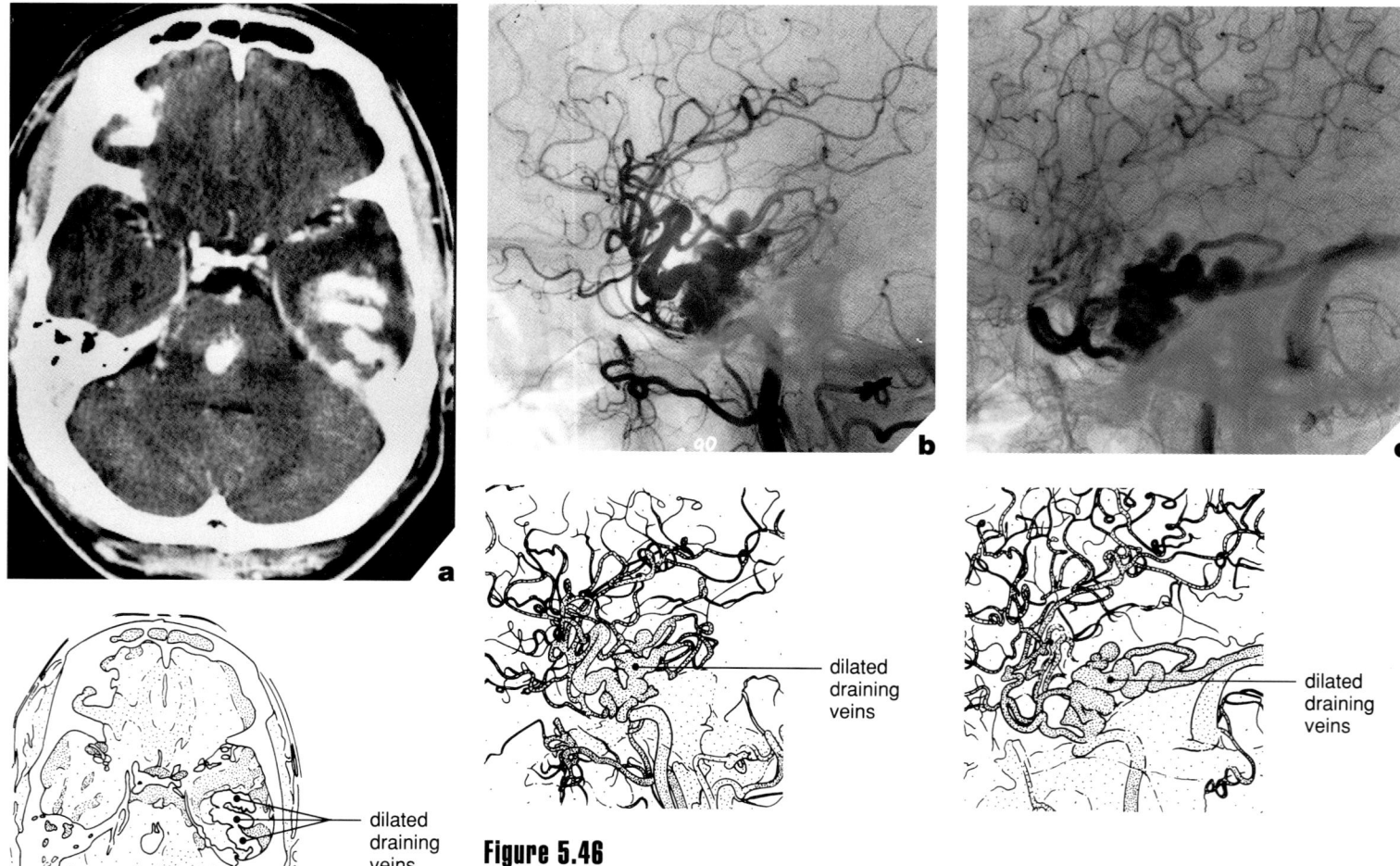

dilated draining veins

dilated draining veins

dilated draining veins

Figure 5.46
AVM. *a* Contrast-enhanced CT of a left temporal lobe AVM shows dilated, tortuous draining veins. *b,c* These vessels are best demonstrated during cerebral angiography.

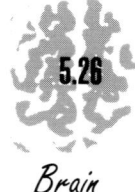

A high jugular bulb represents a developmental variation, which is usually of no clinical significance. However, it may be confused with temporal bone lesions such as a glomus tumor or a metastasis since it enhances on MRI. Dynamic CT is usually characteristic (Fig. 5.52).

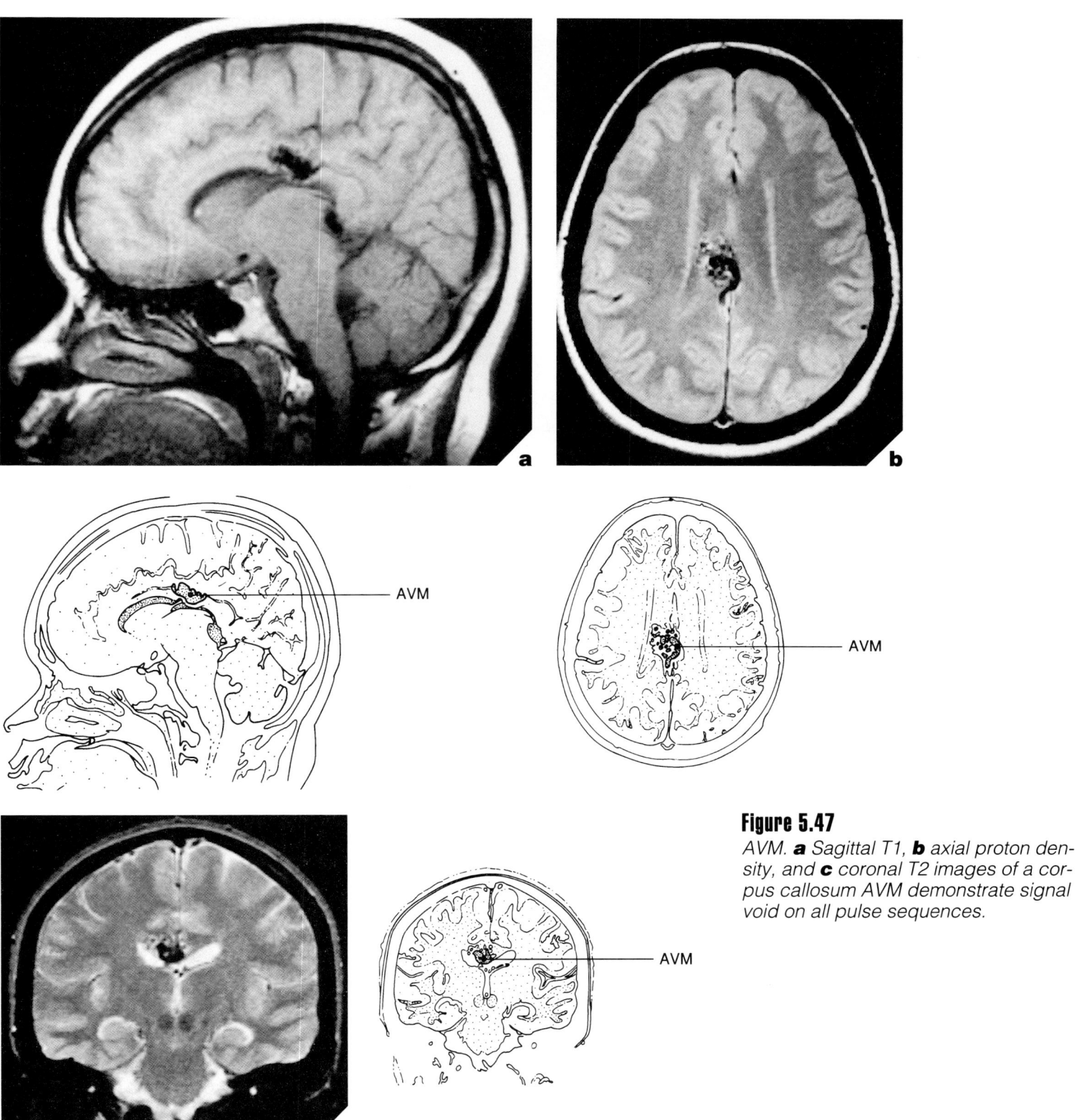

Figure 5.47

*AVM. **a** Sagittal T1, **b** axial proton density, and **c** coronal T2 images of a corpus callosum AVM demonstrate signal void on all pulse sequences.*

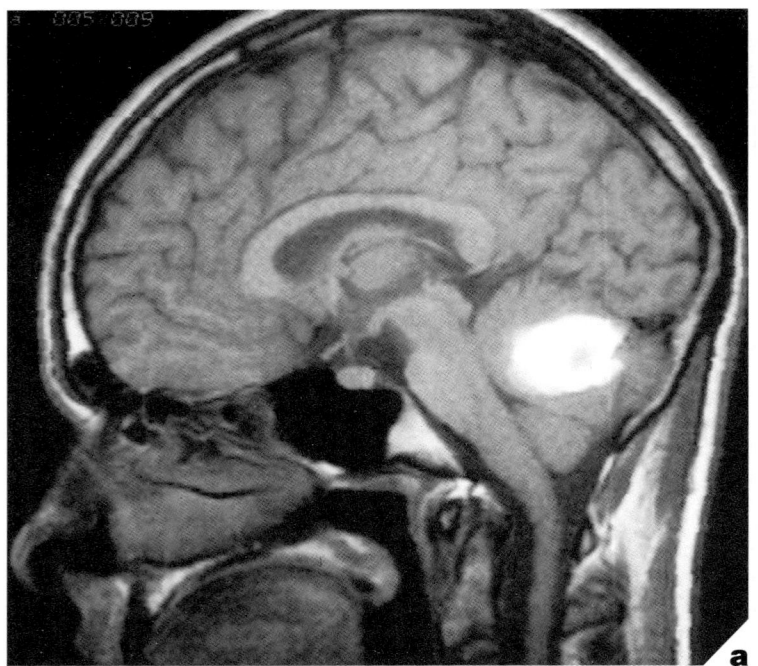

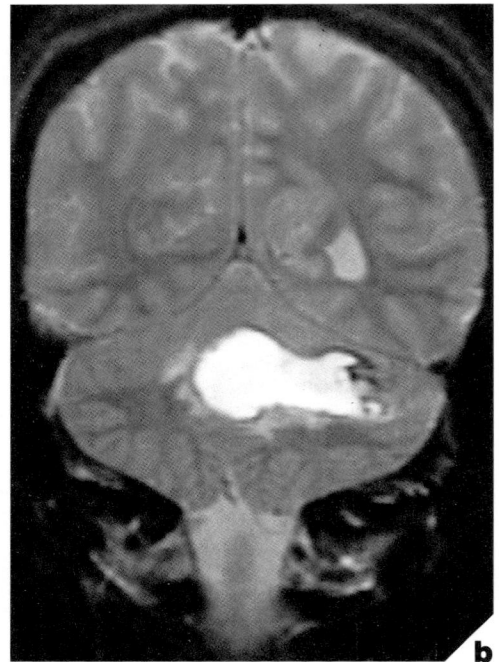

Figure 5.48

Hemorrhagic AVM.
a *Sagittal T1 and*
b *coronal T2 MR
images show an
area of hemor-
rhage in the cere-
bellum. At surgery,
a thrombosed
AVM was demon-
strated.*

a

b

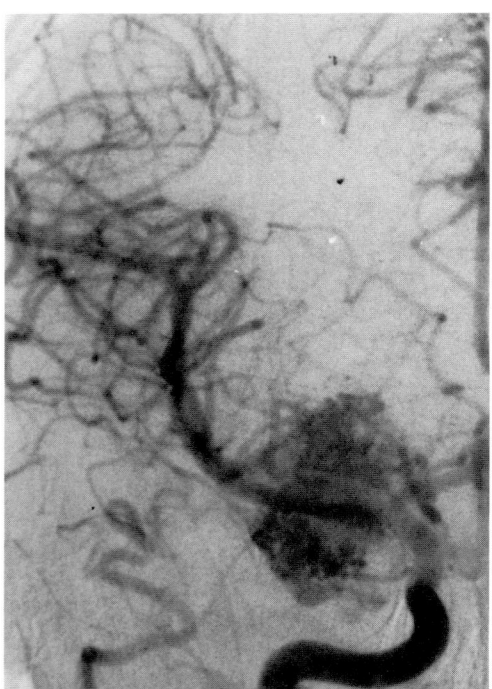

Figure 5.49

*AVM. The nidus of this right basal gan-
glia AVM is composed of innumerable
tiny arterial feeders.*

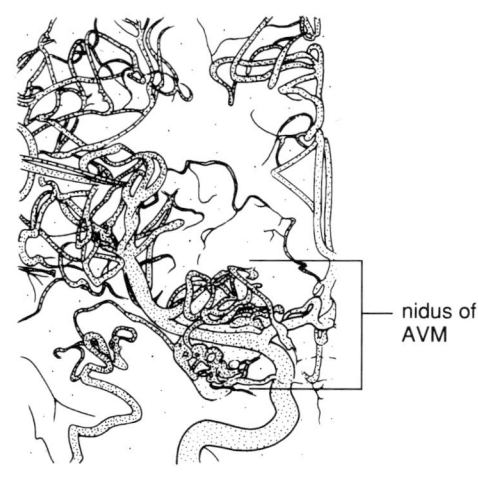

nidus of
AVM

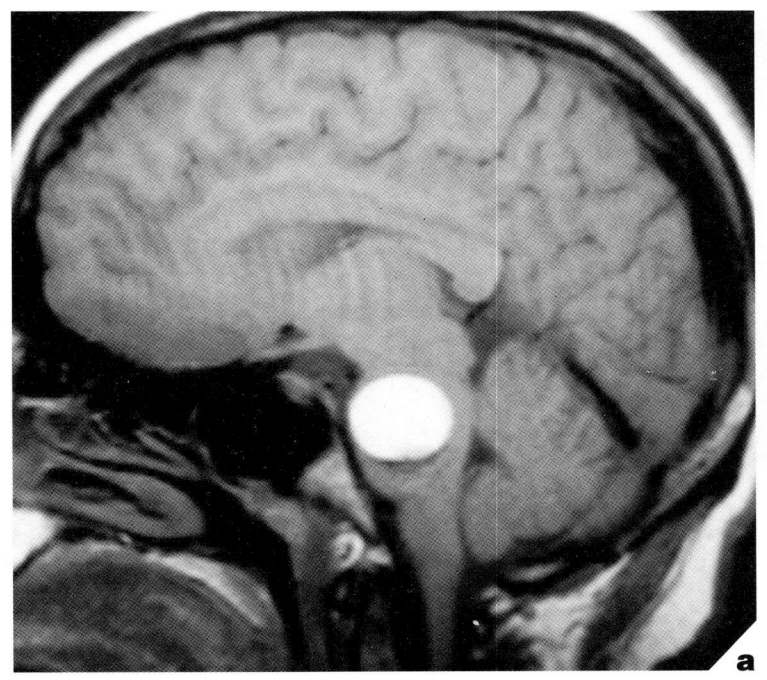

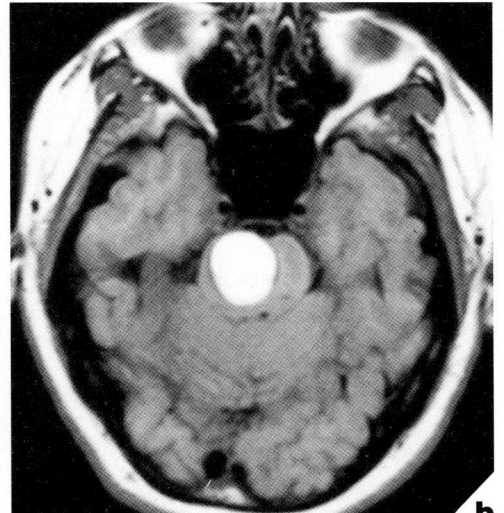

Figure 5.50

*Cavernous angioma. **a** Sagittal and **b** axial T1-weighted images demonstrate a rounded area of hemorrhage in the brainstem, which does not cause significant mass effect.*

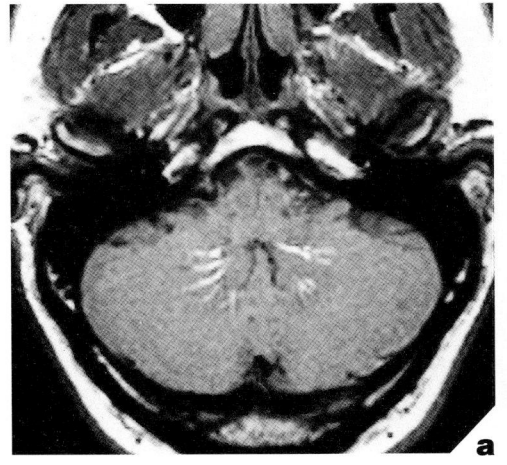

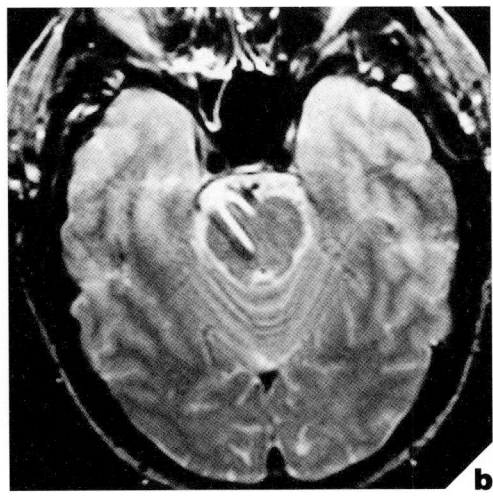

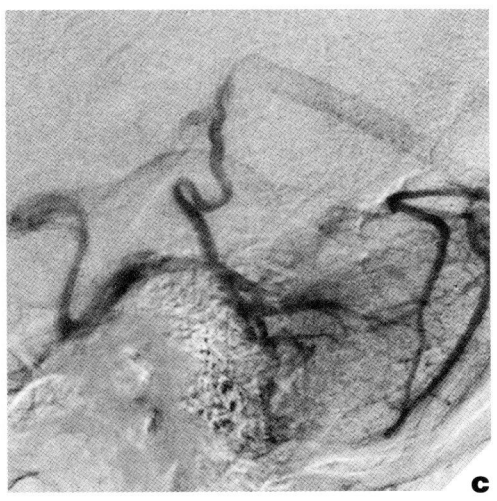

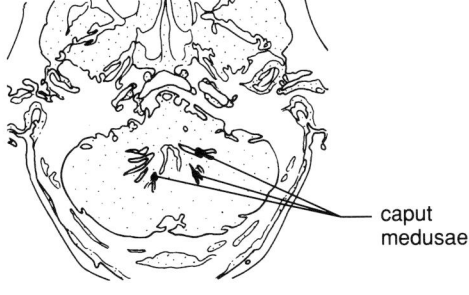

caput medusae

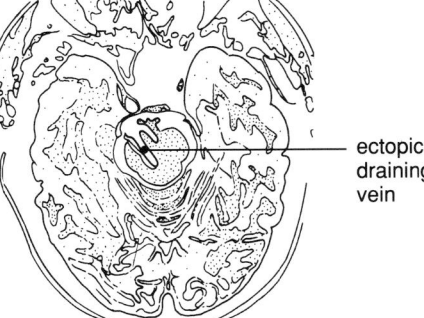

ectopic draining vein

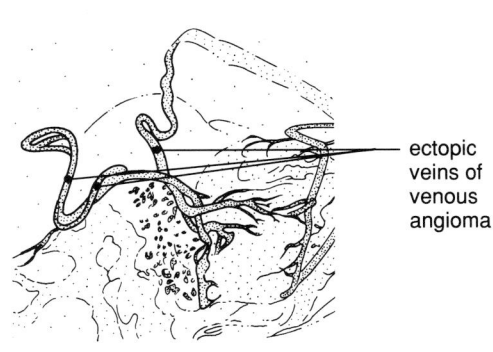

ectopic veins of venous angioma

Figure 5.51

*Venous angioma. **a** Axial T1 and **b** T2 MR images and **c** the venous phase of a posterior fossa angiogram show prominent, anomalous venous channels and a lack of the normal veins of the posterior fossa. No enlarged or abnormal arteries are demonstrated. Unlike the early venous filling of an AVM, the abnormal veins of a venous angioma fill only during the venous phase of an angiogram. Note the "spoke-wheel" pattern of abnormal veins in **a**.*

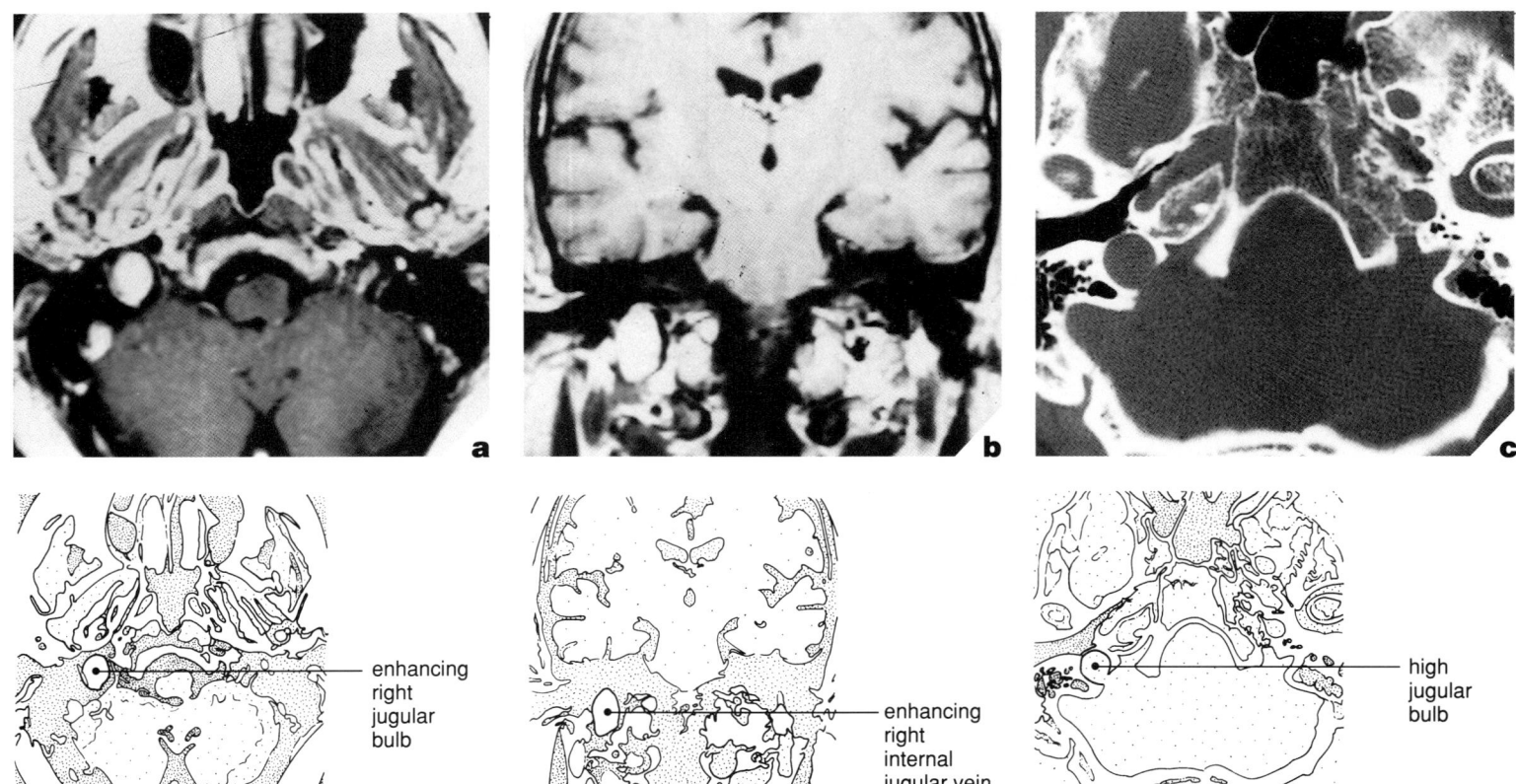

enhancing
right
jugular
bulb

enhancing
right
internal
jugular vein

high
jugular
bulb

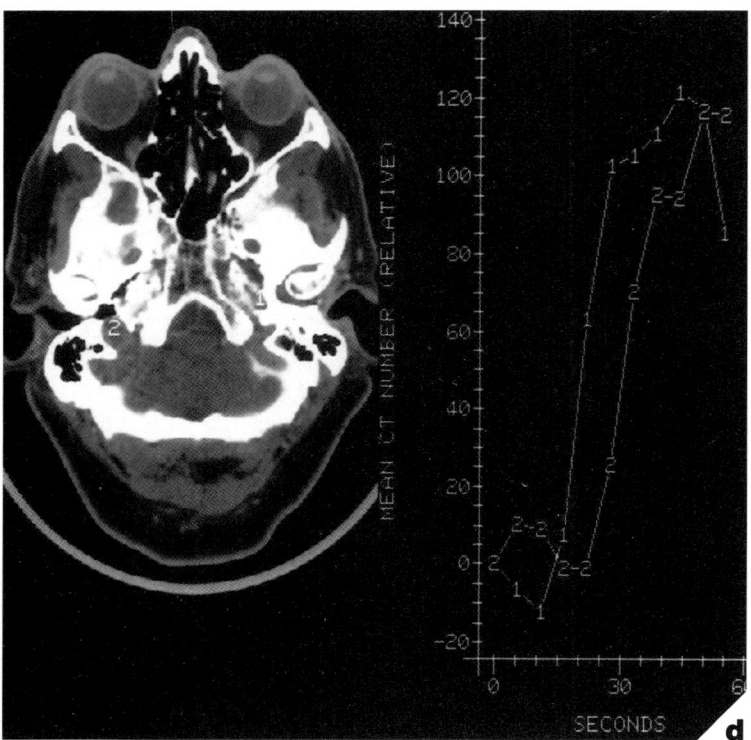

Figure 5.52

High jugular bulb. **a** *Axial and* **b** *coronal Gadolinium-enhanced T1-weighted images show increased signal intensity from enhancement in the region of the right temporal bone.* **c** *Although this alone may be readily identified as representing a high jugular bulb, confirmatory bone windows from a CT scan were also obtained.* **d** *Dynamic contrast-enhanced CT shows that the jugular bulb region (labeled "2") enhances after the carotid artery (labeled "1") does, as expected.*

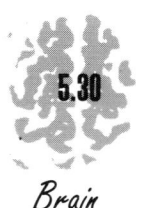

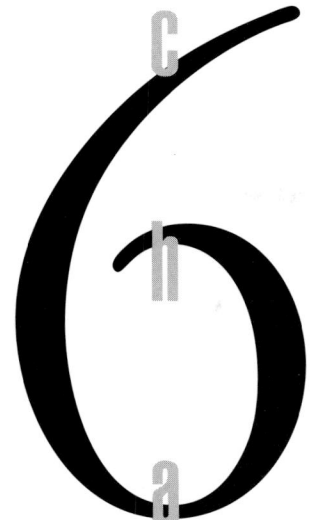

chapter

6

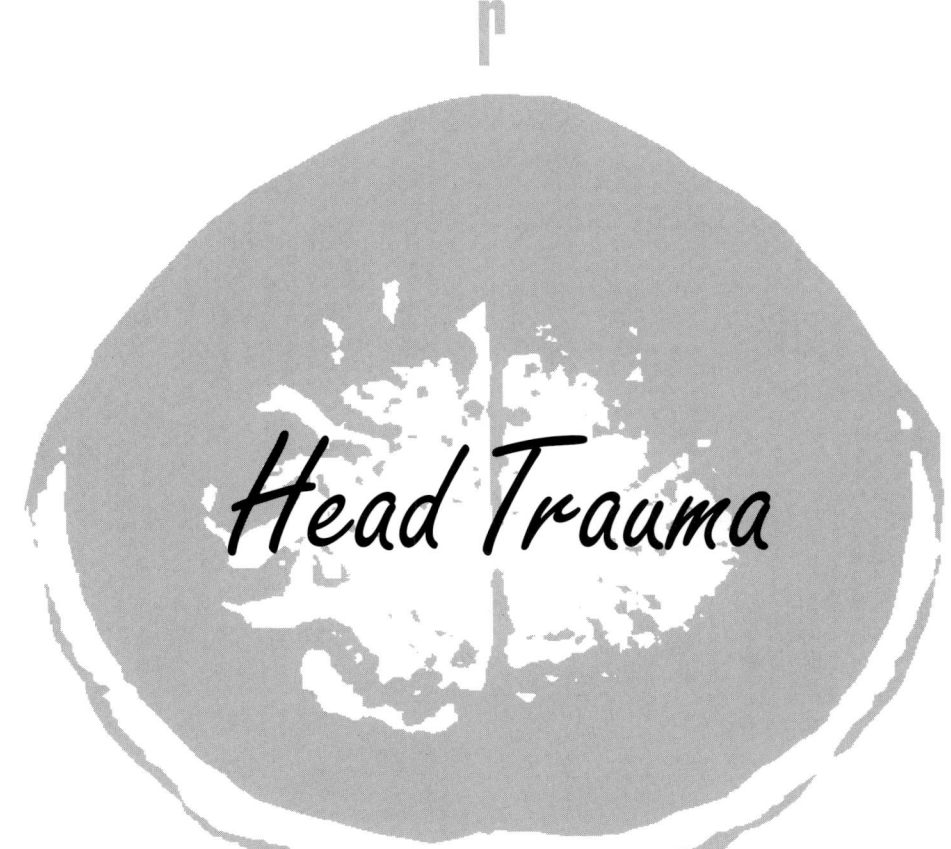

Head Trauma

*h*ead trauma accounts for a tremendous amount of death and disability in the United States. Much head trauma could be avoided by increased use of safety devices such as bicycle and motorcycle helmets, automobile restraining devices, and a generalized public appreciation of the dangers of head injuries. While many severe head injuries are fatal or result in permanent brain damage, prompt surgical intervention is often of great benefit. CT is generally the technique of choice to adequately evaluate for the presence of intracranial hemorrhage and resultant brain compression. Besides its greater availability in an acute setting than MRI, critically ill patients may be monitored more easily during CT scanning. Furthermore, patient motion artifacts are less critical on CT image than MR images. In addition, evaluation of skull fractures and subarachnoid hemorrhage by CT is superior to MRI.

EPIDURAL HEMATOMA

The dura mater forms the periosteum of the inner table of the skull and is therefore very densely adherent to it. Consequently, acute epidural hematomas have a thick, biconvex configuration. Since the dura attaches directly to the inner table of the skull at the site of the cranial sutures, epidural hematomas cannot ordinarily cross sutural lines or the midline supra-

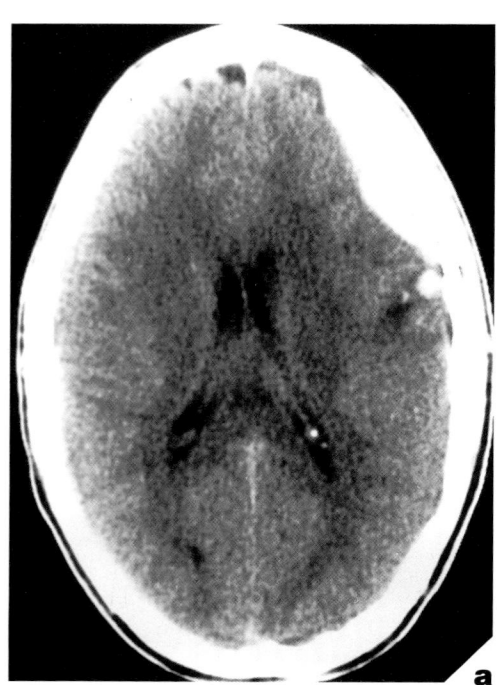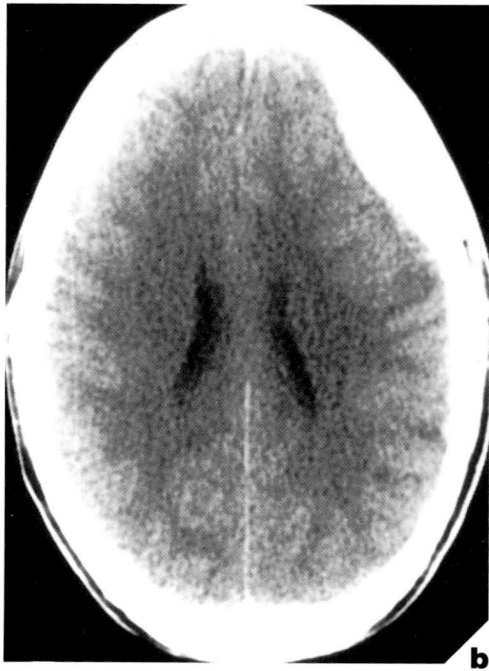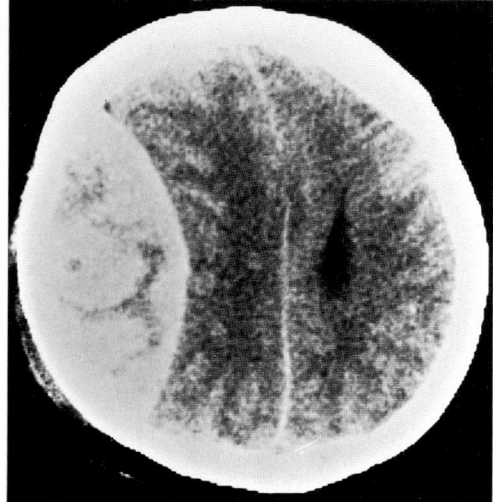

Figure 6.1

*Epidural hematoma. **a,b** Unenhanced CT sections show an extracerebral biconvex region of increased attenuation which compresses the left frontal lobe.*

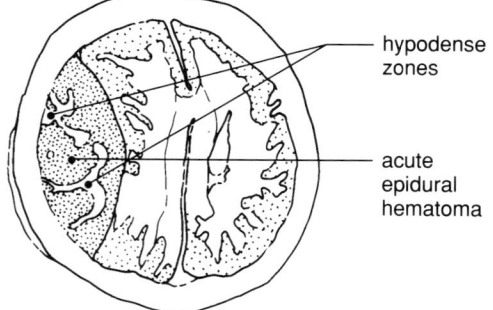

hypodense zones

acute epidural hematoma

Figure 6.2

Hyperacute epidural hematoma. The biconvex configuration is typical of an acute epidural hematoma. Hypodense zones represent areas where coagulation is still incomplete.

tentorially. The typical CT appearance of an epidural hematoma on unenhanced CT is that of an extra-axial, homogeneous biconvex mass of increased density (Fig. 6.1). Hypodense zones may be demonstrated within hyperacute epidural hematomas. These probably represent areas of fresh blood accumulation which have not yet undergone complete coagulation with clot retraction and extrusion of the lower density serum (Fig. 6.2).

Acute epidural hematomas usually result from arterial injury and are frequently associated with skull fractures. Typically, there is a laceration of the mid-dle meningeal artery or its branches. A large venous epidural hematoma can form when one of the dural venous sinuses is injured (Fig. 6.3).

SUBDURAL HEMATOMA

The most common source of subdural blood is tearing of bridging veins. Subdural hematomas may also result from dural lacerations or cortical arterial injuries. On CT, an acute subdural hematoma appears as a sharply defined crescentic area of increased at-

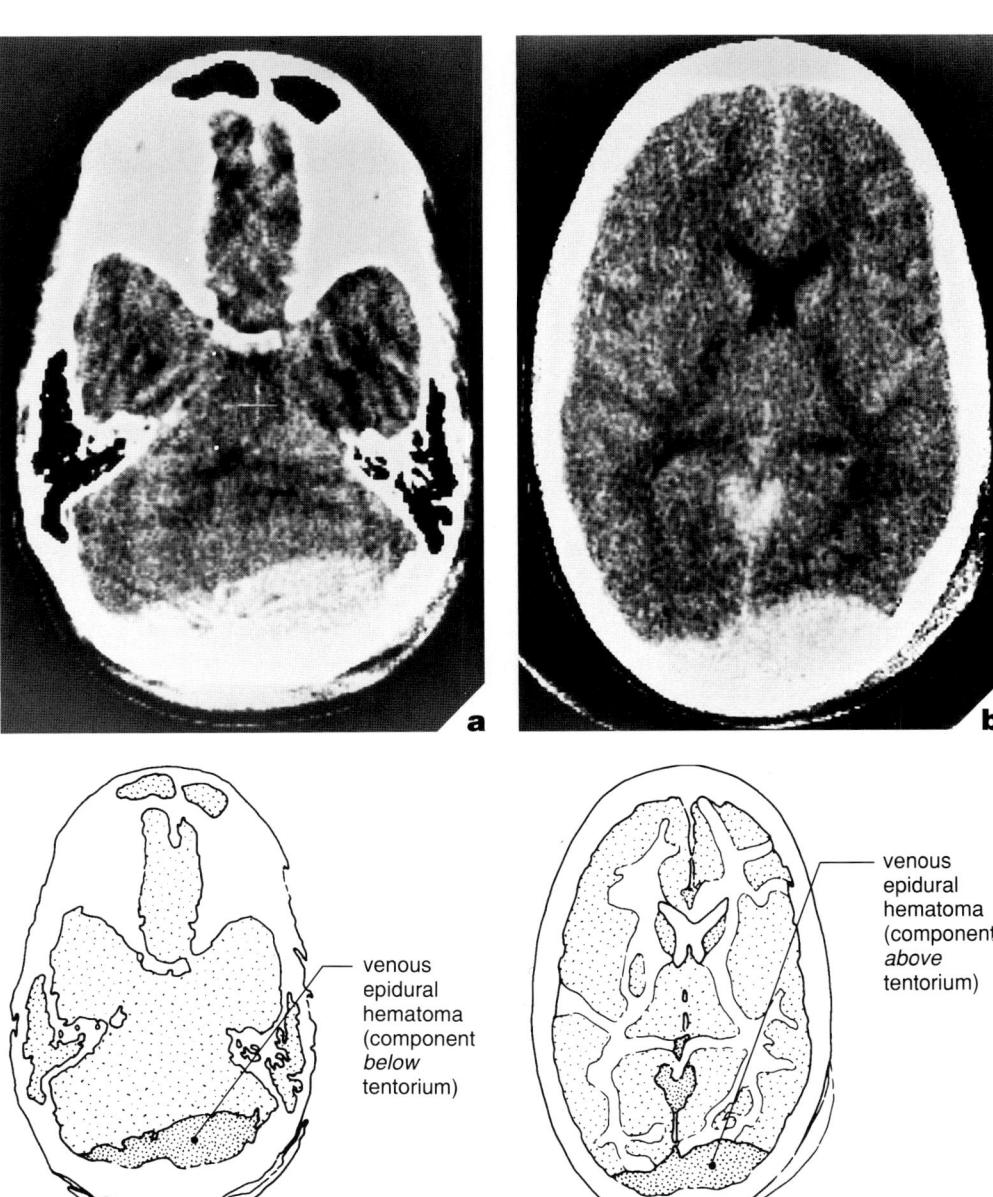

Figure 6.3

Venous epidural hematoma. CT scans through **a** *the posterior fossa and* **b** *just above tentorium show a large epidural hematoma extending from the posterior fossa to the occipital region. This was caused by a laceration of the left transverse sinus. The epidural location of the collection can be recognized by its typical biconvex shape. Incidentally noted in* **b** *is a small subdural hematoma near the free edge of the tentorium.*

venous epidural hematoma (component *below* tentorium)

venous epidural hematoma (component *above* tentorium)

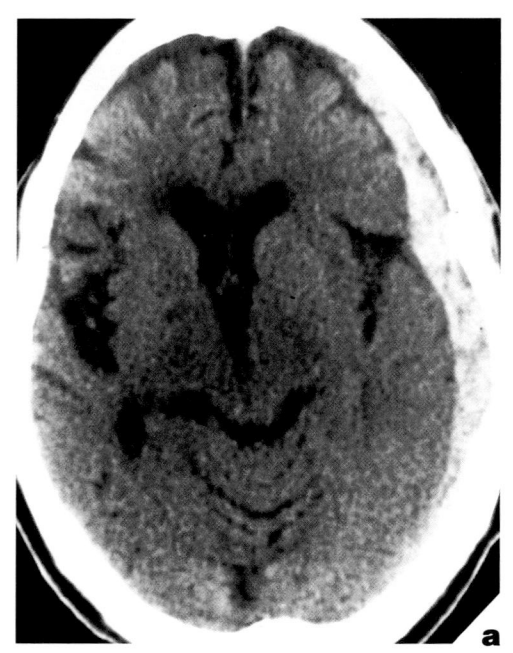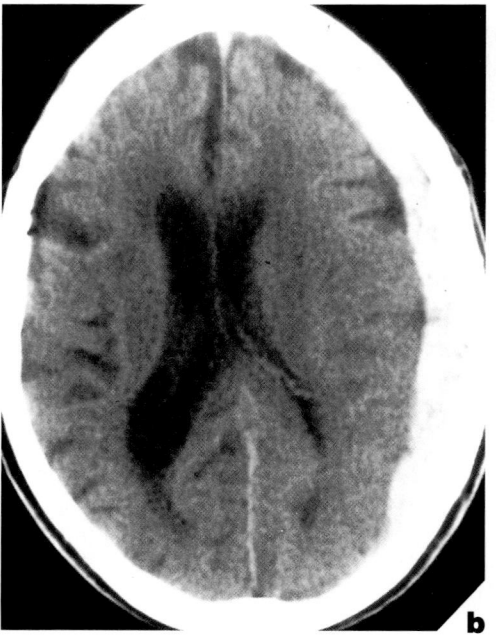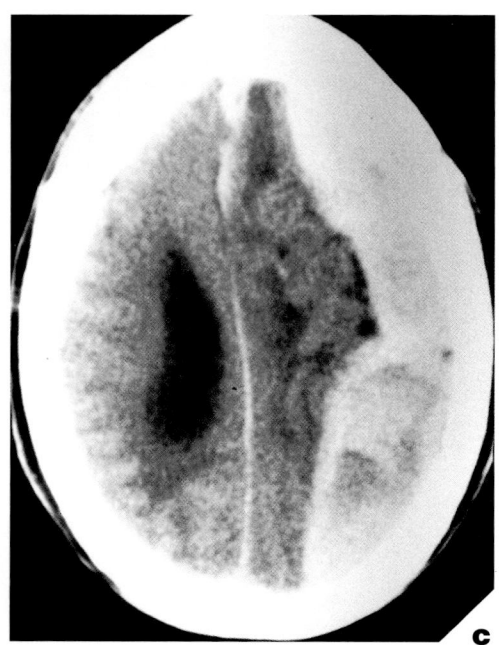

Figure 6.4
Acute subdural hematoma. ***a,b,c*** *CT images show a crescentic hyperdense extracerebral collection. The left cerebral hemisphere and left lateral ventricle are compressed.*

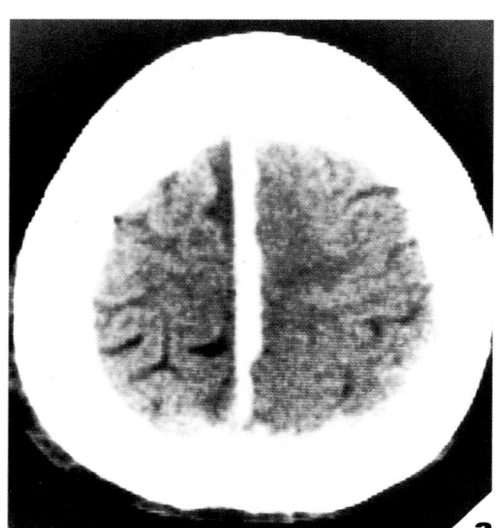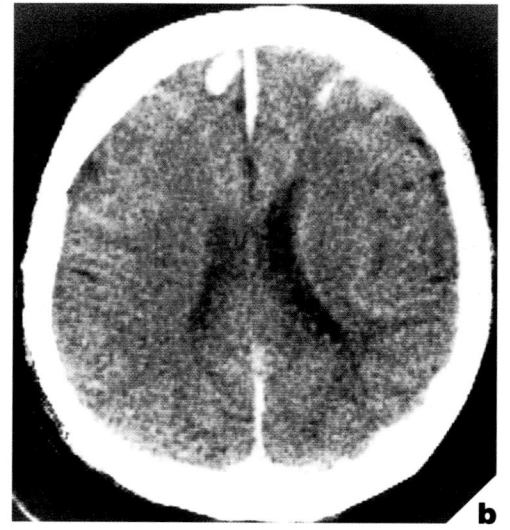

Figure 6.5
Interhemispheric subdural hematoma. ***a,b*** *Axial CT scans show an area of increased attenuation adjacent to the left side of the falx cerebri. The collection is sharply demarcated medially by the falx; the lateral margin, which abuts the medial surface of the left cerebral hemisphere, has an irregular contour. Also noted is a small hemorrhagic contusion in the right frontal lobe and a small amount of subarachnoid blood over the left frontal convexity.*

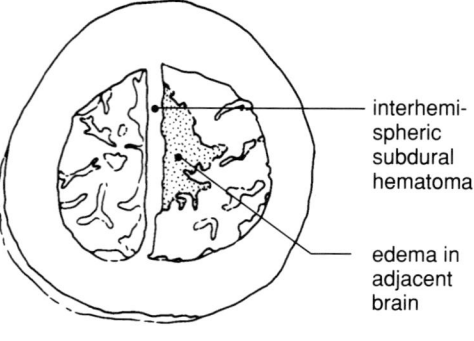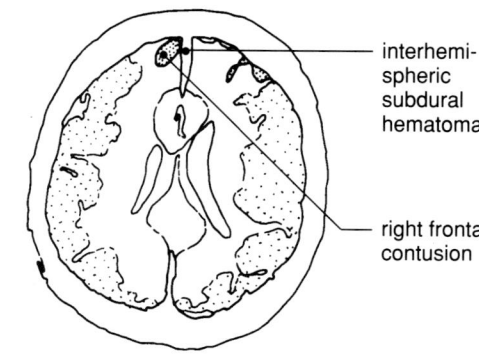

interhemispheric subdural hematoma

edema in adjacent brain

interhemispheric subdural hematoma

right frontal contusion

tenuation conforming to the inner table of the skull (Fig. 6.4). Unlike the convex inner margin seen with epidural hematomas, the inner surface of a subdural hematoma is usually concave in relation to the brain. Because the arachnoid membrane is loosely adherent to the dura, subdural hematomas may extend over large areas while remaining relatively thin. The mass effect associated with a subdural collection is often compounded by underlying cerebral contusion and edema.

Most acute subdural hematomas occur over the lateral convexities; however, they may also occur adjacent to the dural surfaces of the tentorium and falx cerebri, particularly in children. Interhemispheric subdural hematomas appear on CT as areas of in-creased attenuation with a flat medial margin and a lateral extension of variable thickness (Fig. 6.5). Interhemispheric subdural collections are often seen in children who are physically abused. Because of the absence of signal from bone and its multiplanar capabilities, MR is superior to CT in demonstrating convexity subdural hematomas (Fig. 6.6). In general, the precise identification and demarcation of subdural collections is better appreciated with MRI (Fig. 6.7).

The high attenuation of acute subdural hematomas is mainly due to the proteins and the hemoglobin molecules contained within the coagulated red blood cells. Over time there is progressive breakdown of the hemoglobin molecules and the hematoma gradually decreases in density. After a

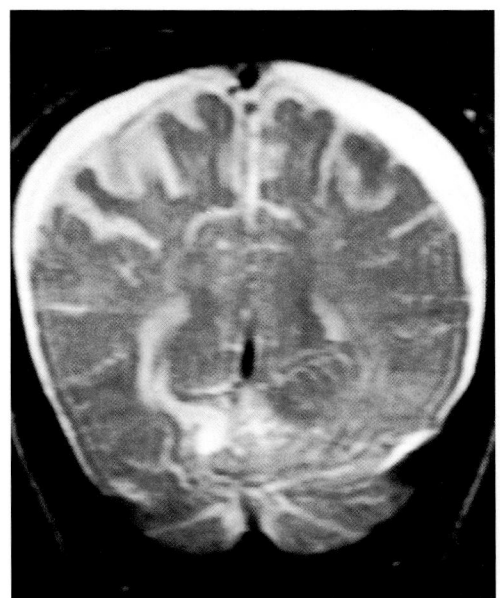

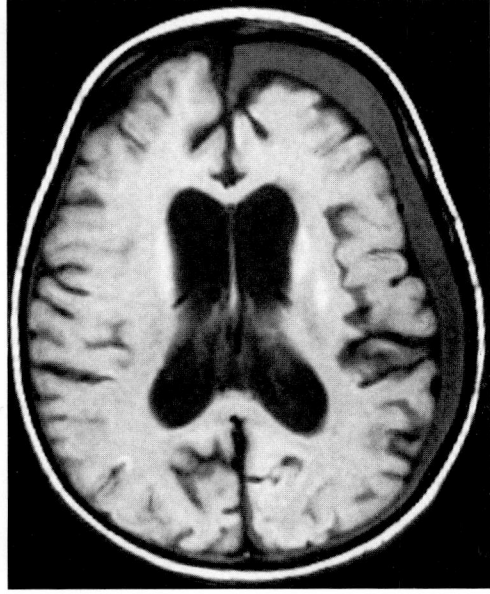

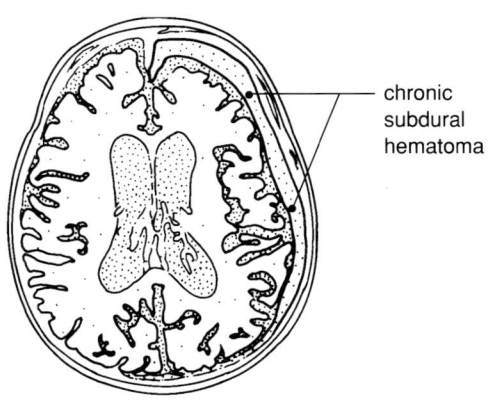

chronic subdural hematoma

Figure 6.6
Bilateral subdural hematomas. T2-weighted MR image shows bilateral crescentic subdural collections compressing the underlying brain. The volume of convexity subdural collections, plus the degree of brain compression, is best appreciated on coronal MR images.

Figure 6.7
Chronic left subdural collection. T1-weighted axial image shows a well-defined hypointense collection of fluid within the left subdural space. Due to its superb contrast resolution, MR generally can separate a subdural collection from the adjacent bone and brain with greater clarity than CT.

variable interval (usually several weeks following the injury), subdural hematomas become hypodense (Fig. 6.8) with respect to the brain, though they usually maintain their crescentic shape.

At some point (usually 10 to 20 days following the injury), a subdural hematoma passes through a brief isodense phase during which it may be difficult to differentiate it from the underlying brain on CT. At this stage, in particular, MRI is vastly superior to CT (Fig. 6.9).

An acute subdural hematoma may sometimes appear isodense or hypodense on CT images. This can occur in patients with anemia or in patients with a laceration of the arachnoid membrane that allows CSF to leak into the subdural space and dilute the blood in the subdural hematoma; layering of CSF and blood within the subdural collection may occur.

A chronic subdural hematoma may sometimes have a biconvex configuration rather than the usual crescentic appearance. Most often this atypical appearance is related to a high protein content in the subdural collection which causes a large volume of water to be drawn into it by osmotic forces. A biconvex subdural hematoma may also develop if the arachnoid is more densely adherent to the dura than usual due to membrane formation. If an acute subdural hematoma does not resolve completely, membrane formation may lead to loculation of the subdural space into multiple compartments; a subsequent injury may cause bleeding into just one of these compartments (Fig. 6.10).

Chronic, slowly progressing subdural hematomas are common in elderly patients due to tears of the bridging veins which are stretched as atrophic changes occur. Approximately 25% of patients with chronic subdural hematomas have bilateral collections.

INTRAPARENCHYMAL HEMORRHAGE AND PENETRATING BRAIN INJURIES

During closed head trauma, the brain is injured by striking the hard, unyielding confines of the skull. The frontal and temporal poles are most frequently injured (Fig. 6.11); injuries of the occipital poles are somewhat less common. Temporal lobe hemorrhage is the most dangerous, since it may cause the medial temporal lobe to herniate through the tentorial incisure, compressing the brainstem. The corpus callosum can be injured in closed head trauma by being thrust against the unyielding falx by an accelerating force. Brain structures also may be injured by striking the tentorial leaflet (Fig. 6.12). Generalized brain edema is a potentially lethal complication of any severe closed head injury.

CT scans are very useful in the evaluation of gunshot wounds (Fig. 6.13) and other penetrating injuries (Fig. 6.14). Various intracranial densities (e.g., blood, bone, metal) may be present following a penetrating injury.

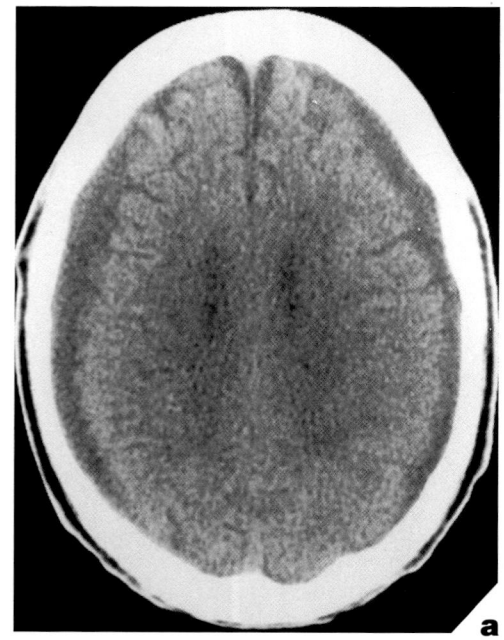
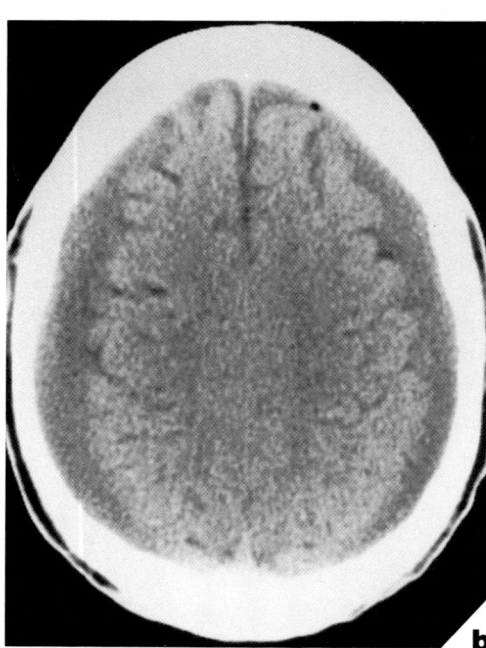

a   b

Figure 6.8
Bilateral chronic subdural collections.
a,b *These chronic subdural collections are hypodense with respect to the brain on unenhanced CT.*

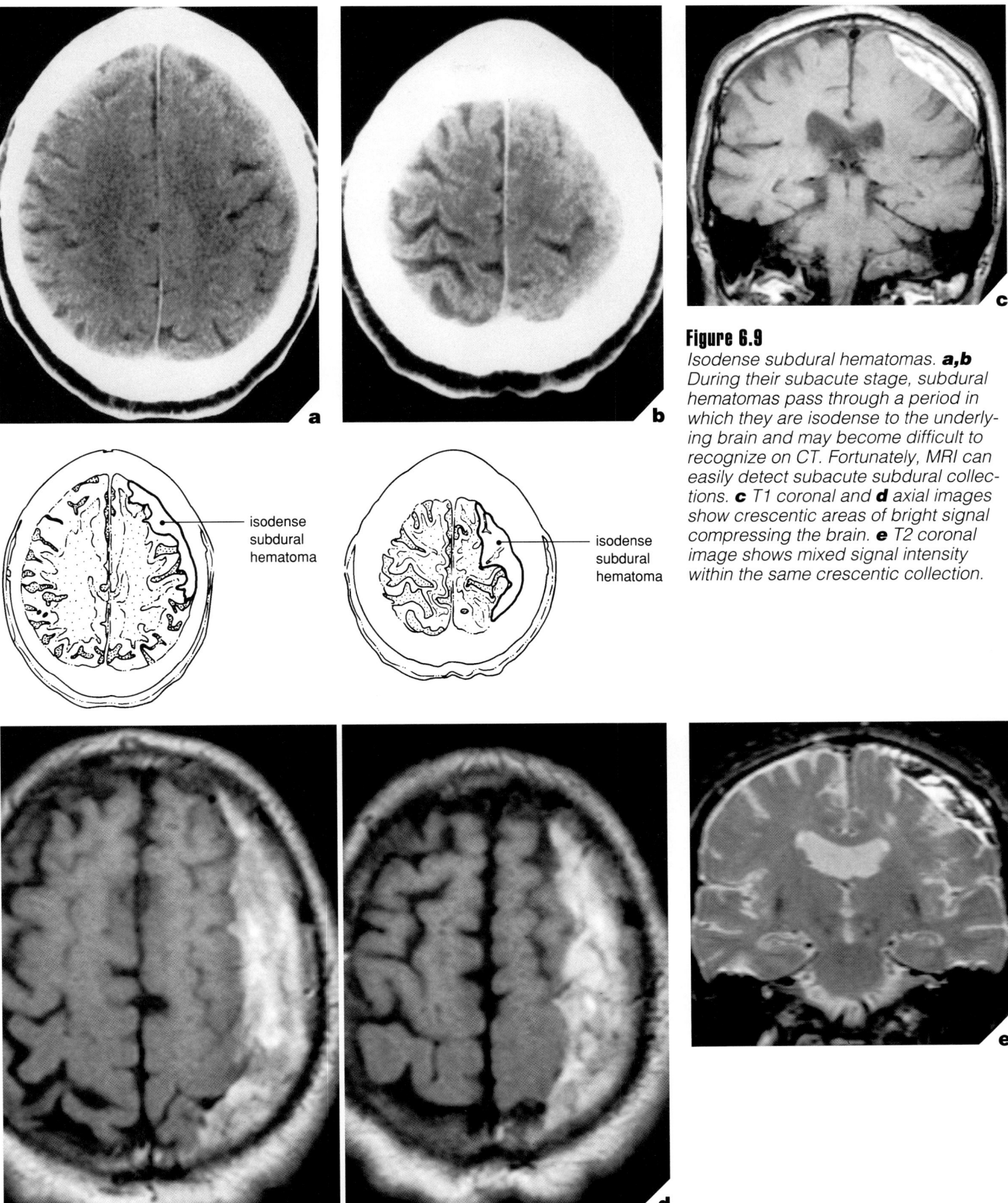

isodense
subdural
hematoma

isodense
subdural
hematoma

Figure 6.9
Isodense subdural hematomas. ***a,b***
*During their subacute stage, subdural
hematomas pass through a period in
which they are isodense to the underlying brain and may become difficult to
recognize on CT. Fortunately, MRI can
easily detect subacute subdural collec-
tions.* ***c*** *T1 coronal and* ***d*** *axial images
show crescentic areas of bright signal
compressing the brain.* ***e*** *T2 coronal
image shows mixed signal intensity
within the same crescentic collection.*

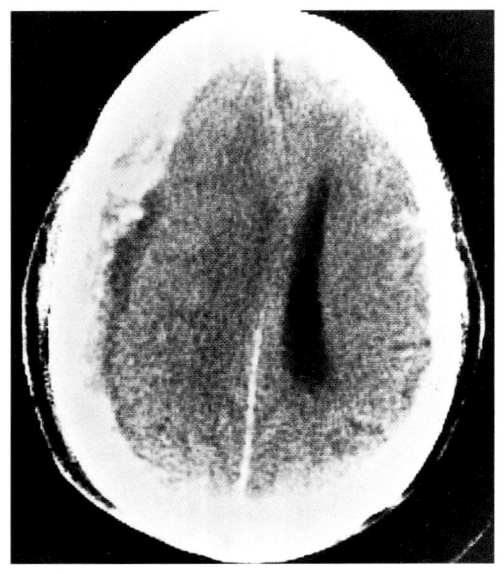

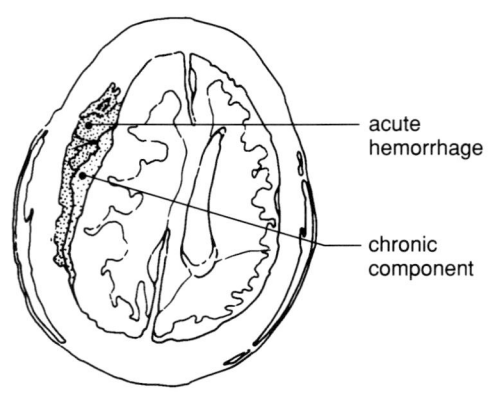

Figure 6.10
Acute bleeding in a chronic subdural hematoma. Membrane formation has created several compartments within the subdural space of this patient with a chronic subdural hematoma. Fresh blood due to a recent injury is present in only one of these loculations.

acute hemorrhage

chronic component

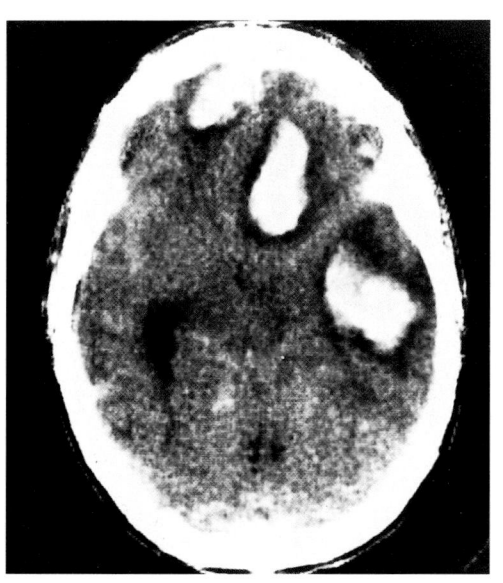

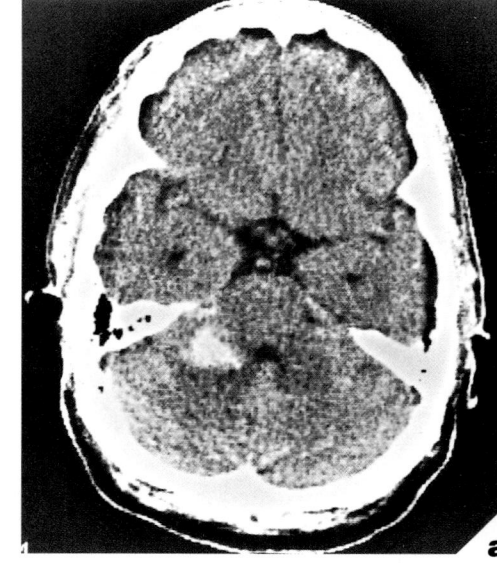

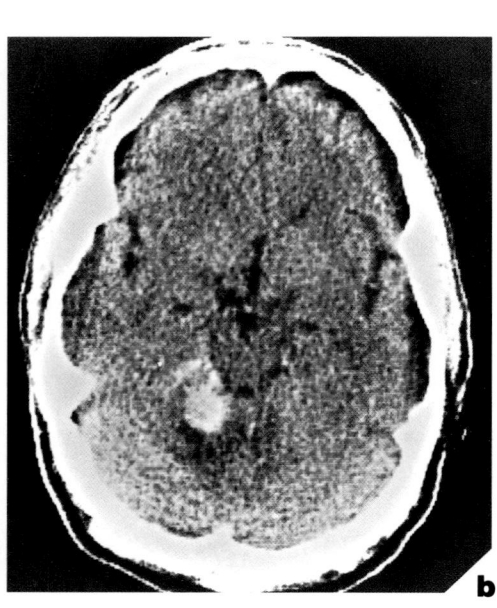

Figure 6.11
Intraparenchymal hemorrhage. There are areas of increased attenuation representing fresh blood in the right frontal pole, left frontal lobe, and left temporal lobe. The right frontal pole was injured by striking the frontal bone; the left frontal lobe was injured while striking the subjacent sphenoid ridge. The areas of decreased attenuation surrounding the hemorrhages represent focal brain edema.

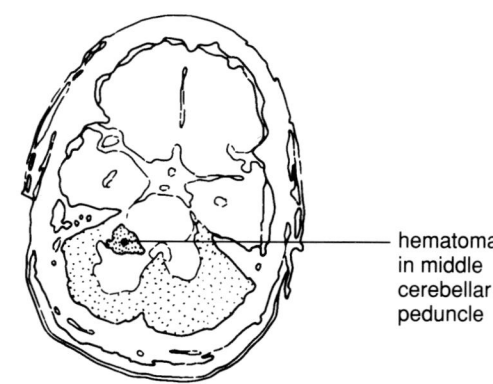

hematoma in middle cerebellar peduncle

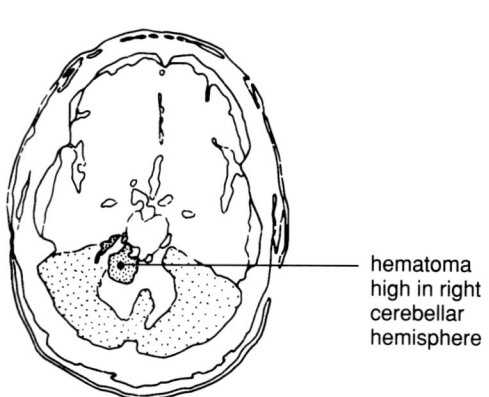

hematoma high in right cerebellar hemisphere

Figure 6.12
*Cerebellar hematoma from striking the tentorium. This patient was in a motor vehicle accident and struck his forehead. **a** An axial section through the posterior fossa shows an area of in-*

*creased attenuation (fresh blood) in the right middle cerebellar peduncle. **b** A more cephalic section shows parenchymal hemorrhage high in the right cerebellar hemisphere.*

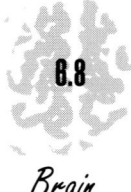

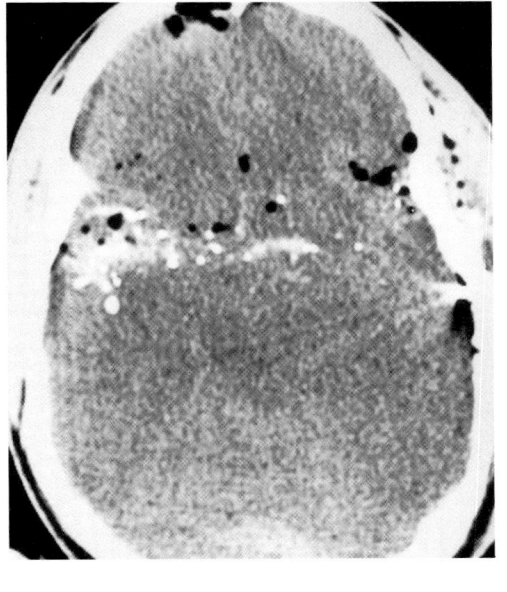

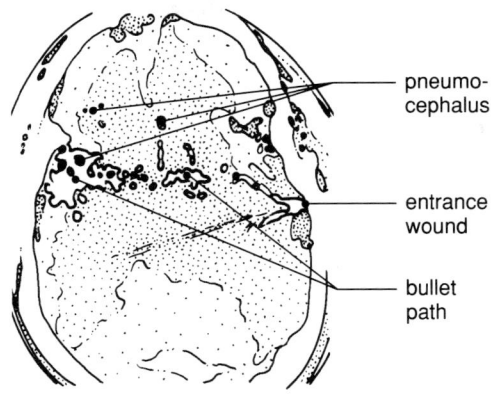

pneumo-
cephalus

entrance
wound

bullet
path

Figure 6.13

Bullet injury. Axial CT scan shows a trail of blood and bone fragments along the path of a bullet which entered through the squamosal portion of the temporal bone on the left (note the scalp swelling) and lodged along the inner table of the opposite side of the skull. Pneumocephalus is evident.

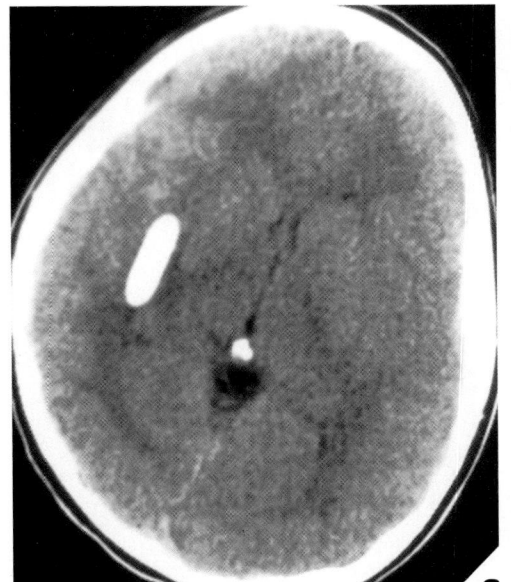

a

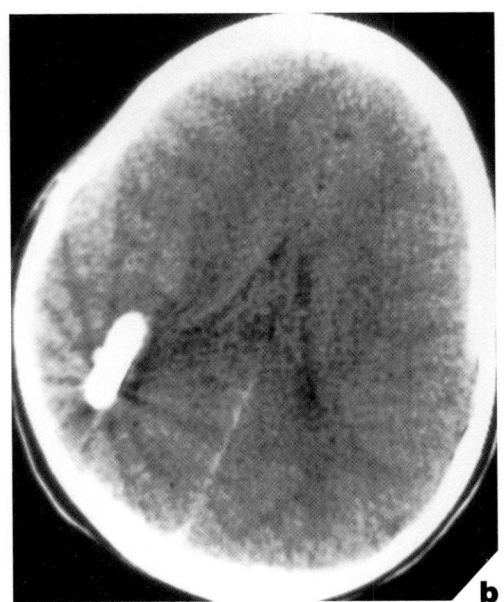

b

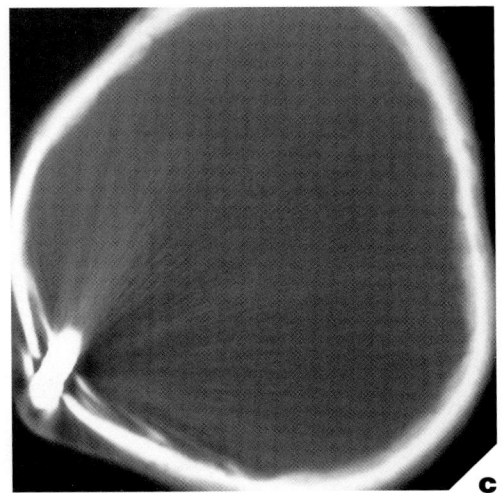

c

Figure 6.14

*Arrow piercing brain and skull. CT scan shows an arrow lodged in the **a,b** right frontal and parietal lobes with its point lodged in the **c** fractured right parietal bone. The arrow entered through the right orbit.*

SKULL FRACTURES

Depressed skull fractures, particularly those involving the lateral convexities, are well evaluated on axial CT sections. The degree of depression, the location and orientation of the fracture fragments are demonstrated best when the fracture is not oriented in the axial plane. Depressed fractures (Fig. 6.15) are the most important type of fracture since brain compression and injury are almost inevitable. Nondepressed fractures (Fig. 6.16) are less significant. Fractures of the anterior cranial fossa, particularly in the region of the cribriform plate, are a common cause of post-traumatic CSF rhinorrhea. This can lead to meningitis. CSF can also leak from fractures involving the frontal sinus, sphenoid sinus, and petrous pyramid. In the latter, there may be communication with the naso-pharynx via the auditory (eustachian) tube. CT with positive contrast cisternography is invaluable in localizing the source of the leak (Fig. 6.17).

Fractures involving the mastoid air cells, the frontal sinus or orbital roofs (Fig. 6.18) are often associated with pneumocephalus. In some cases, the intracranial gas may be the only clue that there is a base of the skull fracture.

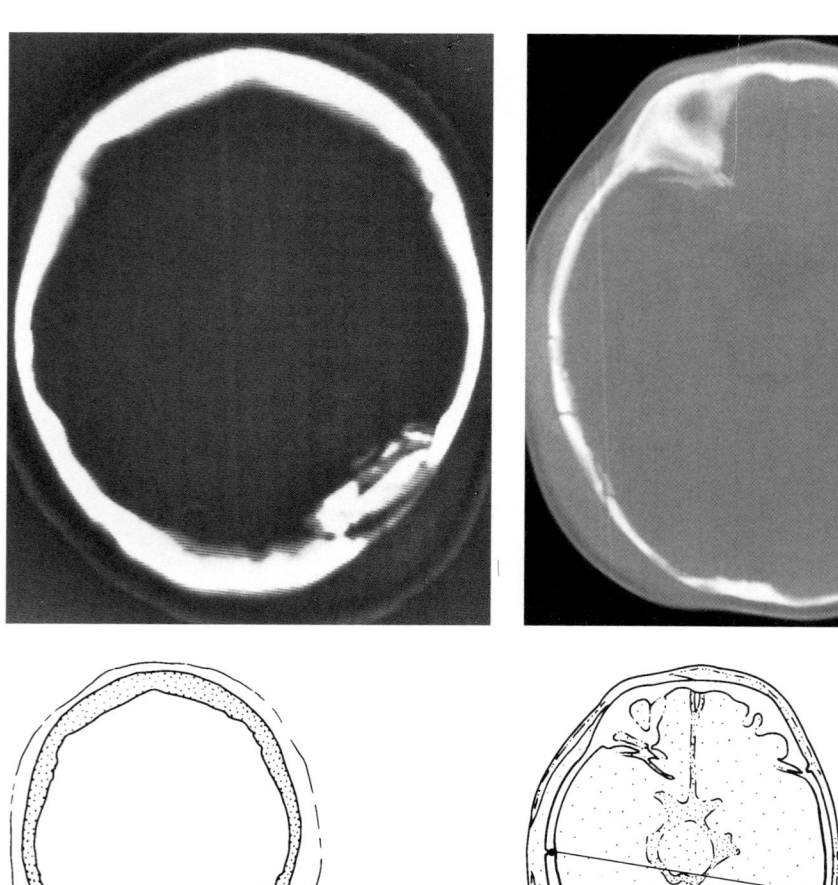

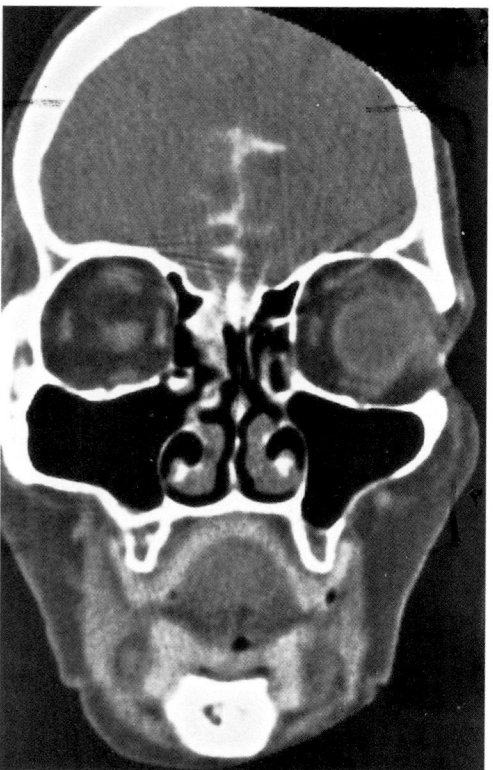

Figure 6.17
Skull fracture and CSF leak. A direct coronal CT scan following the injection of nonionic contrast into the subarachnoid space (positive contrast cisternography) shows contrast material leaking from the subarachnoid space beneath the right frontal lobe into the right ethmoid air cells via a fracture in the cribriform plate.

Figure 6.15
Depressed skull fracture. Bone window of an axial CT scan shows a fracture of the left parietal bone with multiple depressed fragments.

Figure 6.16
Skull fracture. Multiple fractures are seen on this bone window view of a head CT obtained after a three-story fall. The right parietal fracture is not significantly depressed.

POSTOPERATIVE CHANGES

Intracranial air may be introduced at surgery, most commonly when a posterior fossa craniotomy is performed with the patient in a sitting position. Air can also be introduced when large ventricles or cysts are decompressed, or when large extracerebral hematomas are removed. Postoperative pneumocephalus is usually incidental and the air is quickly resorbed.

However, large quantities of air can occasionally act like a mass lesion and cause pressure on the adjacent brain (Fig. 6.19).

Postoperative changes in the brain are usually manifested by areas of low attenuation representing encephalomalacia/tissue loss. Specific patterns of tissue loss relate to the location of the intracranial abnormality which was operated upon and the surgical approach employed.

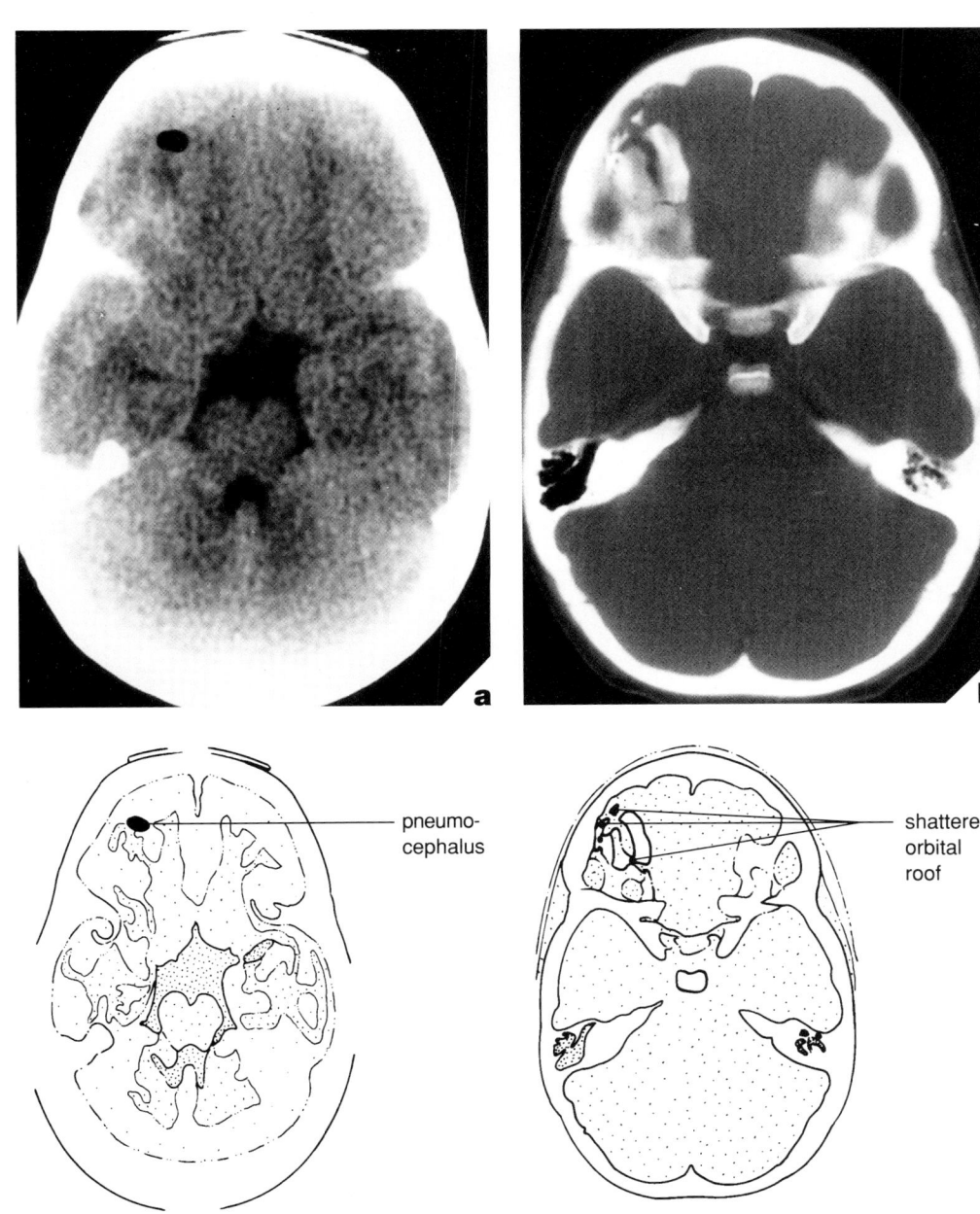

pneumo-
cephalus

shattered
orbital
roof

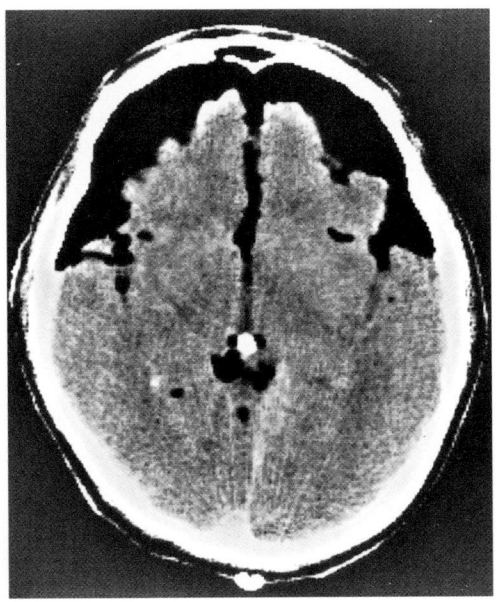

Figure 6.19

Tension pneumocephalus. Following operative removal of a posterior fossa metastasis this patient failed to recover promptly. CT shows a large amount of subdural and subarachnoid air. A craniostomy yielded a large amount of air under pressure, after which the patient's level of consciousness rapidly improved.

Figure 6.18

Supra-orbital fracture with pneumocephalus. ***a*** *An axial, unenhanced CT image shows pneumocephalus in the right side of the anterior cranial fossa.*

There is associated subarachnoid hemorrhage on the right. ***b*** *The bone window reveals comminuted fractures of the right orbital roof.*

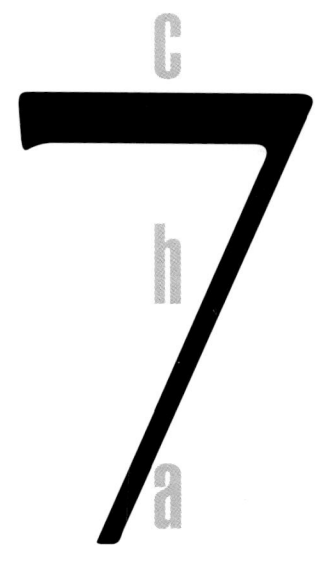

c
h
a
p
t
e
r

7

Hydrocephalus and Degenerative Diseases

the term *hydrocephalus* means enlargement of CSF-containing spaces due to increased CSF pressure. This may occur due to disturbances in resorption, flow, or production of CSF. Because the intact skull, spine, and inelastic dura together form a rigid container, the increased CSF pressure causes characteristic compression and displacement of the adjacent brain, usually resulting in clinical signs and symptoms. *Cerebral atrophy* means enlargement of the CSF-containing spaces due to age-related tissue loss or other degenerative diseases which cause brain substance to be diminished. The resulting ventricular enlargement is compensatory in nature and is not associated with increased CSF pressure. *Hydrocephalus ex vacuo* is an archaic synonym for cerebral atrophy that should be discarded because it is inconsistent

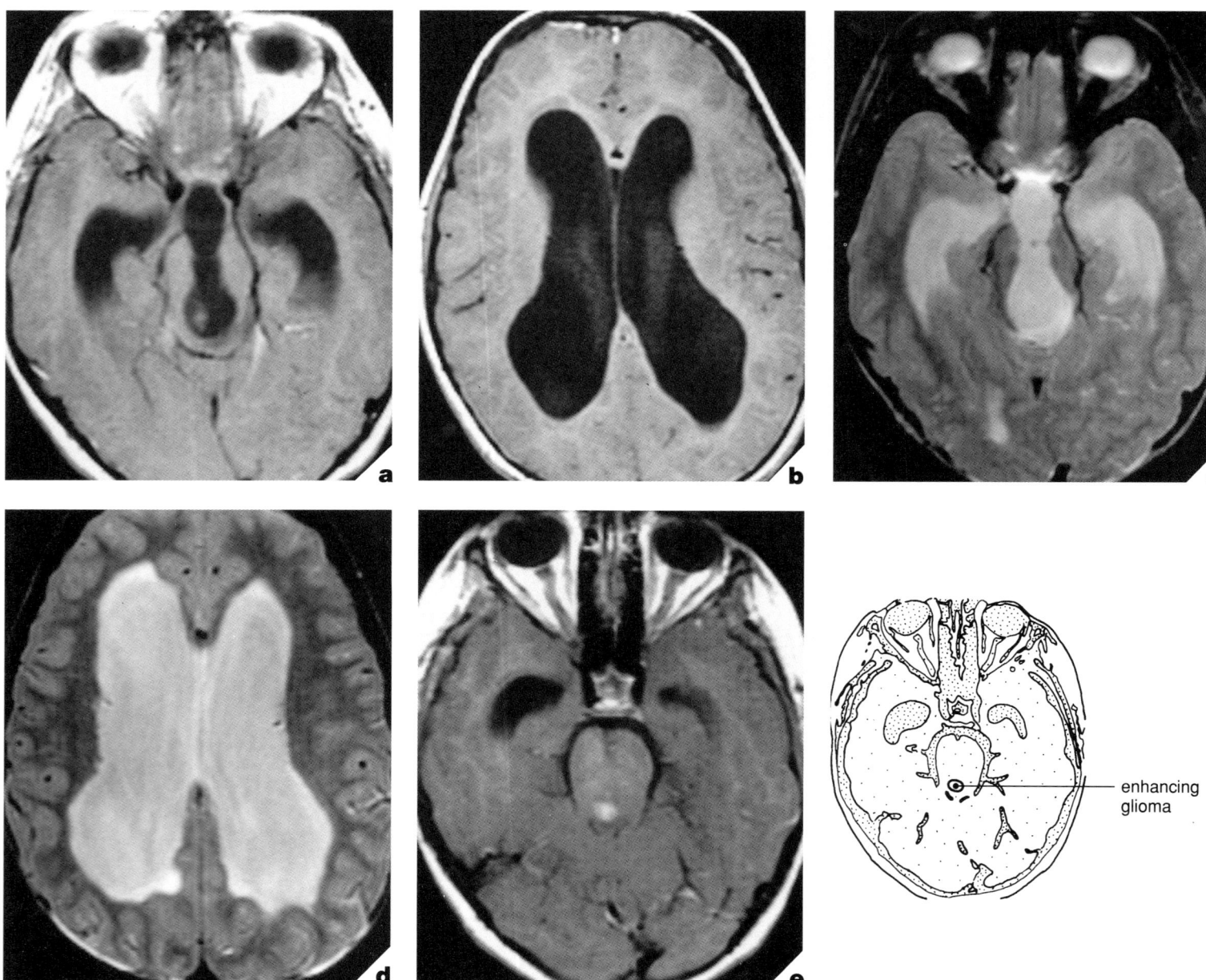

enhancing glioma

Figure 7.1

*Hydrocephalus. Axial **a,b** T1 and **c,d** T2 images show typical features of obstruction of the third and lateral ventricles. The temporal horns are preferentially dilated and the frontal horns are rounded. The third ventricle is ballooned out laterally. In general, the third and lateral ventricles are greatly enlarged and the subarachnoid spaces are compressed. **e** Gadolinium-enhanced T1 image shows a nodule of enhancement in the peri-aqueductal grey matter representing a brainstem glioma. This lesion blocks the Aqueduct of Sylvius.*

with the modern concept of *hydrocephalus* being nearly always caused by obstruction.

HYDROCEPHALUS

Hydrocephalus can result from either obstruction of the pathways between the site of CSF formation and resorption or, very rarely, from overproduction of CSF. Choroid plexus papilloma (see Fig. 4.39) is the only disorder in which overproduction of CSF may contribute to hydrocephalus. However, even in this disorder, hydrocephalus is usually due to obstruction of a CSF pathway by tumor mass or bleeding.

All other forms of hydrocephalus are obstructive. In the 1920s, Dandy introduced the terms *communicating* and *noncommunicating* to differentiate two types of obstructive hydrocephalus. If a vital dye injected into a lateral ventricle could be recovered from the lumbar subarachnoid space, or if air injected via lumbar puncture passed into the ventricular system, Dandy called the disorder communicating (extraventricular obstructive) hydrocephalus. If these studies failed to demonstrate passage of CSF between the ventricles and the lumbar subarachnoid space, the condition was termed noncommunicating (intraventricular obstructive) hydrocephalus. This distinction is not critical since although it is occasionally helpful in

suggesting the etiology of the hydrocephalus, the terminology is somewhat confusing and does not describe the precise site of obstruction.

When the lateral ventricles are obstructed, the temporal and frontal horns become preferentially dilated (Fig. 7.1). The normally slit-like temporal horns become widened in their antero–posterior dimension and thus change their configuration as well as their volume. Likewise, the frontal horns acquire a characteristic rounded shape when obstructed. Overall, the lateral ventricles generally become disproportionally enlarged when compared to the overlying subarachnoid space; indeed, cerebral sulci are often compressed.

Third ventricular obstruction results in a characteristic expansion in its lateral diameter. The lateral margins lose their straight edge and acquire a convex outward bowing (ballooning).

Fourth ventricular changes from hydrocephalus are less common and more subtle than changes in the third and lateral ventricles. The fourth ventricle usually only becomes mildly dilated. However, when obstruction to CSF flow occurs both proximal and distal to the fourth ventricle, there is then marked dilatation of the "trapped" fourth ventricle.

MRI often demonstrates bright-T2 signal abnormality in the periventricular white matter in patients with hydrocephalus. This may be minor (Fig. 7.2) or

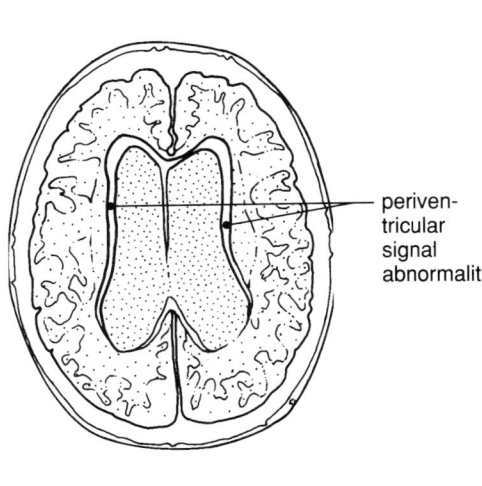

Figure 7.2

Hydrocephalus. Proton density MR image shows minimal periventricular signal abnormality adjacent to the lateral margins of the lateral ventricles in this patient with a partially obstructing colloid cyst.

periven-
tricular
signal
abnormality

profound (Fig. 7.3). Most investigators regard this signal abnormality to represent CSF, which has crossed the ependymal surface of the obstructed ventricle into an intraparenchymal, periventricular white matter location (transependymal spread of CSF).

Enlargement of only one temporal horn—the "trapped" temporal horn—may be seen in cases of an intraventricular mass such as a meningioma (see Fig. 4.40). Unilateral obstruction of a lateral ventricle

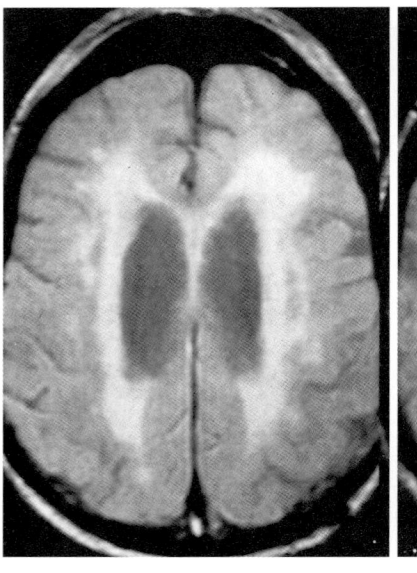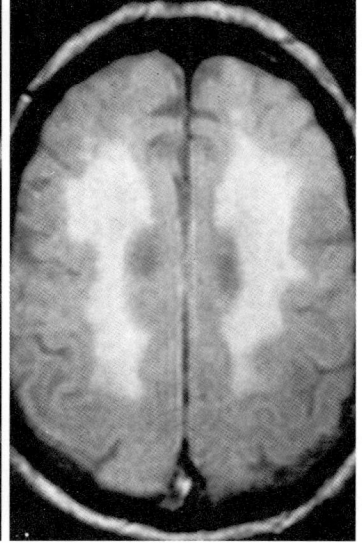

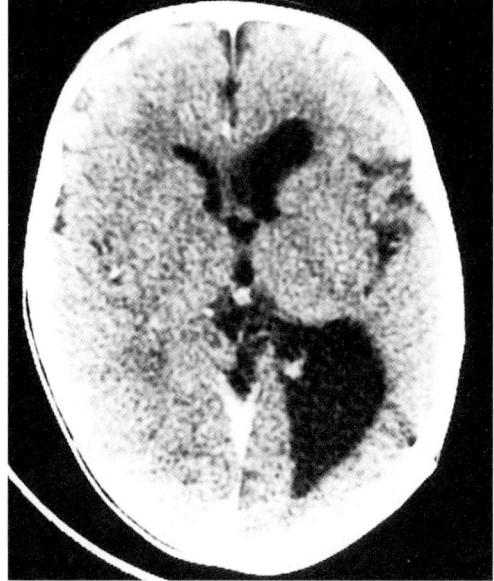

Figure 7.4

Hydrocephalus of one lateral ventricle. CT scan in a 7-month-old boy shows hydrocephalus involving only the left lateral ventricle. At surgery, a congenital web was discovered obstructing the left foramen of Monro.

Figure 7.3

Hydrocephalus with marked transependymal spread of CSF Proton density axial images at the level of the roof of the lateral ventricles show extensive periventricular bright signal abnormality due to CSF accumulating in the periventricular white matter. This patient had long-standing communicating hydrocephalus following subarachnoid hemorrhage.

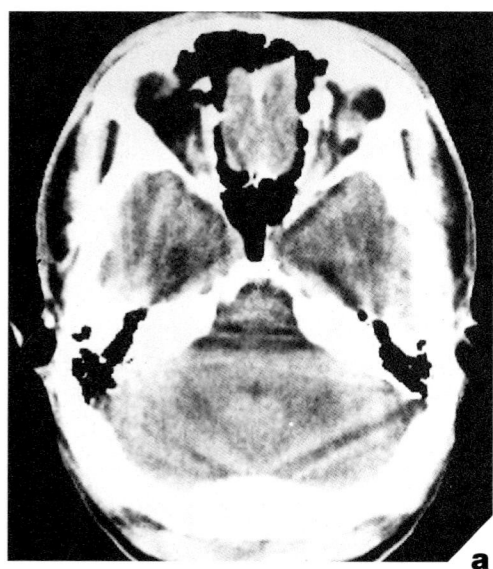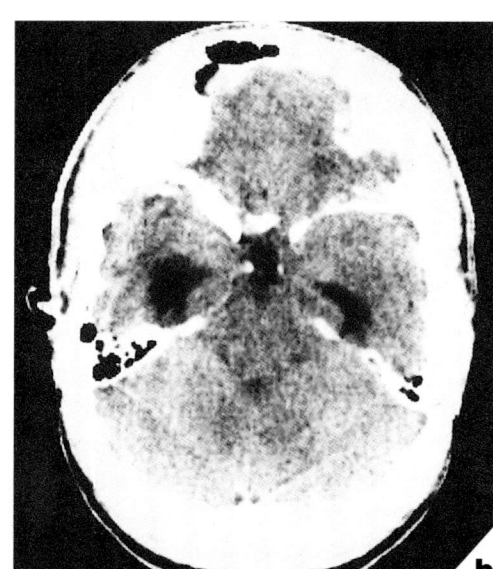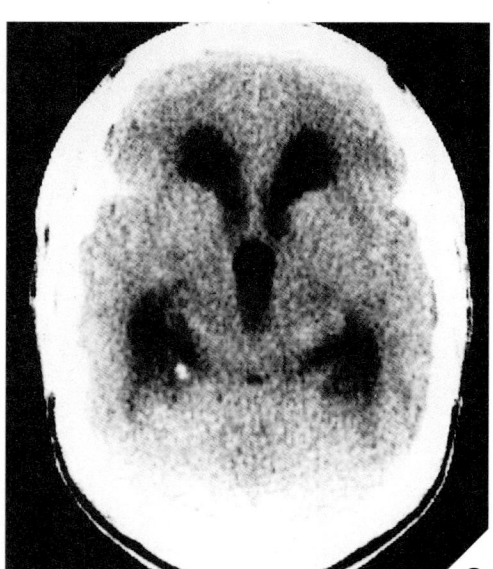

Figure 7.5

*Aqueductal stenosis. **a,b,c** Axial CT sections without contrast reveal moderate enlargement of the third ventricle and both lateral ventricles. The fourth ventricle is small.*

implies that the obstruction is at the ipsilateral foramen of Monro (Fig. 7.4). Colloid cysts of the third ventricle may also obstruct one or both foramina of Monro (see Fig. 4.38). Tumors of the posterior third ventricle and pineal region cause enlargement of the lateral and third ventricles (see Fig. 4.58); however, the remaining CSF spaces are normal. Aqueductal stenosis (Fig. 7.5) is a developmental disorder characterized radiographically by enlargement of the lateral and third ventricles, a small fourth ventricle, and a small subarachnoid space. Brainstem tumors may cause similar findings of dilatation of the third and lateral ventricles.

Obstruction of the outlets of the fourth ventricle may be congenital or acquired. It results in enlargement of the entire ventricular system. Congenital obstruction usually accompanies the Dandy–Walker malformation (Fig. 7.6). Acquired obstruction of the fourth ventricular outlets may be caused by basal meningitis (see Fig. 3.3), subarachnoid hemorrhage, or neoplasms.

Communicating Hydrocephalus

Communicating hydrocephalus, or extraventricular obstructive hydrocephalus, implies that the site of obstruction to CSF flow is distal to the outlets of the

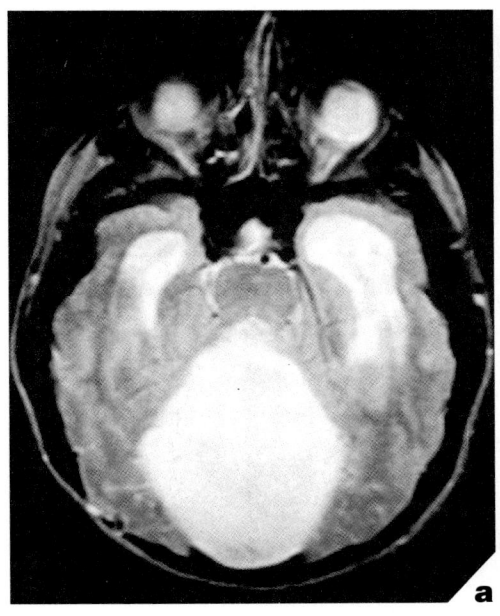

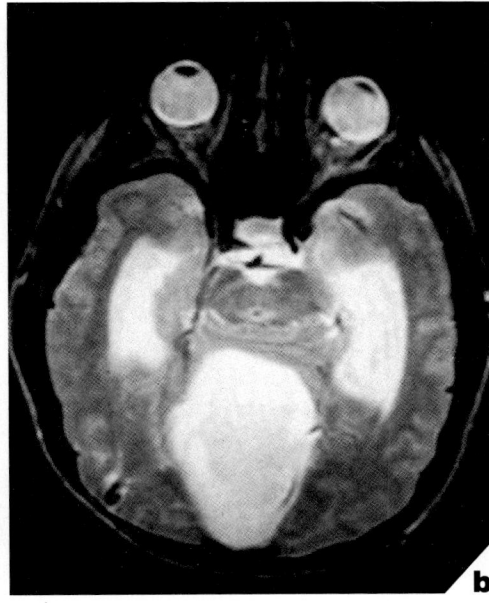

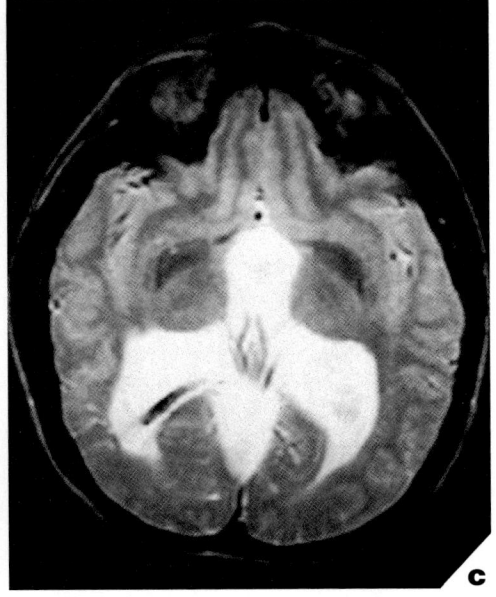

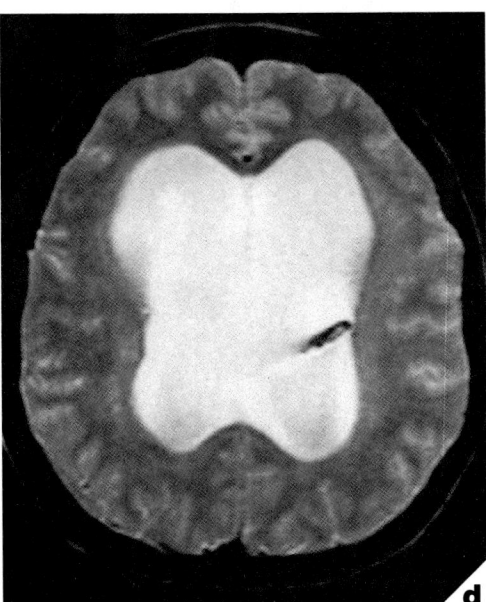

Figure 7.6

Hydrocephalus associated with Dandy–Walker malformation. ***a,b*** *T2-weighted axial images show a large posterior fossa cyst connected to the fourth ventricle. The temporal horns are massively distended.* ***c*** *The third ventricle is ballooned out laterally.* ***d*** *The lateral ventricles, particularly the frontal horns are markedly enlarged and the overlying subarachnoid spaces are compressed.*

fourth ventricle. The causes are varied and include obliteration of the subarachnoid spaces or the arachnoid granulations by infection, subarachnoid hemorrhage, and meningeal carcinomatosis. Uncommon causes include stenosis of the basal foramina due to achondroplasia or Paget's disease. Extracranial venous congestion (e.g., superior vena cava obstruction) and congestive heart failure are also rare causes of communicating hydrocephalus.

Although the site of blockage of CSF flow is distal to the ventricular system, in adults it is usually the ventricles rather than the subarachnoid space which enlarge in communicating hydrocephalus. Since the cranial–spinal cavity is a closed space in adults, according to Laplace's law, the larger diameter ventricular system will expand preferentially to the smaller subarachnoid space. In children with open sutures, communicating hydrocephalus may actually result in proportional enlargement of the subarachnoid space. The frontal convexity subarachnoid space, including the interhemispheric fissure, usually shows the greatest enlargement in children with communicating hydrocephalus (Fig. 7.7). Increased head circumference also helps differentiate this condition from cerebral atrophy.

Normal Pressure Hydrocephalus

Normal pressure hydrocephalus (Fig. 7.8) is a condition of late middle age and the elderly. It is characterized by the clinical triad of gait disturbance, dementia, and incontinence. The normal pressure phase is probably preceded by a hypertensive phase in which a distal block of CSF flow results in elevation of CSF pressure and ventricular enlargement. Gradual removal of CSF by compensatory mechanisms (e.g., increased transependymal resorption of fluid) allows CSF pressure to return to normal although the ventricular system remains enlarged.

Pseudotumor Cerebri

Pseudotumor cerebri, also called benign intracranial hypertension, is a syndrome of unknown pathogenesis in which the CSF pressure is greatly elevated (up to 600 mm H_2O) in the absence of an intracranial mass or hydrocephalus. Most patients are obese young women. The most frequent symptom is headache. The neurological examination is usually normal, except for papilledema. CT and MRI may be normal or may show characteristic, small, slit-like ventricles (Fig. 7.9), and an irregular contour of the optic nerves due to CSF pulsations. A partially empty sella turcica is often present due to CSF herniating through the diaphragma sella.

Clinical correlation is essential since there is considerable overlap between normal and subnormal ventricular size. Serial lumbar punctures, with removal of enough fluid to lower the CSF pressure to normal, may lead to dramatic clinical improvement.

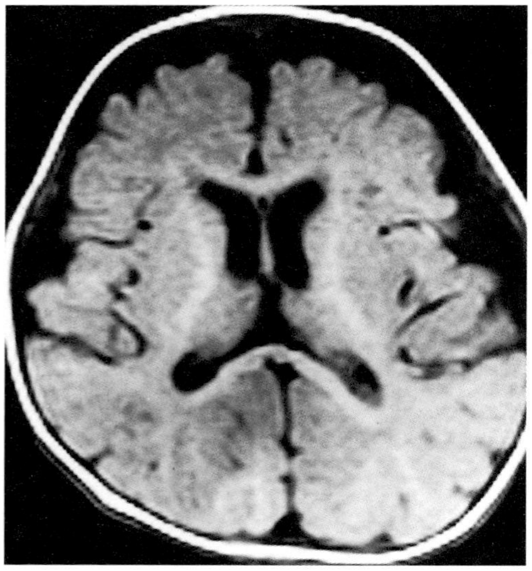

Figure 7.7
External hydrocephalus. There is a dilatation of both the ventricles and subarachnoid spaces in this neonate with communicating hydrocephalus and open fontanelles.

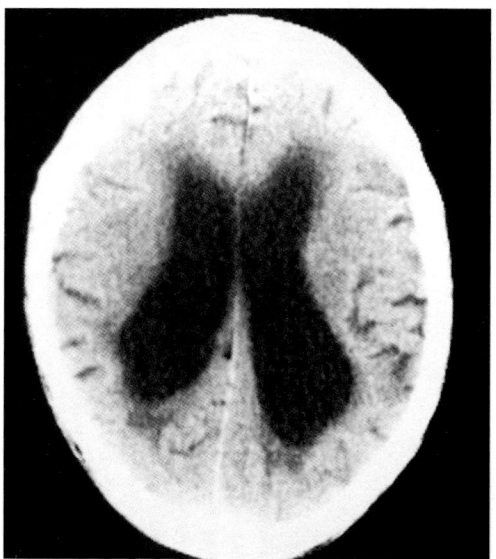

Figure 7.8
Normal pressure hydrocephalus. Axial CT section in this 75-year-old man shows lateral ventricular enlargement without proportionate enlargement of the convexity subarachnoid space.

DEGENERATIVE DISEASES

Cerebral Atrophy

The term *cerebral atrophy* is used to indicate a loss of brain tissue. The atrophy may be diffuse or focal, depending upon its etiology. Usually the changes are irreversible.

Diffuse Cerebral Atrophy

The causes of diffuse cerebral atrophy are numerous and include Alzheimer's disease, cerebrovascular disease, trauma, inflammatory disorders, and degenerative brain diseases. The CT and MRI findings are not specific but show proportionate enlargement of the ventricles and subarachnoid space (Fig. 7.10). The ventricular dilatation is generally symmetrical enlargement of the lateral ventricles without the disproportionate expansion of the frontal and temporal horns seen in hydrocephalus. Moreover, unlike hydrocephalus, the actual configuration of the third and lateral ventricles does not change, only the ventricular volume.

Subarachnoid space enlargement associated with diffuse cerebral atrophy is usually symmetrical. In some individuals, age-related atrophic changes of the subarachnoid spaces predominate in the cranial vertex; in others the sylvian fissures or temporal regions may be primarily involved.

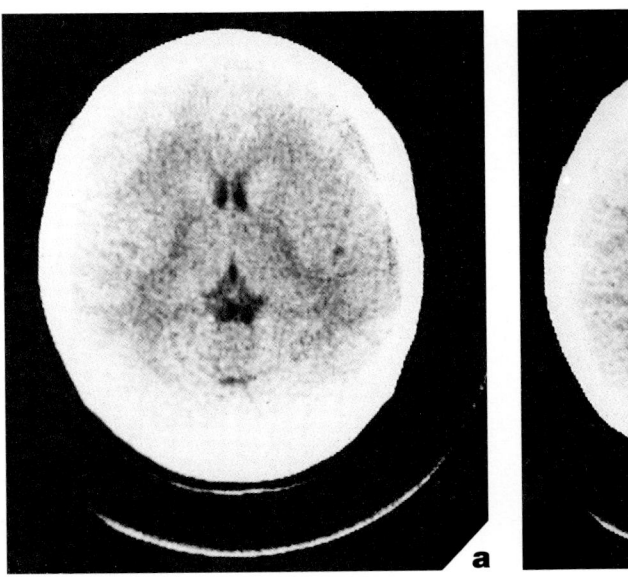
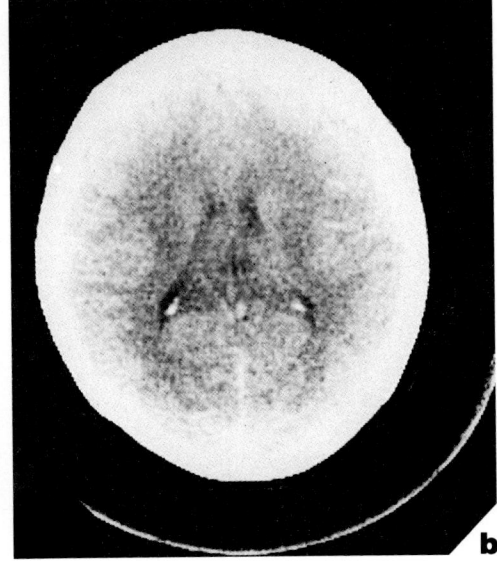

Figure 7.9
*Pseudotumor cerebri. **a,b** Noncontrast axial CT scans in a 40-year-old woman with headaches and papilledema demonstrate small, slit-like lateral ventricles.*

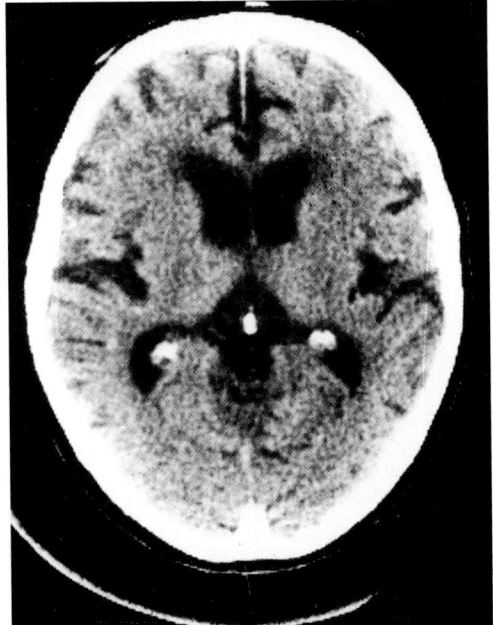
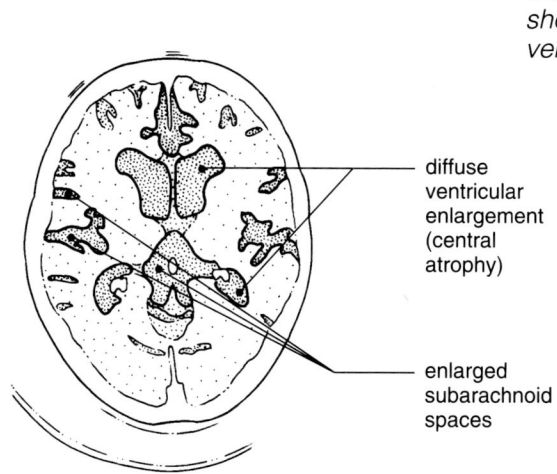

Figure 7.10
Cerebral atrophy. Unenhanced CT scan shows proportionate enlargement of the ventricles and subarachnoid space.

diffuse ventricular enlargement (central atrophy)

enlarged subarachnoid spaces

Focal Cerebral Atrophy

It is sometimes possible to make a specific etiological diagnosis of focal cerebral atrophy. Pick's disease (Fig. 7.11) is a particular form of degenerative brain disease in which the frontal and anterior temporal lobes show severe atrophy with relative sparing of the parietal and occipital lobes and the posterior third of the superior temporal gyrus. Final diagnosis requires the pathologic demonstration of the characteristic argentophilic inclusions (Pick bodies) within neurons.

Huntington's disease is characterized by choreoathetosis and dementia which typically presents in middle age. Transmitted as an autosomal dominant trait, it is one of the most common inherited neurologic diseases. There is gross atrophy of the caudate nucleus, which is reflected on CT and MRI by absence of its usual bulge into the inferolateral border of the frontal horns of the lateral ventricles (Fig. 7.12). This change may be difficult to recognize in borderline cases and in patients with associated diffuse cerebral atrophy.

Degenerative Diseases with Progressive Ataxia

Degenerative diseases with the clinical finding of progressive ataxia comprise a heterogeneous category of disorders for which a completely satisfactory

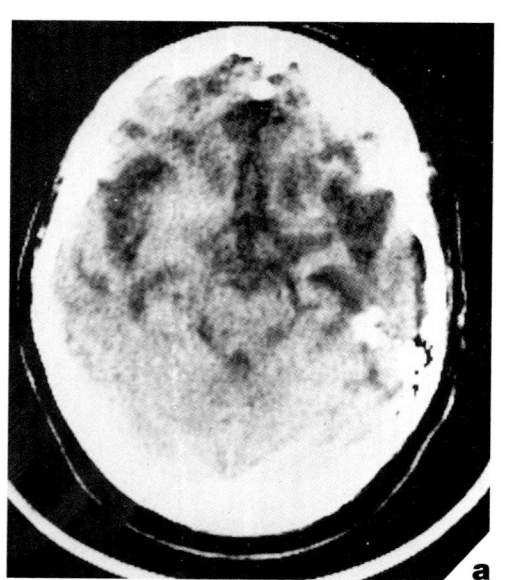
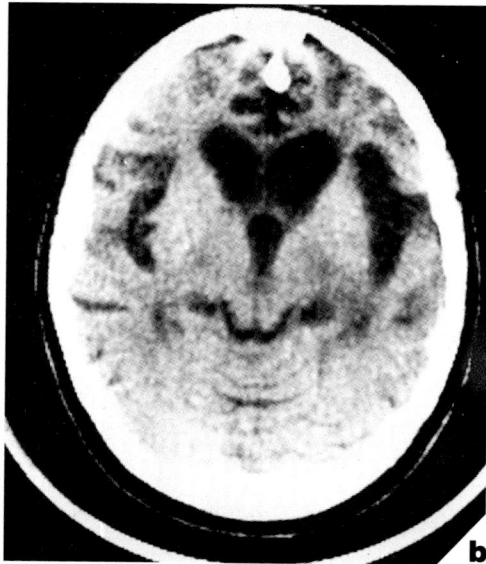

Figure 7.11
*Pick's disease. **a,b** Unenhanced CT scans show marked enlargement of the sylvian fissures and the frontal horns of the lateral ventricles.*

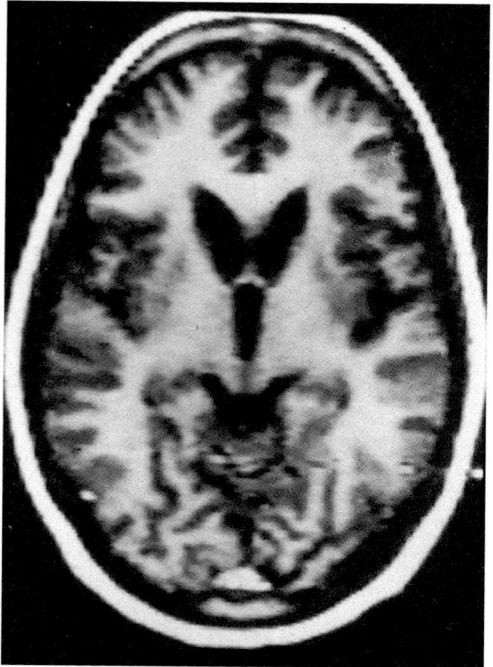
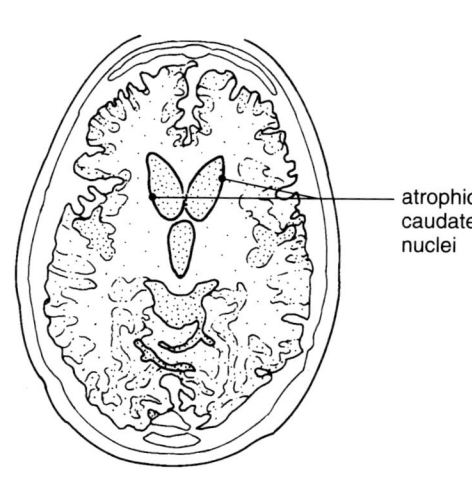

atrophic
caudate
nuclei

Figure 7.12
Huntington's disease. Axial T1-weighted MR image shows absence of the normal concavity of the lateral aspects of the frontal horns, indicating atrophy of the caudate nuclei.

classification has not yet been devised. These disorders include Friedrich's ataxia, spinocerebellar degeneration, cortical cerebellar atrophy, and olivopontocerebellar atrophy (OPCA). While the CT and MRI findings are nonspecific, the presence of disproportionate cerebellar and/or brainstem atrophy suggests the diagnosis of one of these degenerative diseases (Fig. 7.13).

Parkinson's disease is a degenerative disorder of the brain involving the neurons containing melanin pigment in the substantia nigra and smaller centers of dopaminergic activity in the brain. Clinically, there is a static tremor, mask-like face, rigid body movements, and akinesia. MRI may show narrowing of the band of increased T2 signal intensity between the red nucleus and the pars reticularis of the substantia nigra (Fig. 7.14). This is the location of the pars compacta of the substantia nigra and its decreased visualization may be due to loss of the neuromelanin-containing cells within it or to increased iron and other mineral deposition in the adjacent reticular portion of the substantia nigra. Cerebral atrophy is a frequent accompanying finding in patients with Parkinson's disease.

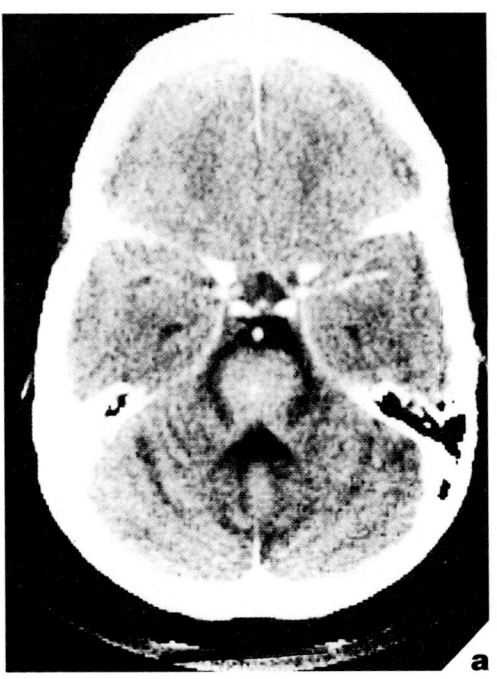
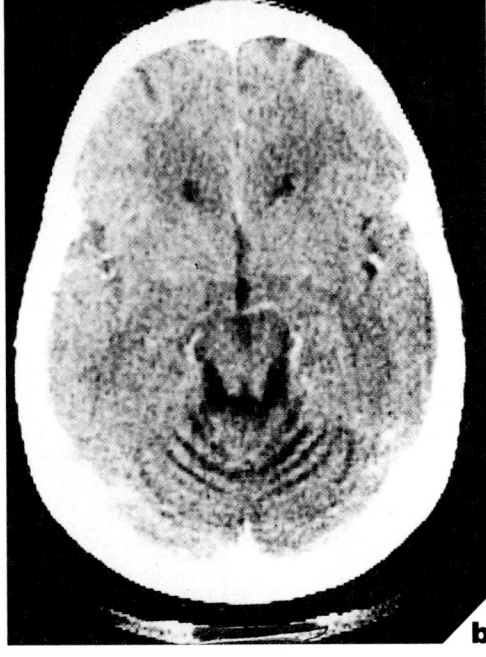

Figure 7.13

*Spinocerebellar degeneration. **a,b** Unenhanced CT scans show atrophy of the brainstem and cerebellum in an 18-year-old male with progressive ataxia.*

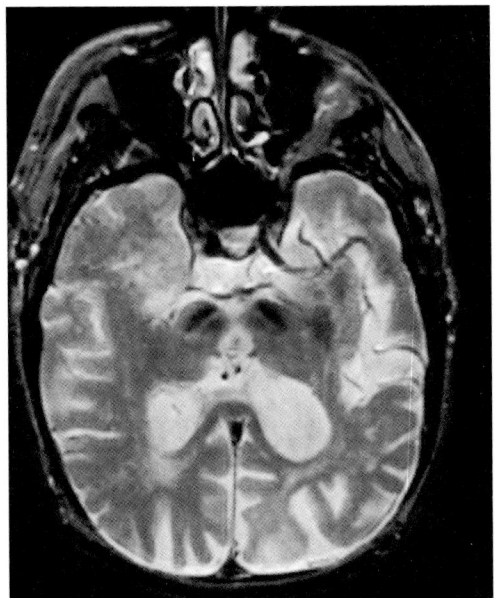
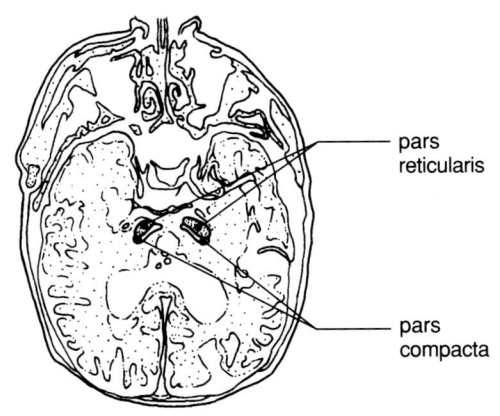

pars
reticularis

pars
compacta

Figure 7.14

Parkinson's disease. T2-weighted axial MR image shows narrowing of the pars compacta of the substantia nigra. This may be due to cellular loss within this dopaminergic center or due to increased mineral deposition in the pars reticularis.

Hydrocephalus and Degenerative Diseases

part two

s
p
i
n
e

In contrast to the tremendous variety of primary brain abnormalities, most spinal diseases result from extrinsic compression of neural elements by their surrounding bony or cartilaginous structures. Imperfections in human evolution have left our spines with a great susceptibility to degenerative disease. Spinal trauma often has disastrous clinical consequences.

As with the brain, advances in spinal imaging have been nothing short of miraculous. After so many frustrating years of evaluating myelographic shadows, MRI has finally allowed us to visualize the spinal cord directly. Intervertebral disc disease, although still poorly understood, can now be evaluated with much more confidence. Spinal neoplasms can be detected easier and with greater sensitivity.

While the spinal images that follow are certainly impressive in their quality and scope, it remains a formidable challenge to convert these radiologic advances into tangible reductions in patient morbidity and mortality, which is the ultimate goal of all radiologic procedures.

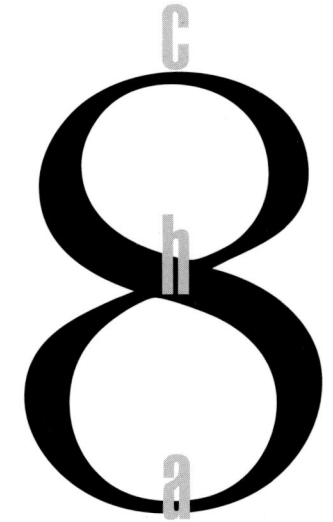

Chapter 8

Congenital Malformations of the Spine

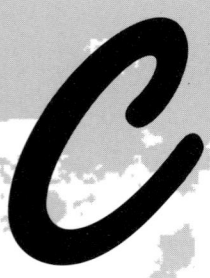ongenital malformations of the spine are usually caused by embryologic defects in neural tube formation. Most commonly these defects affect fusion of midline structures and are termed *spinal dysraphism*.

lated defect in a single part of the spine. It includes disorders of segmentation and other anomalies of vertebral bodies and posterior elements, diastematomyelia, tethered spinal cord, and meningomyelocele, and its less severe variants. Usually these disorders present in early childhood, although some may be clinically silent or not present with signs or symptoms until adulthood.

SPINAL DYSRAPHISM

Spinal dysraphism may result in extensive, complex abnormalities involving the spinal cord, meninges, and bony structures, or it may be limited to an iso-

Primary Bony Abnormalities

Structural abnormalities of the spine are often detected by the scoliosis or angulation of the spine

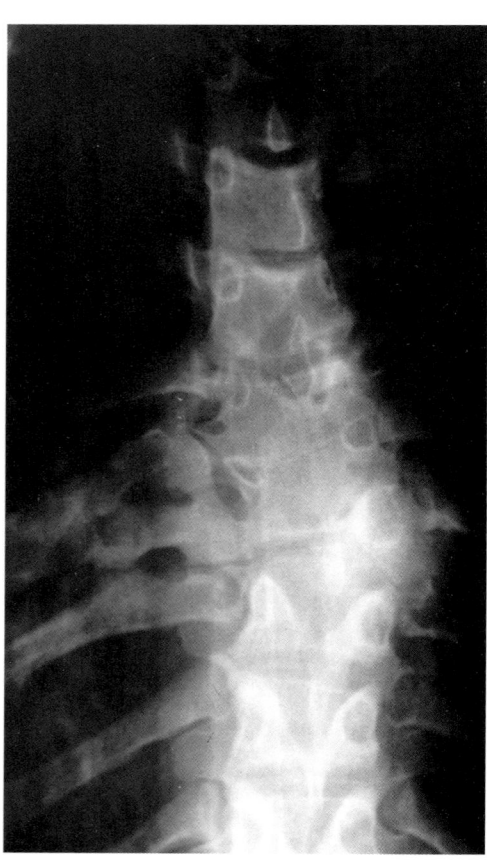

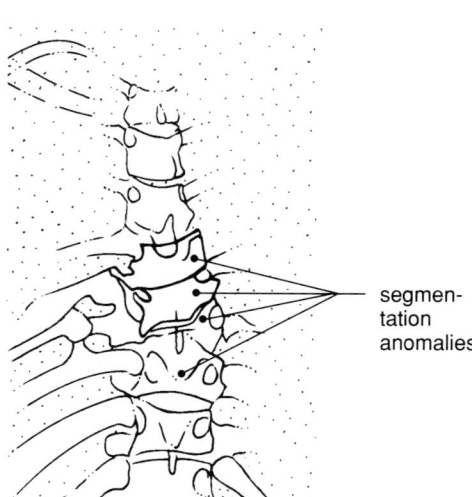

segmentation anomalies

Figure 8.1
Block vertebrae and hemivertebra. Fusion, hypoplasia, and segmentation abnormalities are evident in the mid-thoracic spine with a resultant scoliosis. There are associated rib anomalies and chest deformity.

which they produce (Fig. 8.1). Butterfly vertebrae, hemivertebra, and anomalies of segmentation may occur. Such segmentation anomalies in the cervical spine are known as the Klippel–Feil syndrome (Fig. 8.2); there may be an associated elevated scapula (Sprengel deformity).

Various other structural defects may occur involving the vertebral body, posterior elements, or both.

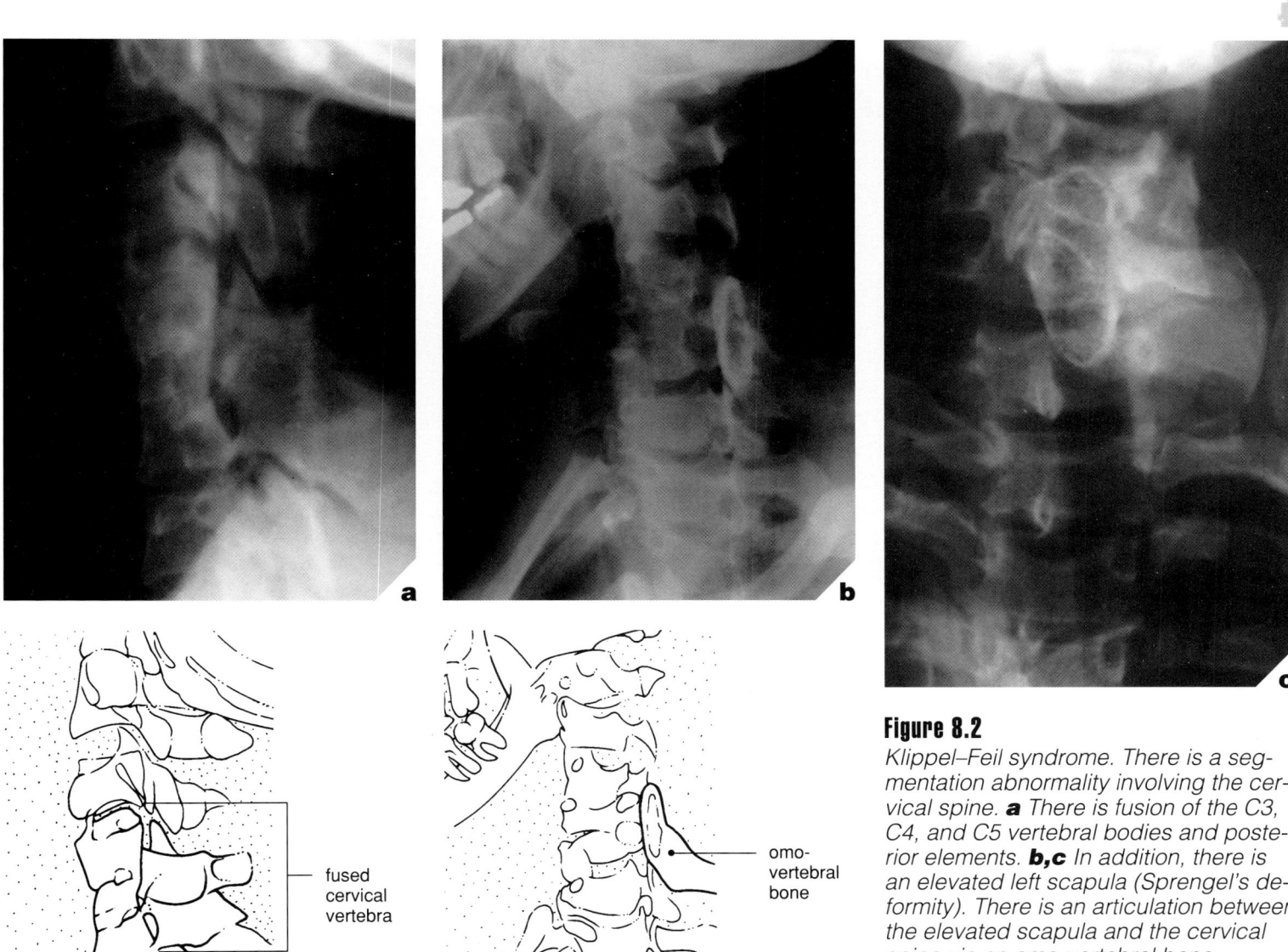

fused cervical vertebra

omo-vertebral bone

Figure 8.2

*Klippel–Feil syndrome. There is a segmentation abnormality involving the cervical spine. **a** There is fusion of the C3, C4, and C5 vertebral bodies and posterior elements. **b,c** In addition, there is an elevated left scapula (Sprengel's deformity). There is an articulation between the elevated scapula and the cervical spine via an omo-vertebral bone.*

Butterfly vertebra (Fig. 8.3), hemivertebra, and mild or severe failures of the posterior elements to fuse together (spina bifida) may be isolated abnormalities or they may be associated with malformations of the neural elements and meninges such as diastematomyelia, meningomyelocele, and tethered spinal cord.

Complete or partial absence of the sacrum (Fig. 8.4) occurs as part of the "caudal regression syndrome." This syndrome is associated with abnormalities of the lumbar and lower thoracic spine, genitourinary tract, lungs, and an imperforate anus. It occurs with increased frequency in infants of diabetic mothers.

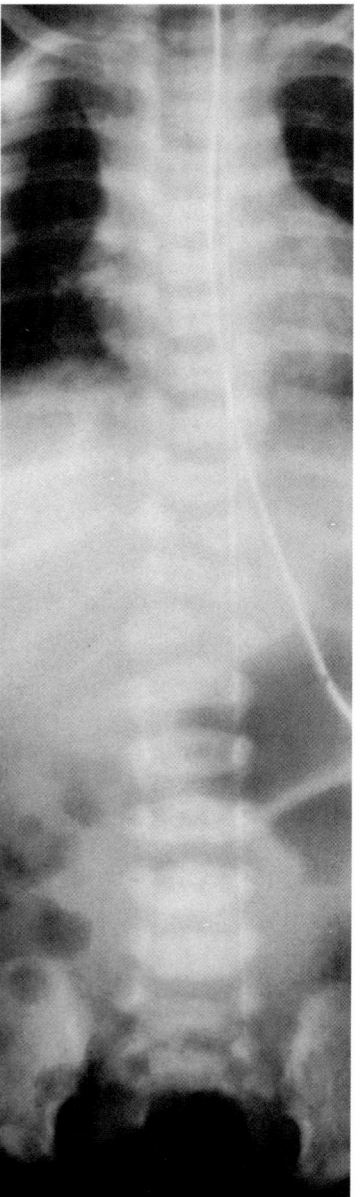

Figure 8.3
Butterfly vertebra. There are sagittal clefts in the deformed T10 through T12 vertebral bodies.

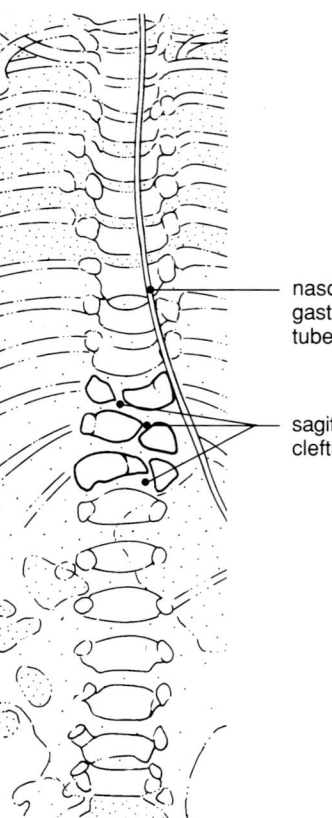

naso-gastric tube

sagittal clefts

Figure 8.4
Caudal regression syndrome. There is congenital absence of the sacrum in this infant of a diabetic mother.

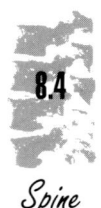

Spinal Lipoma

Spinal lipoma is the most common type of midline congenital mass. Fatty deposits are frequently associated with important malformations such as a meningomyelocele. Spinal lipomas frequently occur within the filum terminale or at the termination point of the conus medullaris (Fig. 8.5). Although some spinal lipomas produce symptoms by virtue of spinal

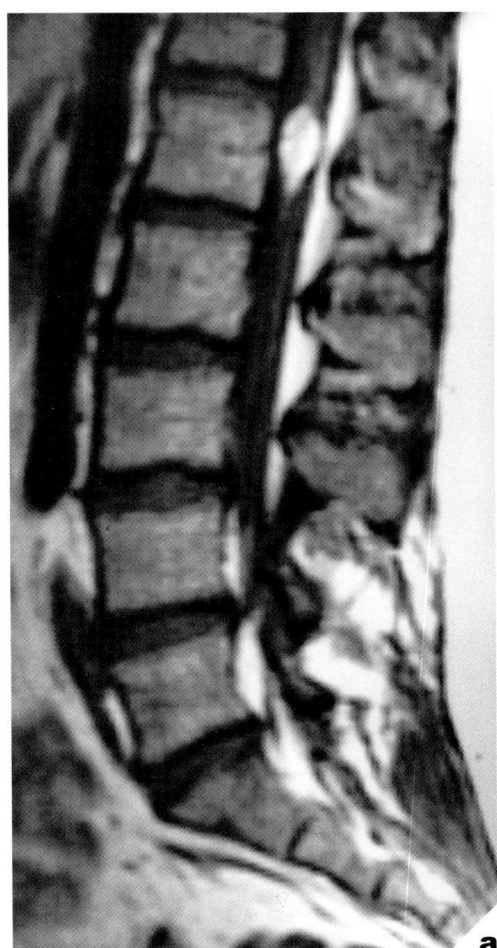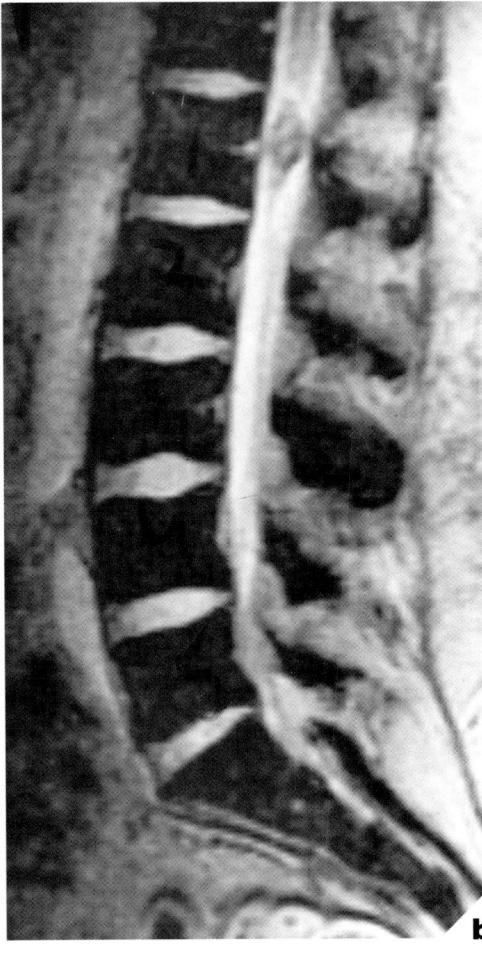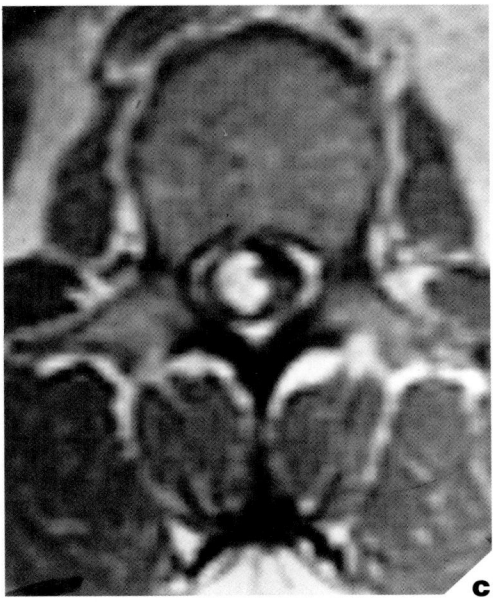

Figure 8.5

*Lipoma of the conus medullaris. **a** Sagittal T1, **b** T2, and **c** axial T1-weighted MR images demonstrate an intradural mass attached to the distal end of the conus medullaris. The mass has the bright-T1, intermediate T2 signal characteristics of fat.*

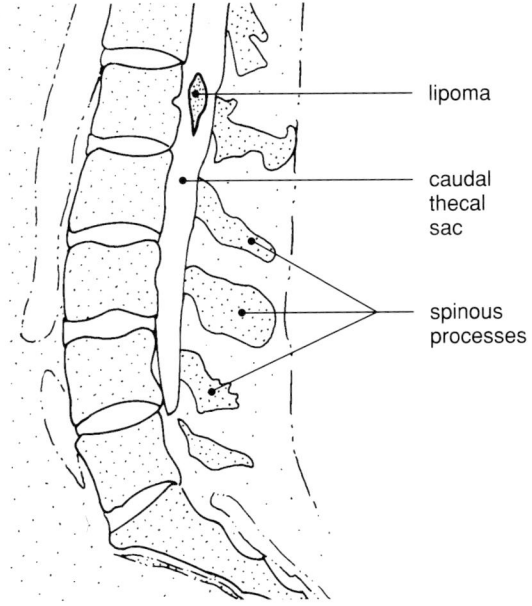

lipoma

caudal thecal sac

spinous processes

cord or nerve root compression, many, particularly lipomas of the filum terminale (Fig 8.6), are completely asymptomatic and merely represent an incidental finding.

Spinal lipomas are readily identifiable by MRI due to their bright-T1 signal characteristics. The lipomas may be intradural or extradural. Diffuse fatty deposition in the extradural spaces may occur with Cushing's disease or other endocrinological abnormalities (see Chapter 12) and result in compression of the spinal cord or thecal sac.

Meningomyelocele

Failure of closure of the neural tube results in a spectrum of abnormalities best described by naming the

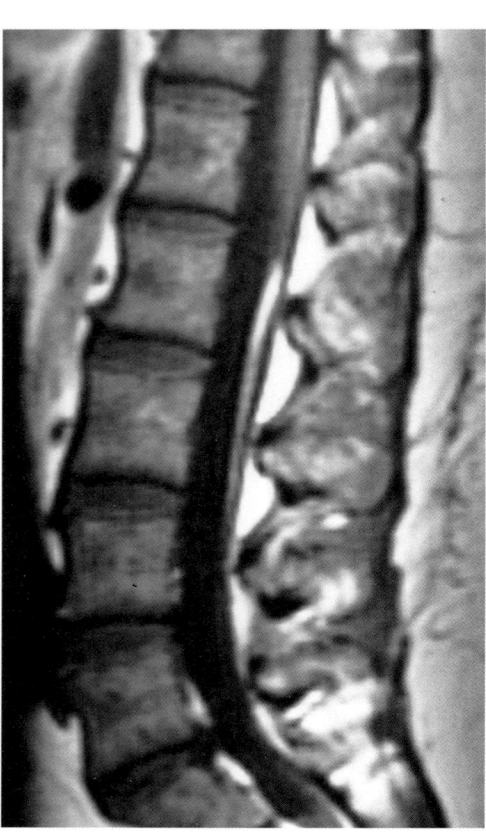

Figure 8.6
Lipoma of the filum terminale. Sagittal T1-weighted image of the lumbar spine demonstrates a linear band of bright signal within the filum terminale which represents a filolipoma. There is no associated meningomyelocele.

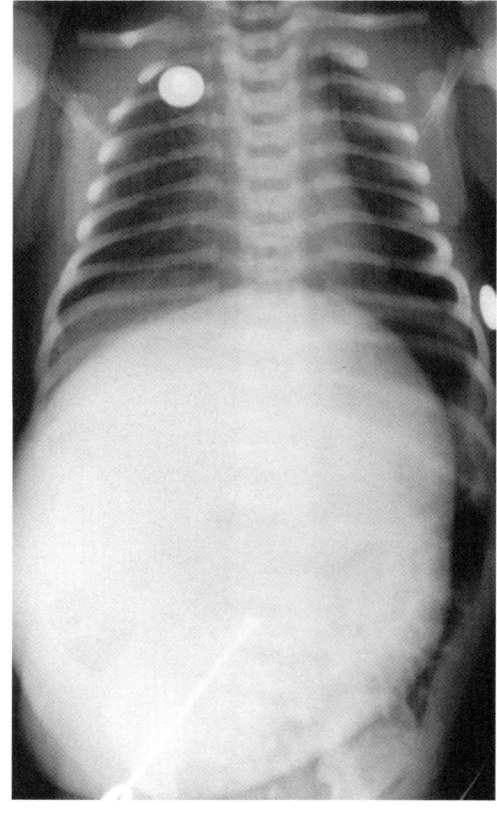

Figure 8.7
Meningomyelocele. PA radiograph of the abdomen and chest in a neonate demonstrates a huge soft tissue mass behind the pelvis and abdomen, surrounded by air.

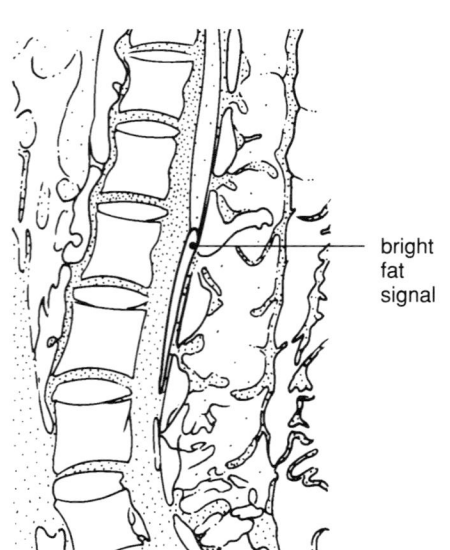

bright
fat
signal

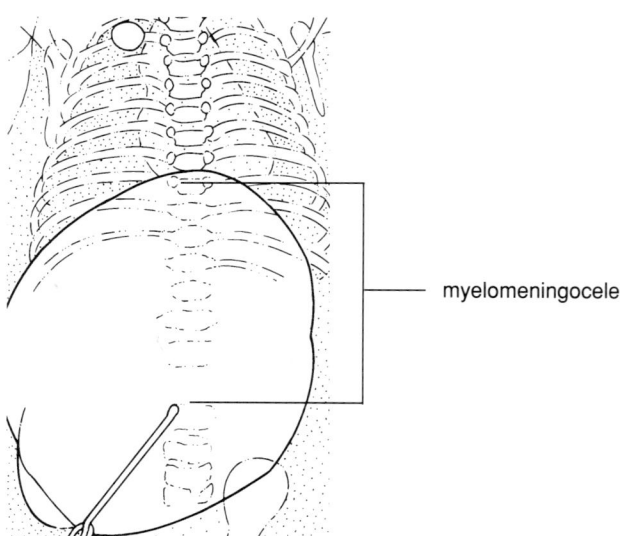

myelomeningocele

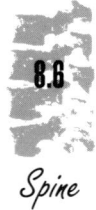

components of the neural axis which herniate. Thus, a meningocele represents a protrusion of dura and arachnoid mater outside the spinal canal, usually associated with a large CSF-containing cavity. Usually the meninges and their contained CSF herniate posteriorly, but anterior or lateral meningoceles are common in patients with neurofibromatosis.

A meningomyelocele (Fig. 8.7) represents herniation of both meninges and neural tissue outside the spinal canal. The Arnold–Chiari malformation (Chiari II) is a spectrum of anomalies of the brain and spine which are associated with a lumbo-sacral meningomyelocele. A wide spina bifida deformity is generally present on plain films of the spine at the site of the meningomyelocele. There is often tethering of the spinal cord at an abnormally low posi-

tion. The cerebellum and medulla are displaced caudally, often to the level of C2 or lower. The fourth venticle is elongated and displaced below the foramen magnum. Syringomyelia is commonly associated with the Arnold–Chiari malformation. Clinically, patients have lower extremity motor and sensory deficits, bladder and bowel dysfunction, and symptoms from hydrocephalus. This disorder is illustrated in Chapter 1.

A meningomyelocele is frequently associated with tethering of the spinal cord (Fig 8.8), hydromyelia, and diastematomyelia. There is an abnormally low termination point of the spinal cord, below the level of L2. The distal portion of neural tissue forms a plaque which is adherent to the posterior wall of the thecal sac.

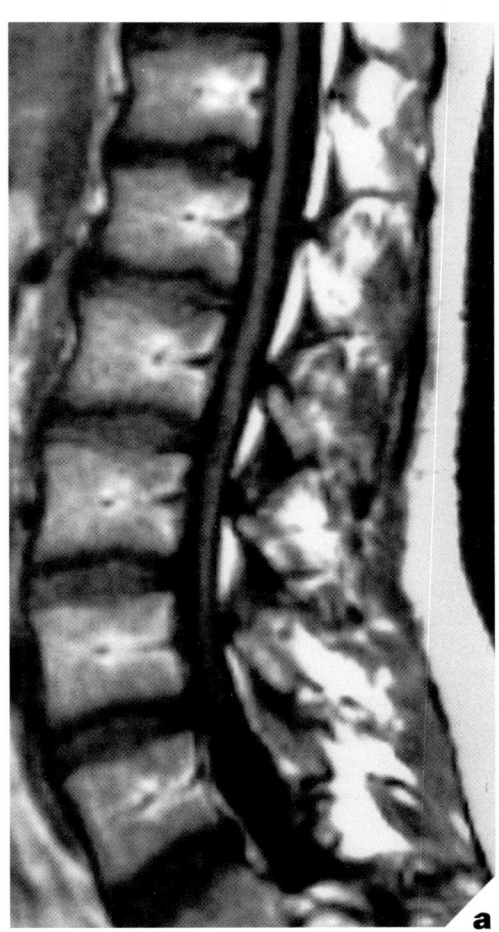 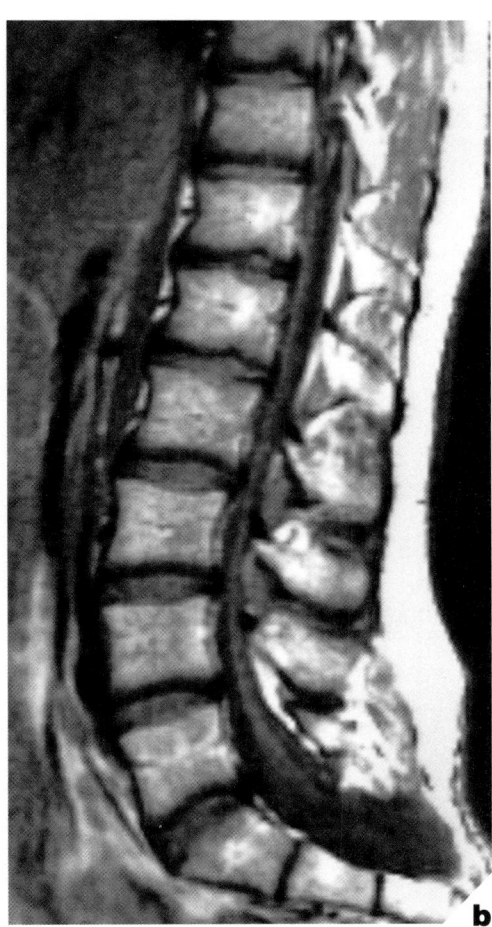 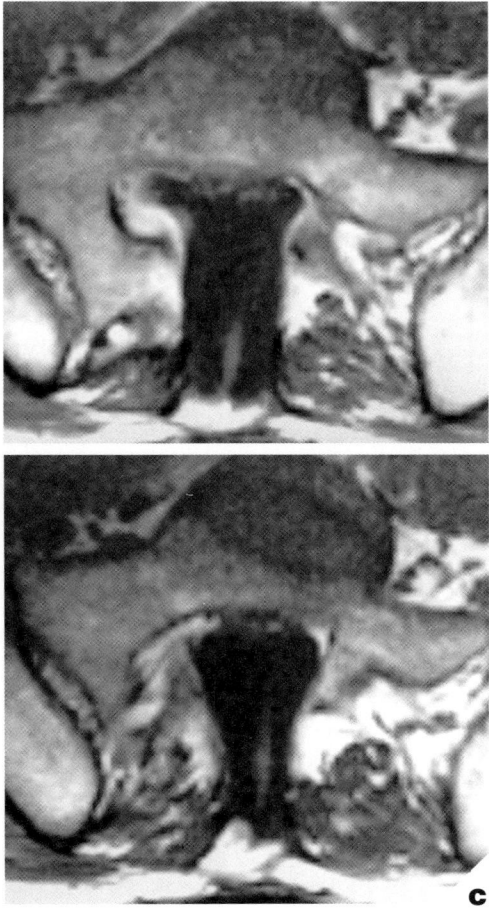

Figure 8.8

Meningomyelocele with tethered spinal cord. **a,b** Sagittal and **c** axial T1-weighted MR images of the lumbar spine demonstrate a large collection of CSF protruding through a defect in the caudal portion of the spinal canal. The spinal cord extends far inferiorly into this collection where it attaches along the dorsal surface of the thecal sac.

Tethering of the spinal cord without an associated meningomyelocele may present clinically as the "tight filum terminale syndrome." This is a disorder of childhood typically presenting with sensorimotor findings in the lower extremities and bladder dysfunction. MRI or myelography show a thickened filum terminale and the tip of the conus medullaris lying below L2.

A lipomeningomyelocele (Fig 8.9) is identical to a simple meningomyelocele except for the presence of a lipoma attached to the distal end of the filum terminale. There is usually a wide sacral spina bifida and tethering of the spinal cord. CT and MRI show characteristic fat density or signal intensity, respectively.

A myelocele represents herniation of neural elements outside the spinal canal without accompanying meninges. There is a plaque of neurovascular tissue at the skin surface. A lipomyelocele contains fat along the surface of the neural placode.

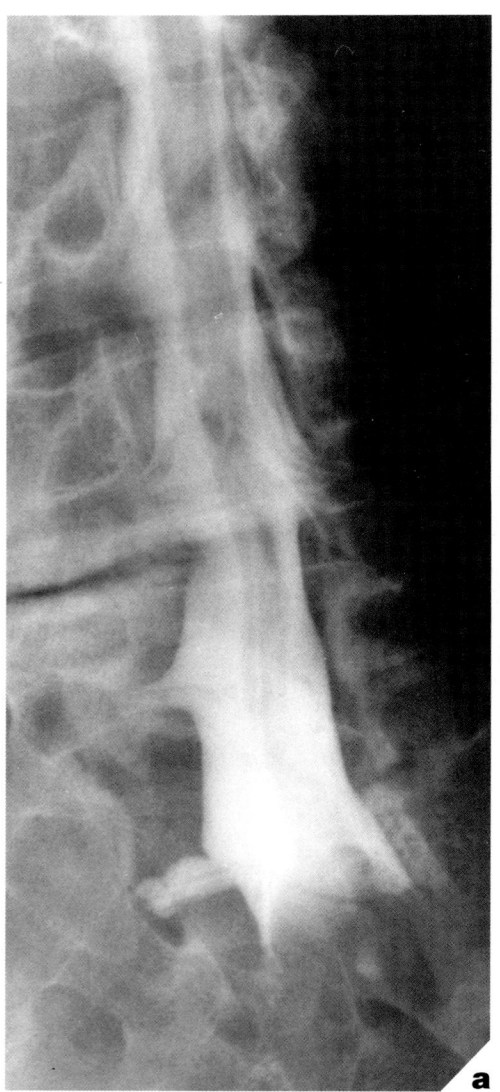

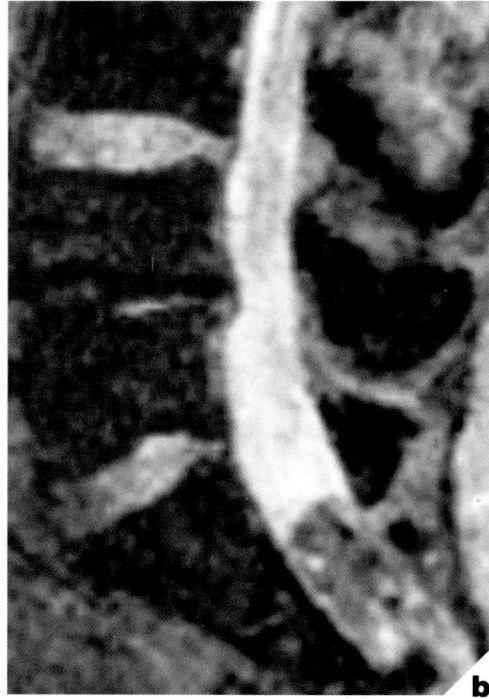

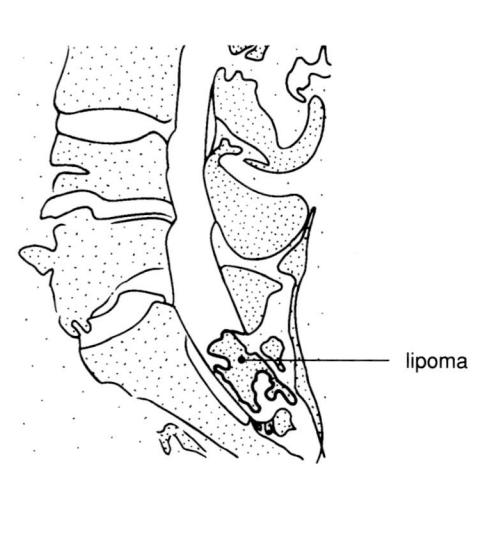

lipoma

Figure 8.9

*Lipomeningomyelocele with tethered spinal cord. **a** Lumbar myelogram demonstrates marked caudal extension of the spinal cord to the level of S1/S2 where there is a large intradural mass. **b** This mass has intermediate T2-weighted signal characteristics on sagittal MR images. **c** Postmyelographic CT scans confirm the low level of the spinal cord and **d,e** demonstrate fatty density within the intradural mass at the level of S1/S2. There is an asymmetrical spina bifida deformity at this level which is commonly demonstrated in patients with lipomeningomyelocele.*

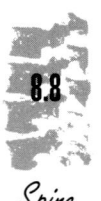

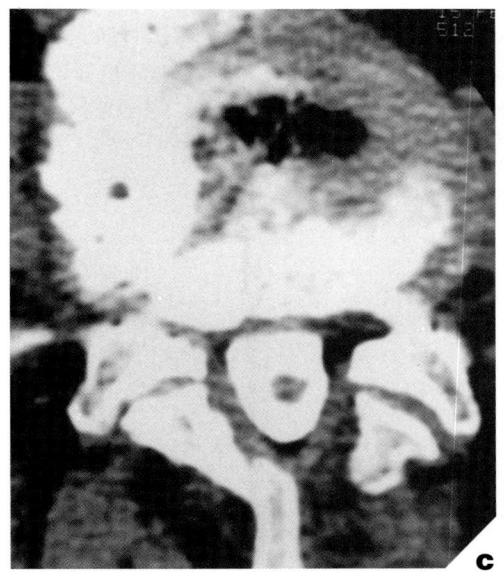

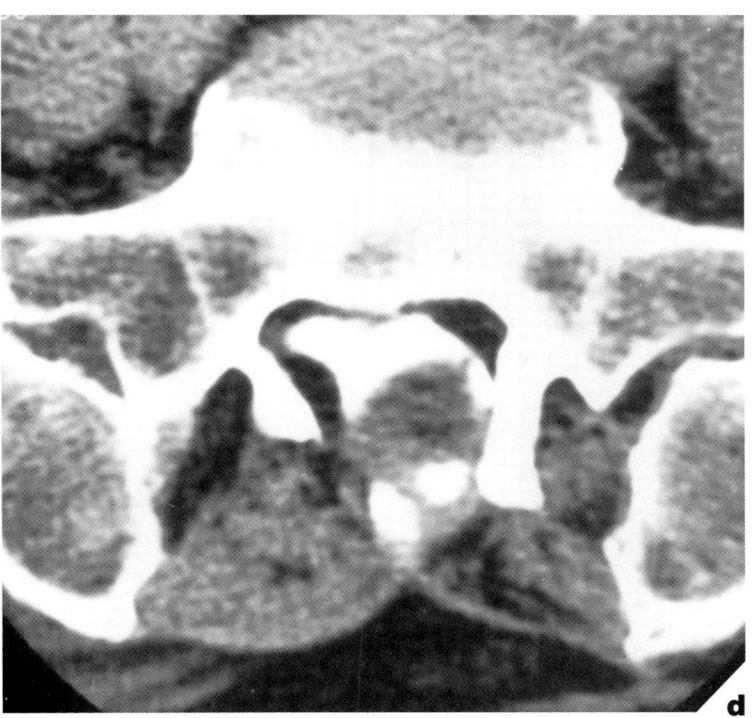

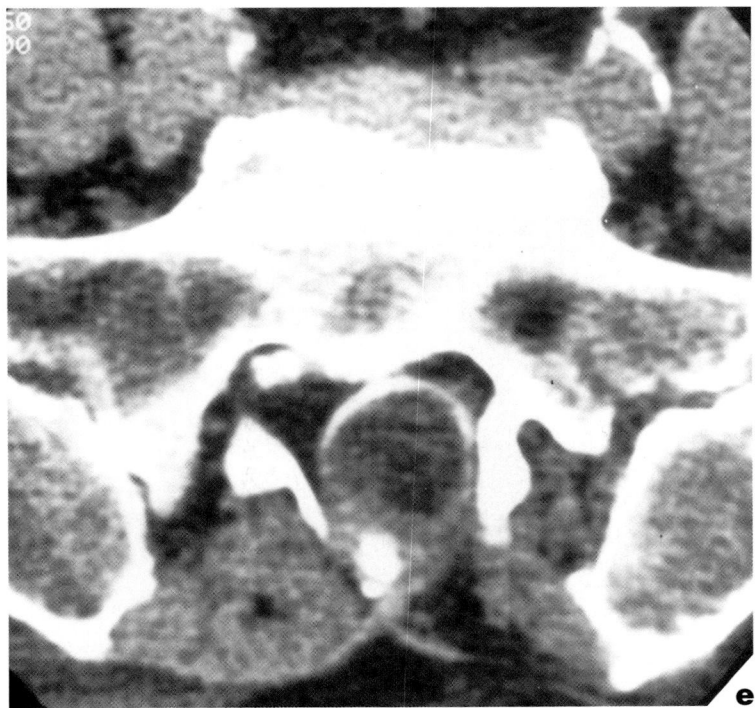

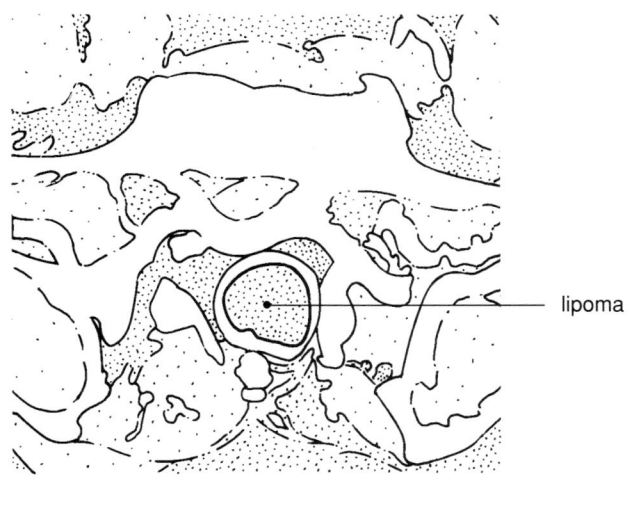

lipoma

Diastematomyelia

Diastematomyelia (Fig 8.10) is a severe form of spinal dysraphism in which there is a complete sagittal cleft within the spinal cord that extends for a vari-able length and results in the production of two hemicords. There are usually associated bony deformities of the spine at the level of the diastematomyelia which include a sagittally oriented bony

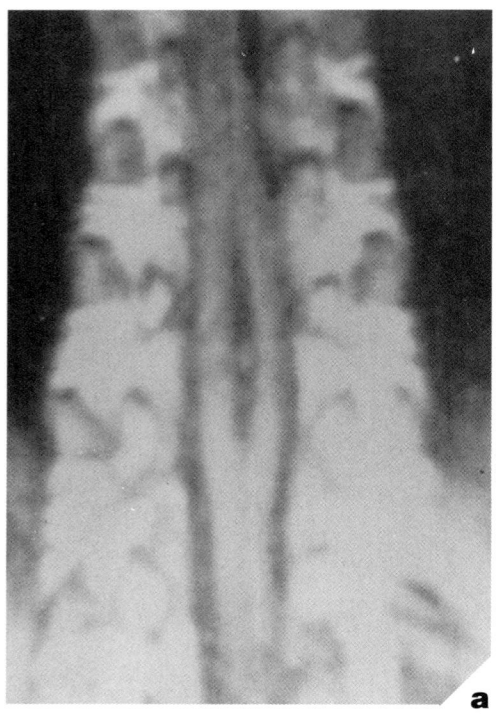

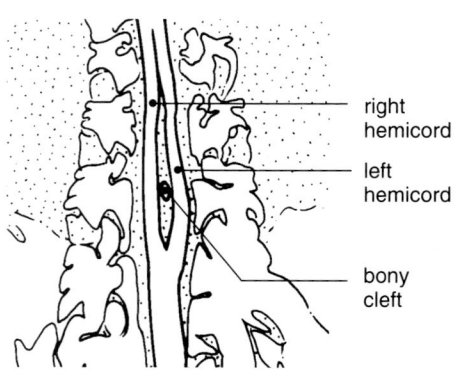

right hemicord

left hemicord

bony cleft

Figure 8.10

*Diastematomyelia. **a** Sagittal and **b** axial T1-weighted MR images demonstrate a complete sagittal cleft within the lower thoracic spinal cord. A small bony cleft is demonstrated centrally. The two hemi-cords reunite distally. **c** Postmyelo-graphic CT scan shows the presence of separate arachnoid and dural tubes for each hemicord. There is an associated spina bifida deformity.*

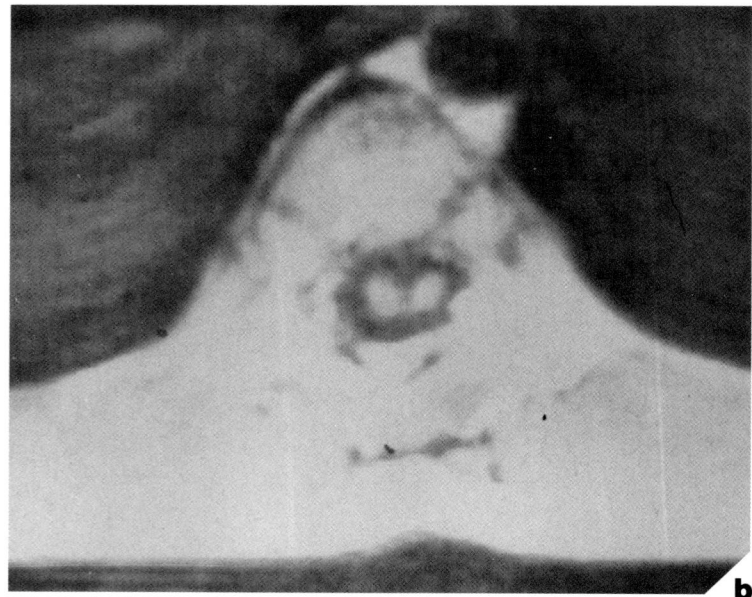

a

b

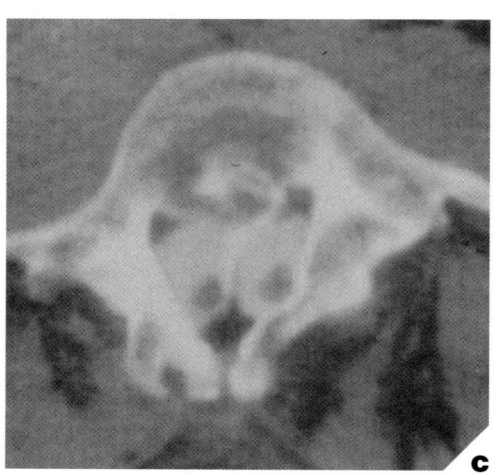

c

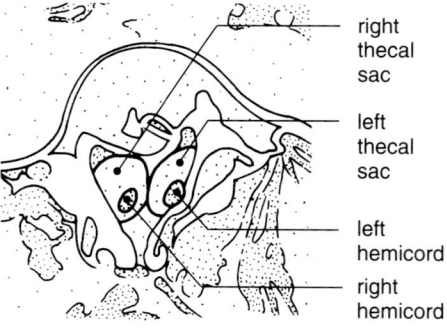

right thecal sac

left thecal sac

left hemicord

right hemicord

spicule attached to the vertebral body, segmentation anomalies, spina bifida, and scoliosis. When present, the bony spicule lies at the inferior margin of the split spinal cord.

Diastematomyelia should be distinguished from diplomyelia; in diplomyelia there is a true duplication of the spinal cord rather than a separation. In most cases of diastematomyelia, the two hemicords reunite in the lower thoracic region or at the conus medullaris. Each hemicord may lie within its own separate dural and arachnoid tube. Slightly more commonly, both hemicords lie adjacent to each other within a single coaxial arachnoid and dural tube. These may be distinguished by CT myelography (Fig. 8.10c) although the presence of a bony spur on plain films usually indicates the presence of separate arachnoid and dural

tubes for each hemicord. Rarely, there may be syringomyelia within one or both hemicords (Fig 8.11).

SYRINGOHYDROMYELIA

Syringohydromyelia (Fig. 8.12) represents a cystic collection, usually containing CSF, which lies within the spinal cord. The cystic collection may represent dilatation of the central canal (hydromyelia) or a cystic collection not lined by ependyma occurring within the spinal cord itself (syringomyelia). Practically, it is usually best to describe any such cystic dilatation as *syringohydromyelia*. The cyst may extend cephalad to involve the brainstem (syringobulbia). Often there are multiple septations within the cyst.

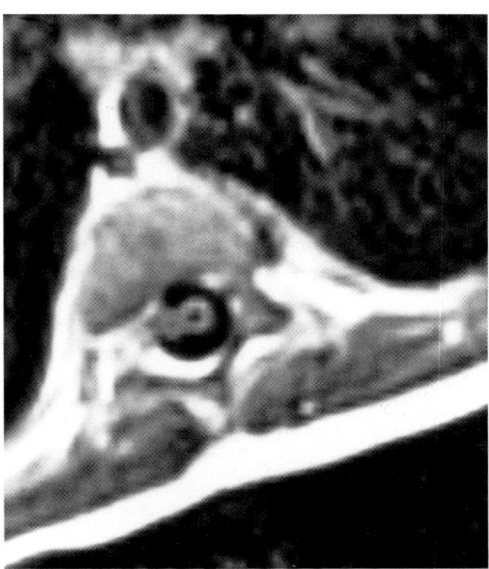

Figure 8.11
Diastematomyelia with syringomyelia in both hemicords. Axial T1-weighted MR image demonstrates the presence of two asymmetric hemicords lying adjacent to each other in the lower thoracic spine. There is a small syrinx within the right hemicord and a larger syrinx within the left hemicord.

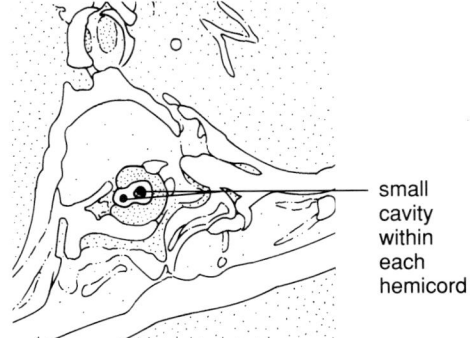

— small cavity within each hemicord

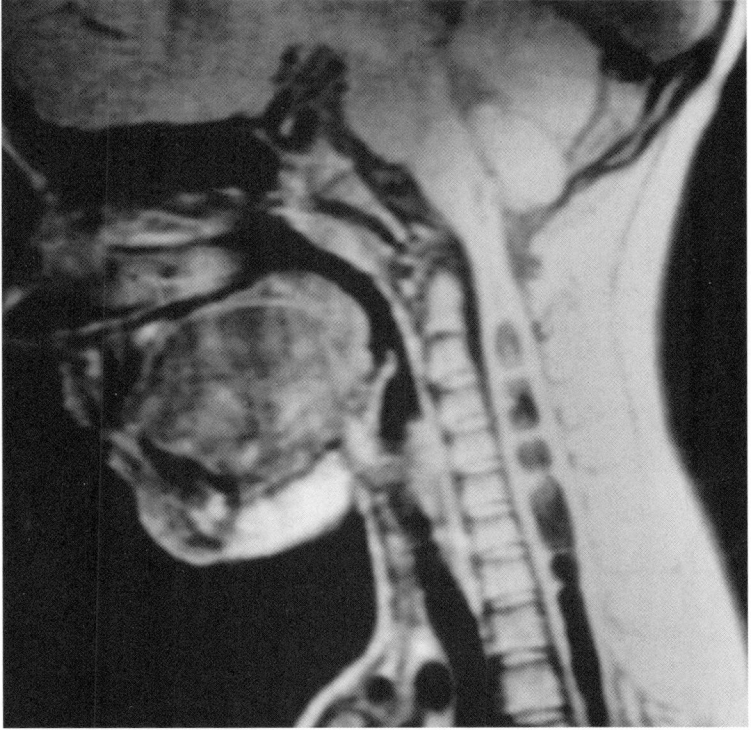

Figure 8.12
Syringohydromyelia. There is a large, multiseptated cystic cavity within the cervical spinal cord below the level of C2. The spinal cord is markedly enlarged.

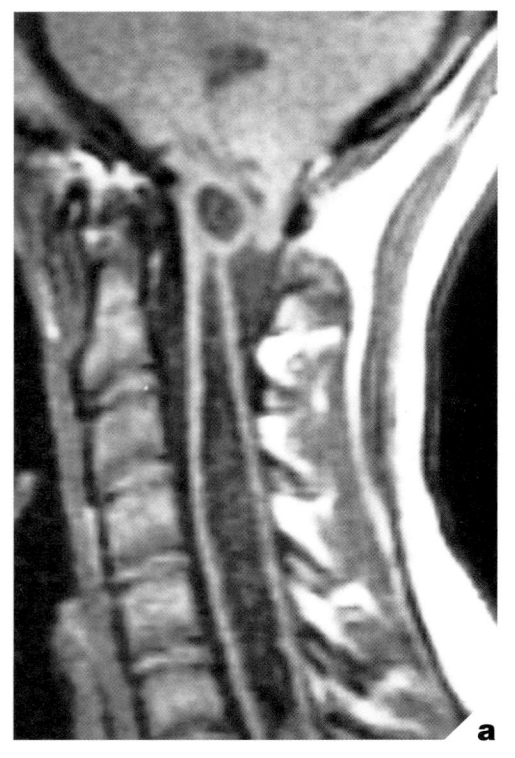

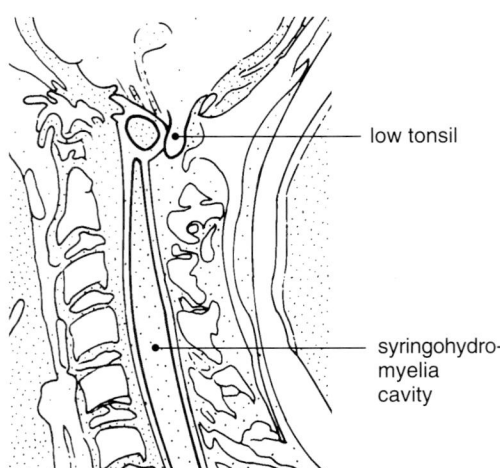

low tonsil

syringohydro-
myelia
cavity

Figure 8.13
*Syringohydromyelia and syringobulbia
associated with Chiari I syndrome.
a Sagittal and **b** axial T1- and **c** T2-
weighted images of the cervical spine
show a large cystic cavity within the cervical spinal cord and lower brainstem.
The cavity demonstrates dark-T1, bright-
T2 signal and is isointense to CSF on all
sequences. The cerebellar tonsils extend
1 cm below the foramen magnum.*

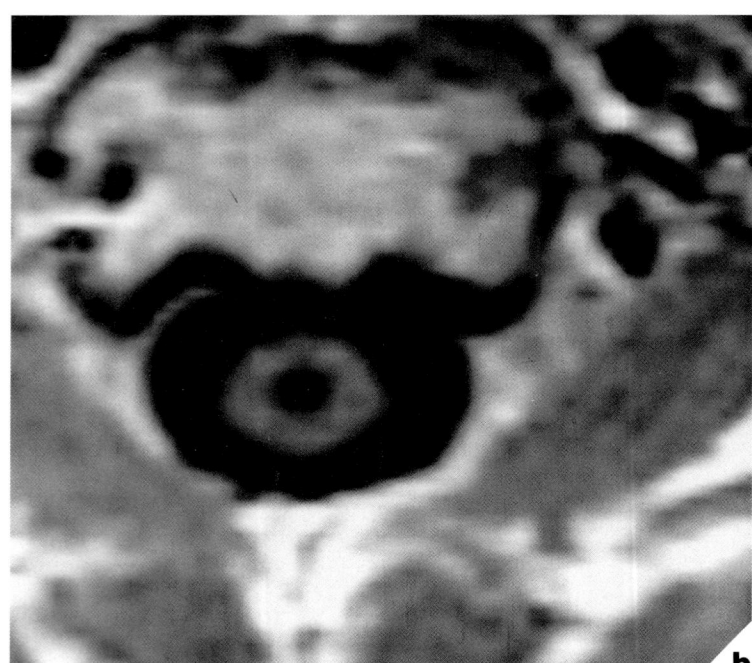

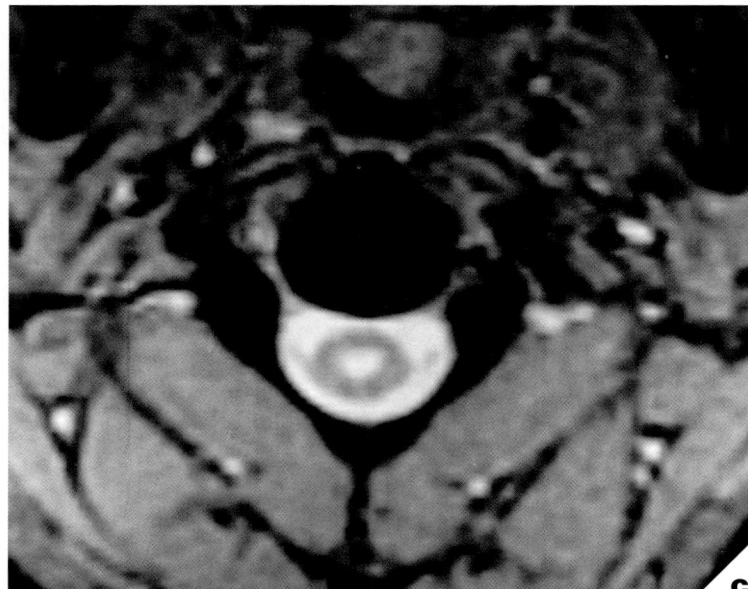

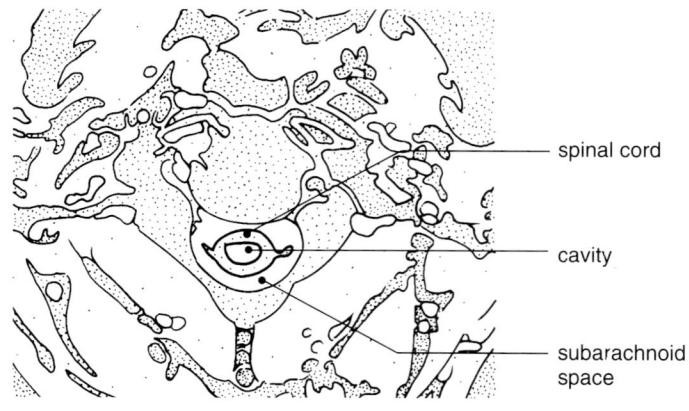

spinal cord

cavity

subarachnoid
space

Syringohydromyelia is commonly associated with cerebellar tonsillar ectopia (Chiari I malformation) (Fig. 8.13) or Arnold–Chiari malformation (Chiari II). It is best diagnosed by MRI. CT and myelography may show nonspecific widening of the spinal cord. Delayed CT images following myelography often show contrast within the cyst (Fig. 8.14).

Syringohydromyelia may also occur following trauma, be related to spinal cord neoplasms, or occur independently and without any other findings (Fig. 8.15).

SPINAL ARACHNOID CYSTS

Spinal arachnoid cysts (Fig. 8.16) represent loculated, extramedullary focal CSF collections. They may or may not communicate with the surrounding subarachnoid space. Spinal cord or nerve root compression may occur; there may be a complete block to flow of contrast medium at myelography.

Perineural expansion of the subarachnoid space (Tarlov's cysts) (Figs. 8.17, 8.18) is a frequent finding at myelography. Unless there is nerve root or thecal sac compression, these collections are usually of no clinical significance. Subarachnoid cysts along nerve root sleeves are often associated with erosion and subsequent widening of neural foramina, particularly in the sacrum. These erosions may be quite large.

MISCELLANEOUS CONGENITAL SPINAL DISORDERS

Hurler's syndrome (Fig. 8.19) is a type of mucopolysaccharidosis (MPS I-H) in which there is urinary excretion of dermatan and heparan sulfates due to a deficiency of α-L-iduronidase. The vertebral bodies have an oval shape with a characteristic antero-inferior beak seen on lateral views.

Achondroplasia (Fig. 8.20) represents an anomaly of endochondral bone formation which results in congenital spinal stenosis due to short pedicles and a narrow interpedicular distance. The vertebral bodies have a characteristic central anterior beak, most prominent in the thoraco-lumbar junction. There is a marked decreased height of the vertebral bodies; they are shorter in height than the intervertebral discs.

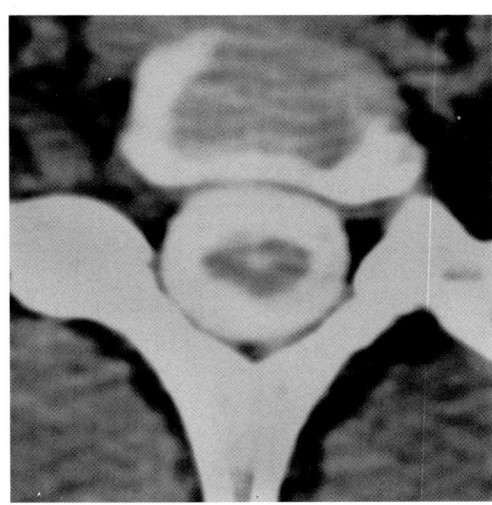

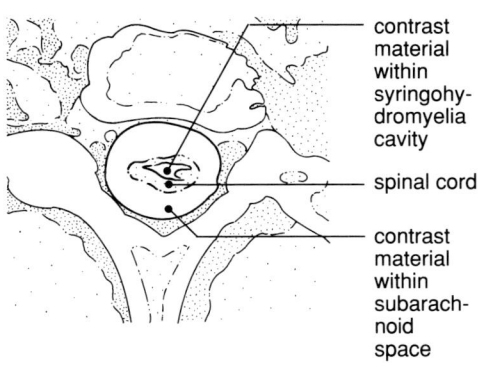

contrast material within syringohydromyelia cavity

spinal cord

contrast material within subarachnoid space

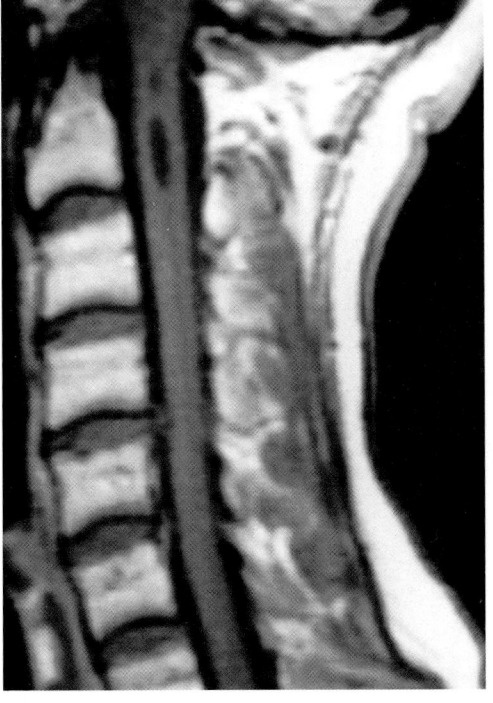

Figure 8.14
Syringohydromyelia. A CT scan of the cervical spine performed 6 hours following myelography demonstrates the presence of contrast material within a central cavity in the cervical spinal cord. No contrast material was demonstrated within the cavity on a CT scan obtained immediately following myelography.

Figure 8.15
Syringohydromyelia. Sagittal T1-weighted image shows a small septated cavity at the level of C2 without any other associated abnormalities.

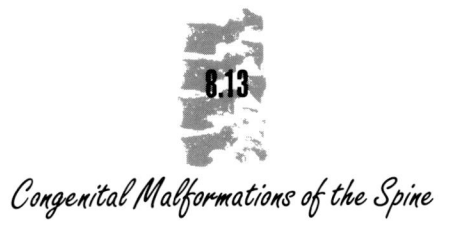

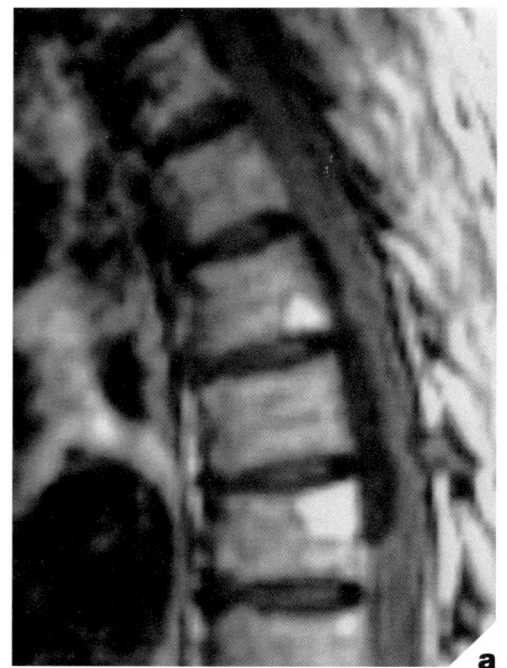

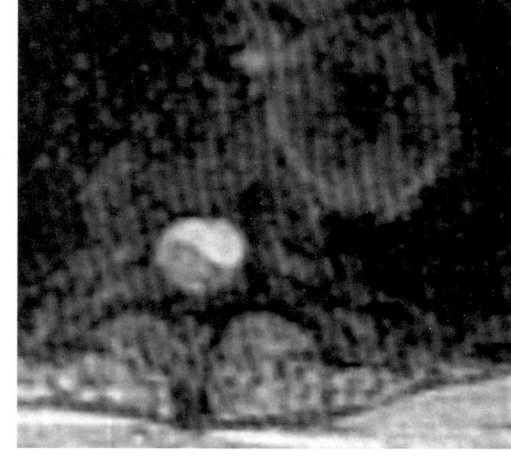

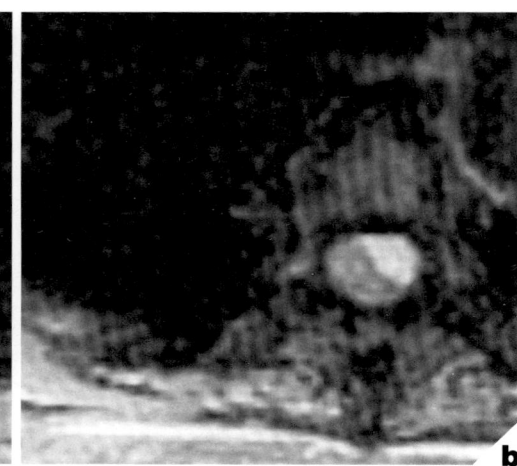

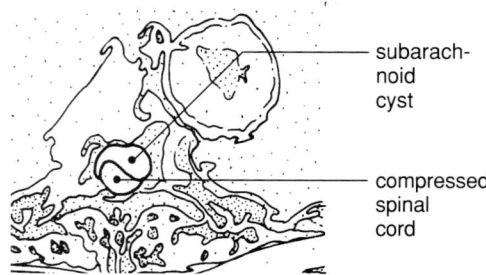

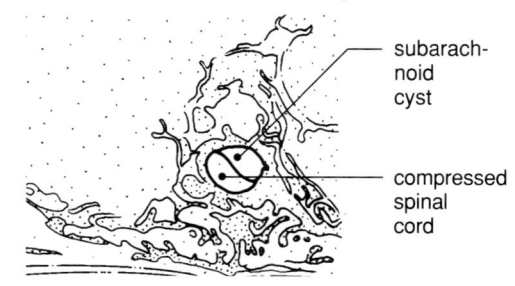

subarach-
noid
cyst

compressed
spinal
cord

subarach-
noid
cyst

compressed
spinal
cord

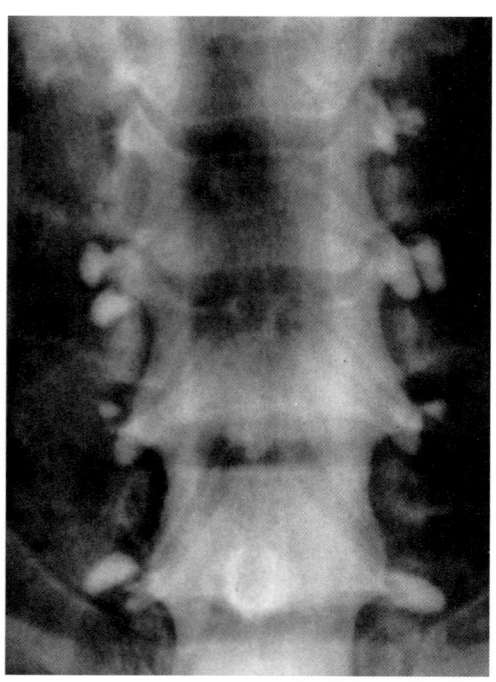

compressed
spinal
cord

subarach-
noid
cyst

Figure 8.16

*Spinal arachnoid cyst. **a** Sagittal T1-
and **b** axial T2-weighted MR images
demonstrate an extramedullary mass
anterior and to the left of the thoracic
spinal cord. The spinal cord is com-*
*pressed. The mass is isointense to CSF
on both pulse sequences, smoothly
marginated and well defined and represents an arachnoid cyst.*

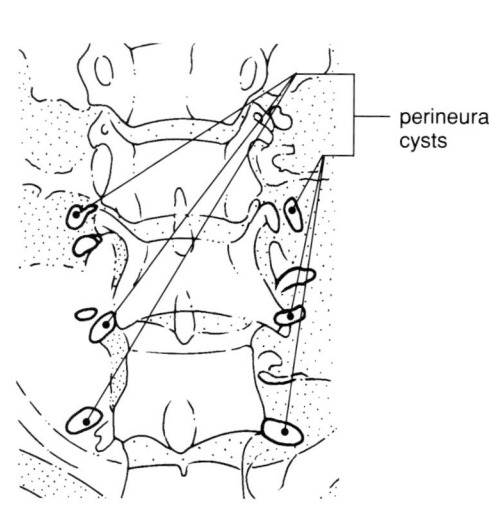

perineural
cysts

Figure 8.17

*Perineural (Tarlov's) cysts. Cervical
myelographic film demonstrates the
presence of numerous sac-like exten-
sions along the pathways of the cervical
nerve roots.*

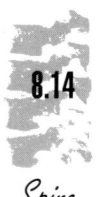

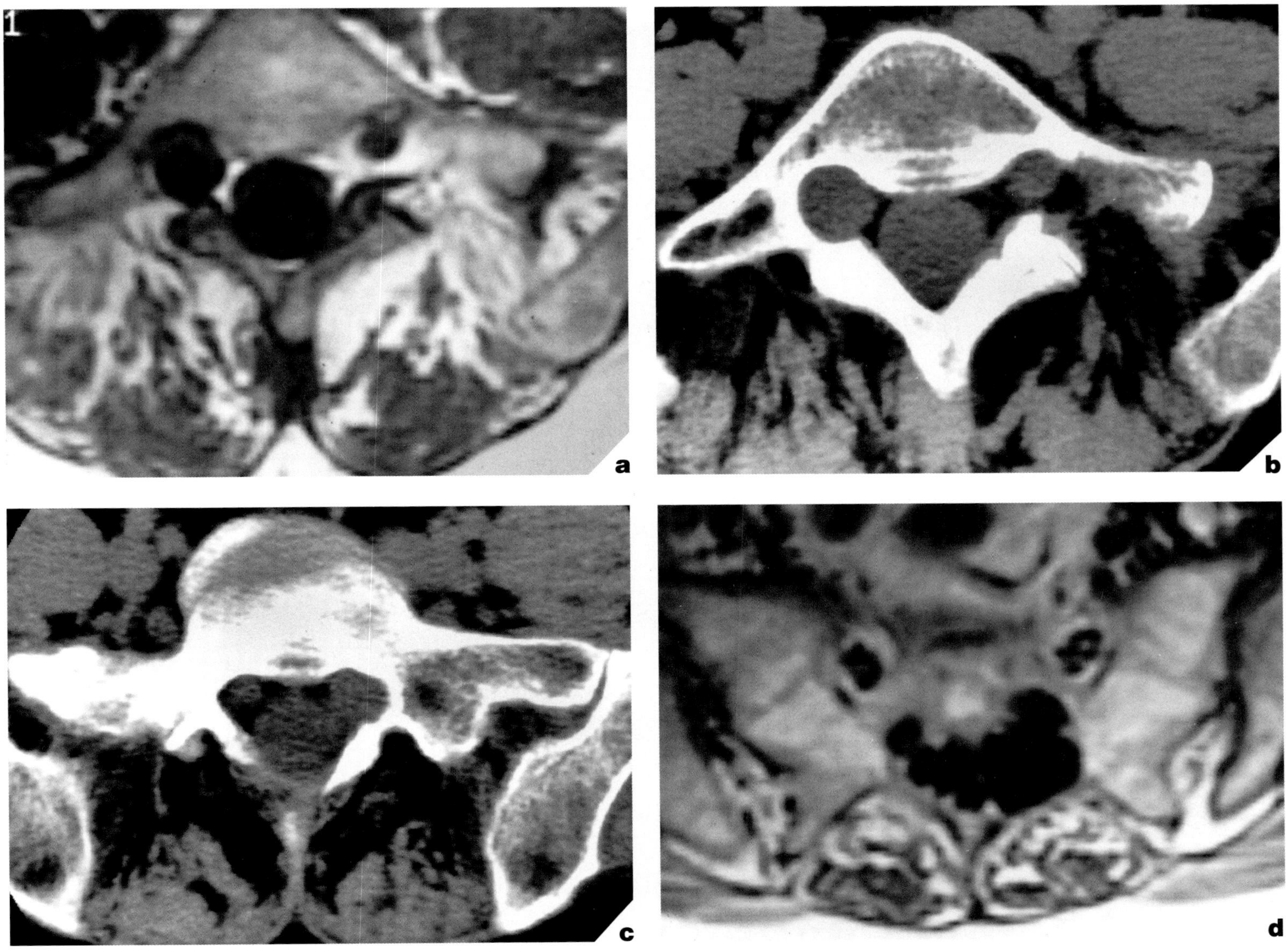

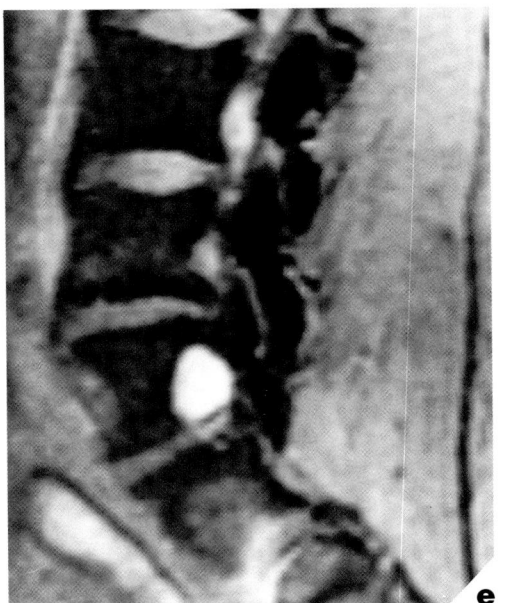

Figure 8.18

Lumbo-sacral subarachnoid cysts. **a** *T1-weighted axial MRI and* **b** *axial CT scan at the level of S1 show dilatation of the S1 nerve root sleeves, especially on the right.* **c,d** *Additional perineural cystic collections of CSF are seen,* **e** *including a large perineural cyst of the right L5 nerve root sleeve is also demonstrated by sagittal T2-weighted MRI.*

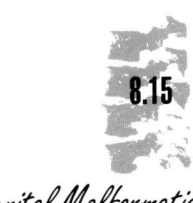

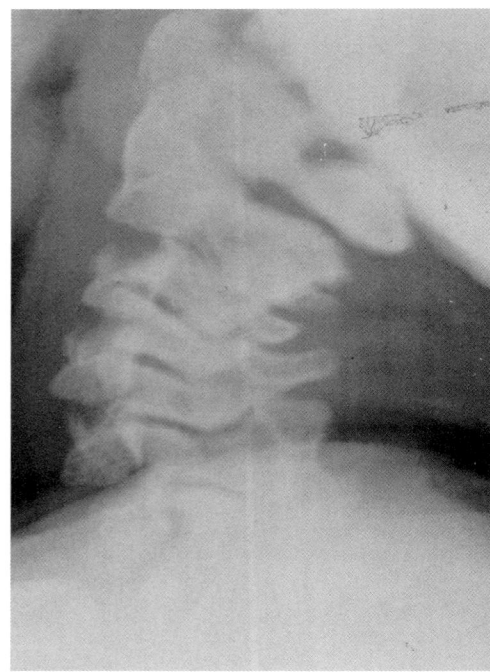

Figure 8.19
Hurler's syndrome. Lateral plain film of
the cervical spine shows characteristic
"beaks" extending from the antero-
inferior margin of oval-shaped cervical
vertebral bodies.

antero-
inferior
vertebral
body
"beaks"

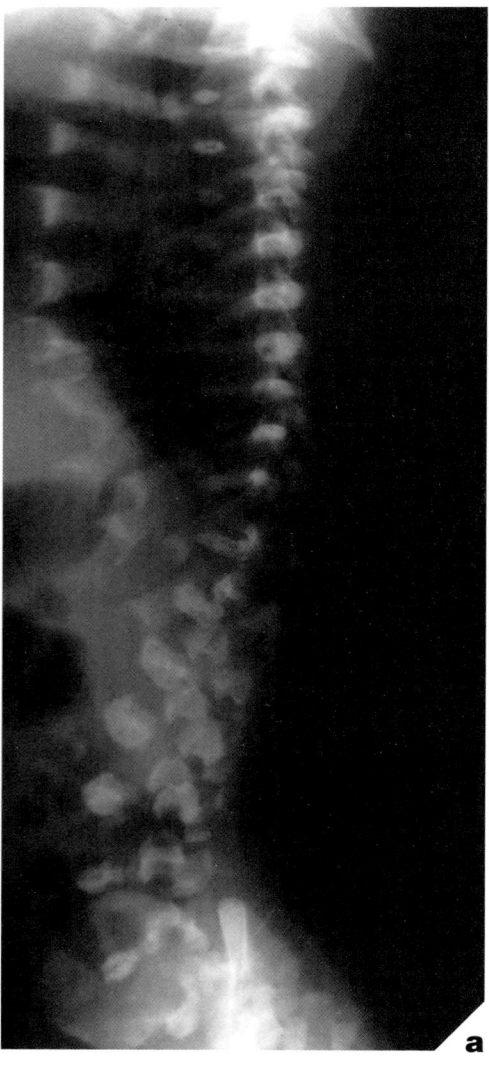

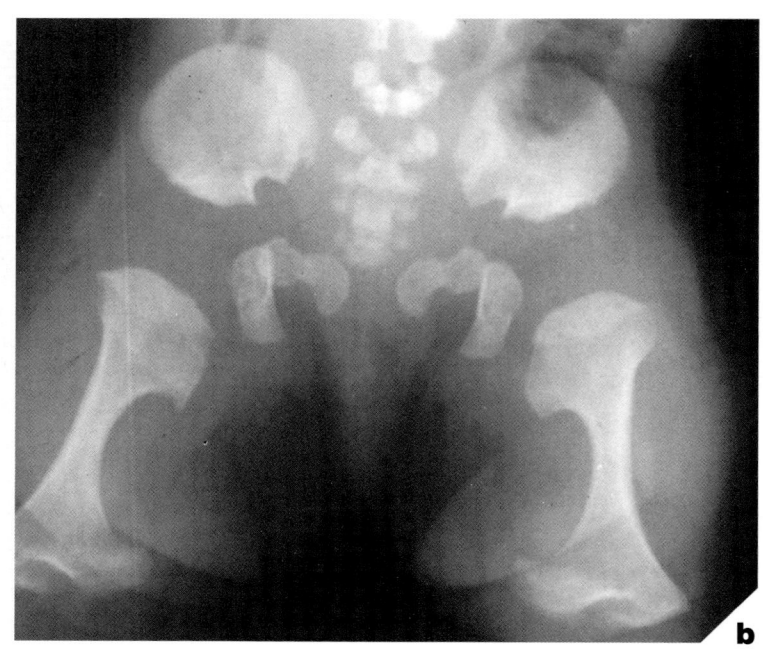

Figure 8.20
Achondroplasia. **a** Lateral view of the spine shows characteristic loss of height of the vertebral bodies and central, anterior
beaks. The intervertebral disc spaces are taller than the vertebral bodies,the reverse of normal. **b** AP view of the sacrum
which includes the pelvis and femora shows a narrowed interpedicular distance at L5. There is rounding of the iliac wings,
short sciatic notches and horizontal acetabular roofs. (Note
the short, stubby femoral shafts and flared metaphyses, characteristic findings in achondroplasia.)

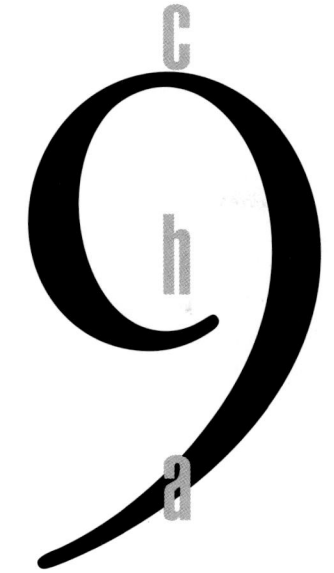

c
h
a
p
t
e
r

9

Inflammatory Diseases of the Spine

*i*nflammatory diseases of the spine represent an important but often overlooked category of neuropathology. The incidence of spinal infections has recently increased, mostly due to the AIDS epidemic. Failure to consider inflammatory processes in the evaluation of low back pain is a common pitfall of neuroradiologic and clinical practice. Fortunately, there are many characteristic features of infectious spondylitis which can be looked for and properly evaluated.

Infectious disorders of the spine usually initially involve a vertebral body endplate. The anterior two-thirds of the vertebral endplates are typically affected; there is usually sparing of the posterior elements. Once organisms breech the vertebral endplate, they pass unrestricted into the adjacent intervertebral disc and opposite vertebral body endplate. This creates a much different appearance on magnetic resonance imaging, computed tomography, and plain radiographs of the spine than neoplastic diseases which typically do not invade the intervertebral disc. Furthermore, neoplastic processes tend to involve primarily the pedicles and posterior portions of the vertebral bodies; these areas are usually spared by spinal infections.

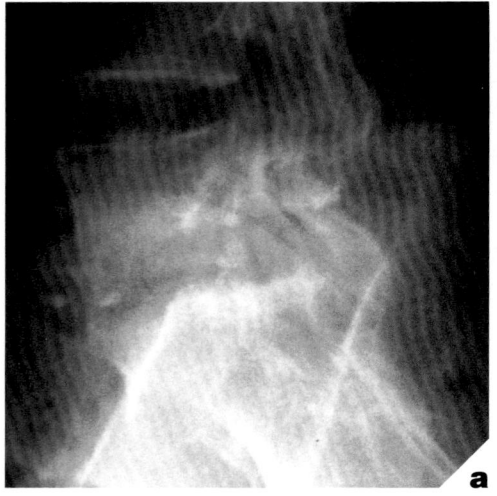

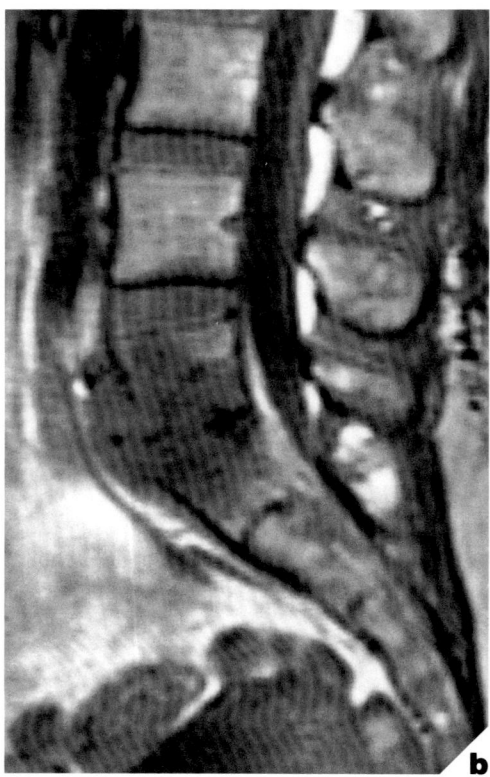

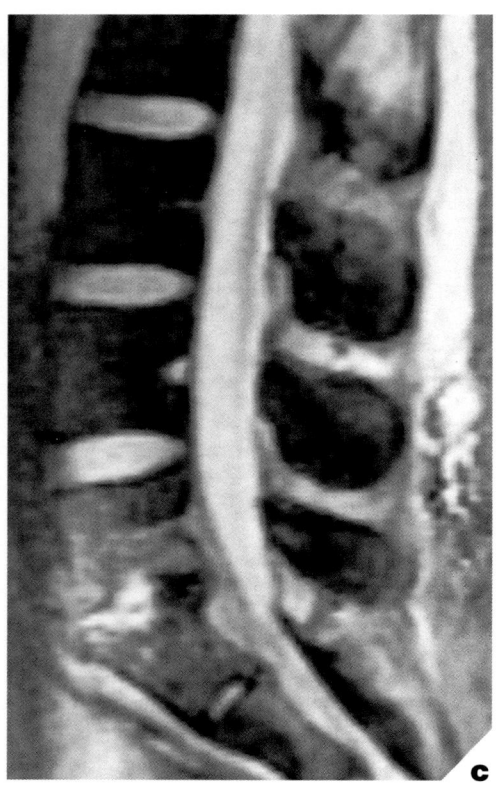

Figure 9.1

*Discitis, osteomyelitis and epidural abscess. **a** A plain film lateral view shows loss of height of the L5/S1 intervertebral disc space plus marked irregularity of the inferior end plate of L5. **b** T1 and **c** T2 sagittal MR images show dark-T1, bright-T2 signal abnormality within the L5/S1 intervertebral disc and within the adjacent vertebral endplates. There is considerable signal abnormality within the anterior portion of the entire L5 ver-tebral body. **d,e** CT scans obtained following instillation of intrathecal contrast material show marked irregularity and destruction of the superior endplate of S1. There is a large intraspinal extension of soft tissue compressing the caudal thecal sac and represents an epidural empyema. Epidural empyema is also demonstrated on **f** axial T1-unenhanced and **g** Gadolinium-DTPA-enhanced images as a diffuse, enhancing epidural mass.*

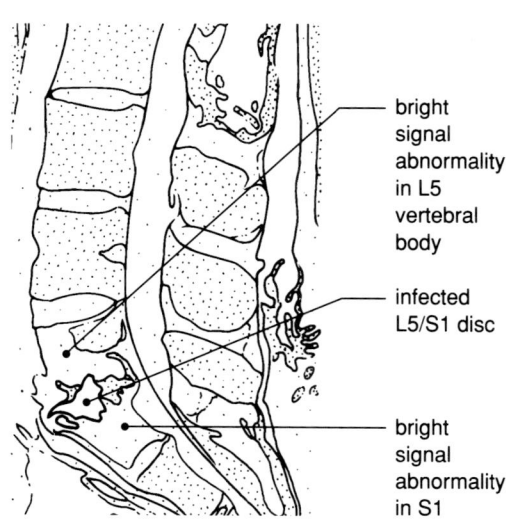

bright signal abnormality in L5 vertebral body

infected L5/S1 disc

bright signal abnormality in S1

BACTERIAL INFECTIONS

Discitis/Osteomyelitis

Loss of height and integrity of the disc plus marked irregularity of the adjacent endplates is the hallmark of infectious discitis (Fig. 9.1). This is well evaluated by most imaging modalities. Plain films show loss of height of the disc space with irregularity and rarefaction of the adjacent endplates. A paraspinal or prevertebral soft tissue mass may be seen when a soft tissue abscess develops. MRI is the most sensitive method since it detects dark-T1, bright-T2 signal abnormalities within the intervertebral disc and vertebral endplates in the early stages of the disease. A nuclear medicine (Technetium) bone scan is also more sensitive than plain films in the detection of early infectious spondylitis. Computed tomography excels in its ability to accurately delineate endplate destruction and paraspinal abscesses.

Staphylococcus aureus is the most common cause of bacterial infection of the spine. Other common bacterial organisms include *Streptococci, E. Coli,* and *Pseudomonas. Salmonella* is common in patients with sickle cell disease.

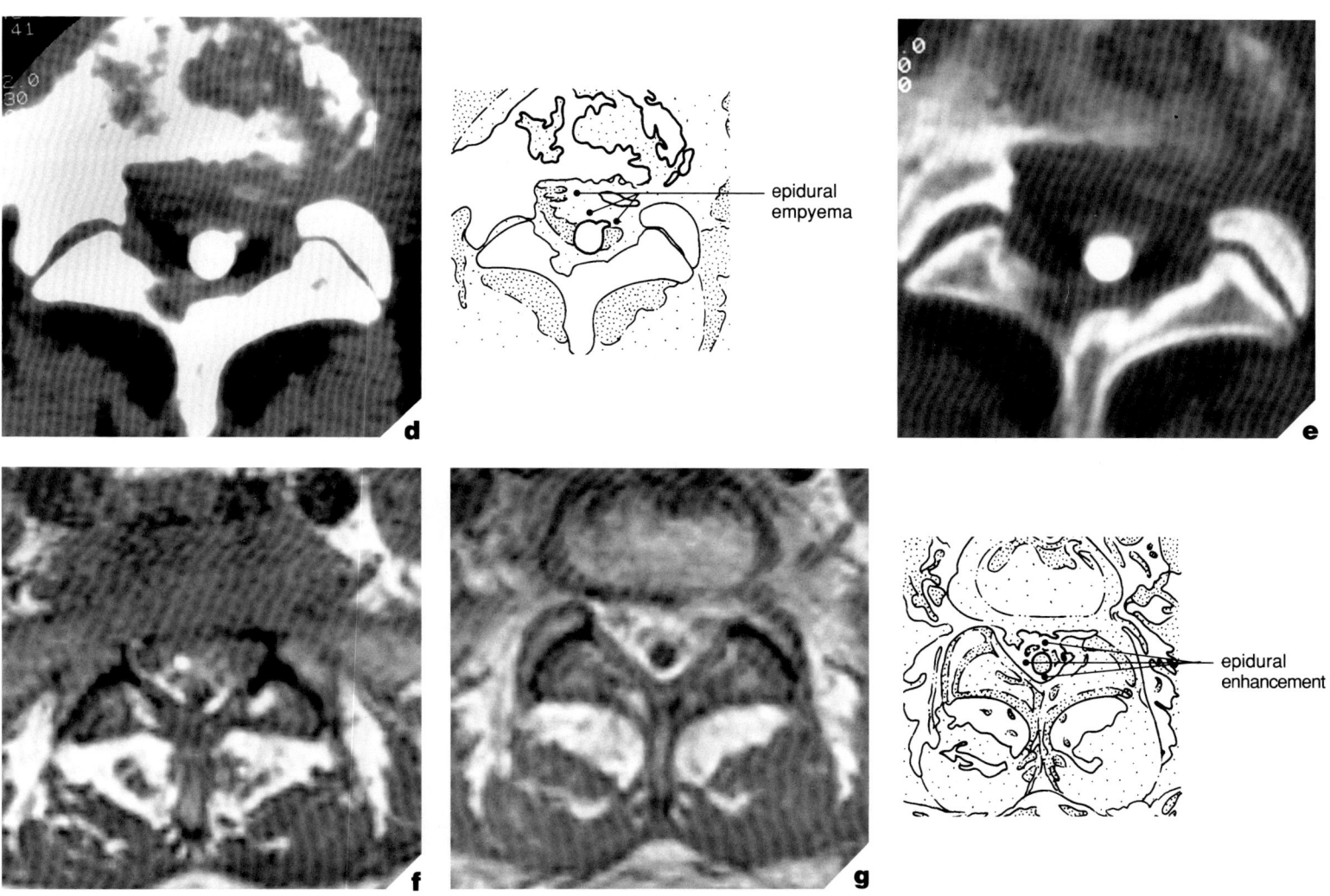

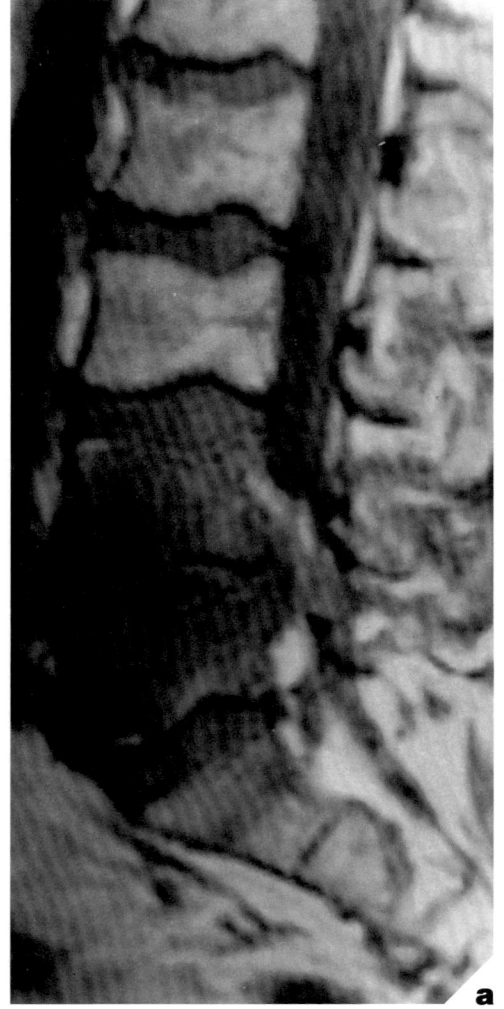

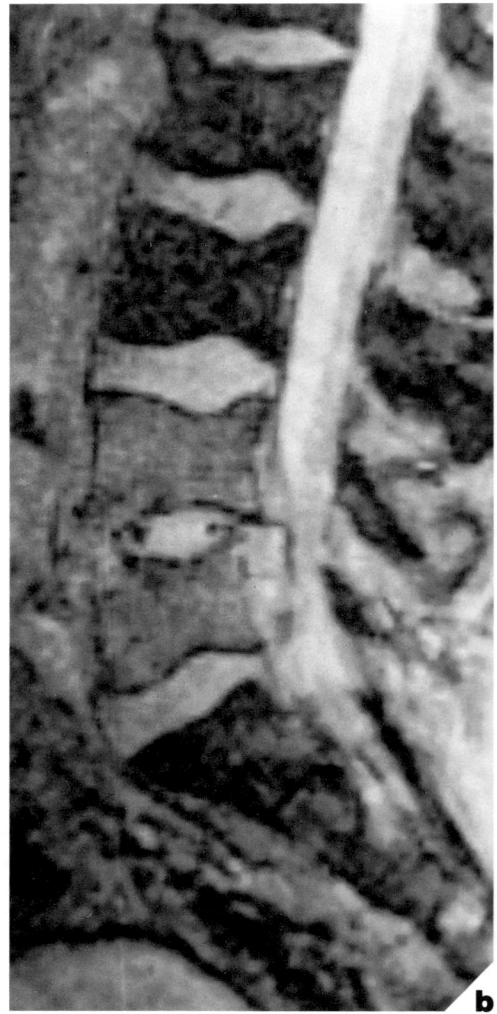

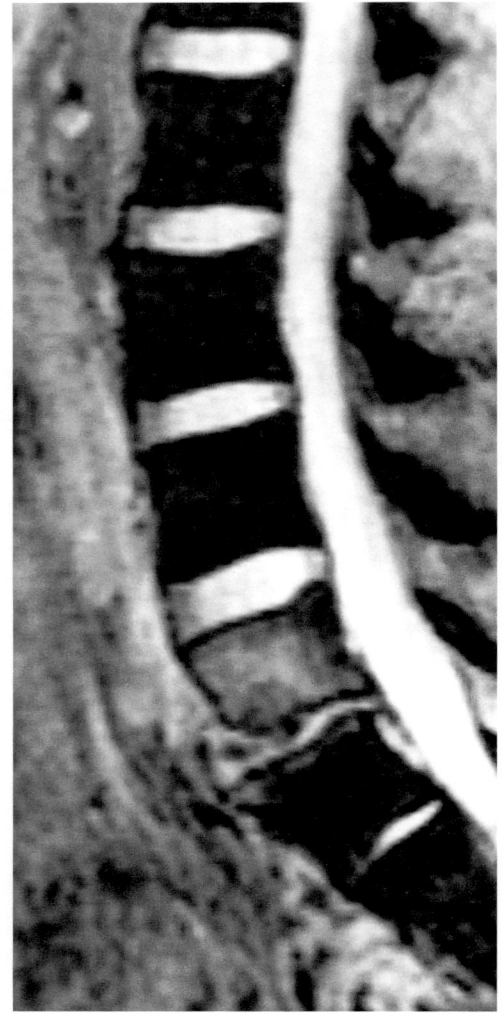

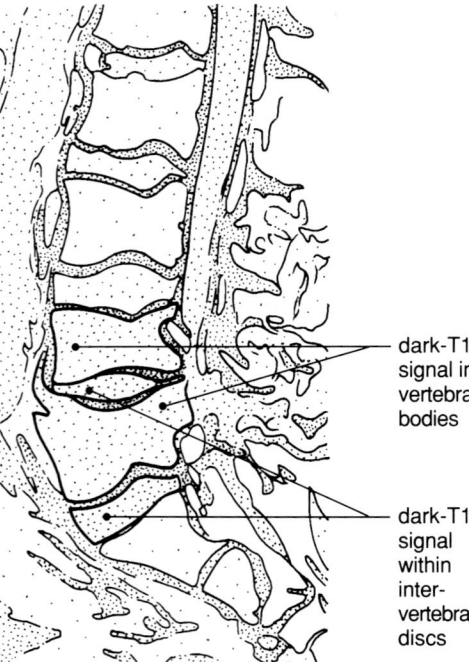

dark-T1 signal in vertebral bodies

dark-T1 signal within inter-vertebral discs

Figure 9.2

Osteomyelitis/discitis. **a** *Sagittal T1 and* **b** *T2 MR images demonstrate dark-T1, bright-T2 signal abnormality within the L4 and L5 vertebral bodies representing osteomyelitis. In addition, dark-T1 signal abnormality is seen within the L4/5 and L5/S1 intervertebral discs indicating discitis.*

Figure 9.3

Osteomyelitis/discitis. T2-weighted sagittal MR image demonstrates decreased height of the L5/S1 intervertebral disc, endplate irregularity and T2-bright signal abnormality within the L5 vertebral body. There is extension of infectious tissue anteriorly at the level of L5/S1 into the paraspinal soft tissues.

The causes of bacterial infections of the spine include hematogenous extension from nearby or remote infections including skin lesions, retroperitoneal abscesses, and pharyngeal abscesses. Organisms may be directly introduced by trauma, spinal puncture, or surgery.

Although intervertebral disc infection is nearly always present early, osteomyelitis of one or more vertebral bodies may become the dominant feature (Figs. 9.2, 9.3). There may be collapse of the vertebral body, usually producing a wedge-shaped deformity.

Spinal Abscess

Paravertebral abscess formation frequently occurs. The diagnosis may be confirmed by CT-guided needle aspiration. When discitis or vertebral osteomyelitis extends into the spinal canal, an epidural abscess (see Fig. 9.1d) is formed. This may result in spinal cord or nerve root compression and usually requires prompt surgical drainage. Occasionally, an epidural abscess will form without any associated discitis or vertebral osteomyelitis.

Intradural empyema and inflammatory arachnoiditis may occur secondary to epidural empyema formation, spinal puncture, or surgery. This may be difficult to distinguish from epidural empyema.

SPINAL TUBERCULOSIS

Spinal tuberculosis results in fairly characteristic radiographic changes, often allowing a specific diagnosis to be suggested. It usually results from extension of pulmonary or renal tuberculosis. Myobacterium tuberculosis typically first involves the anterior portion of a vertebral body and then extends anteriorly to create a paraspinal abscess (Fig 9.4). The my-

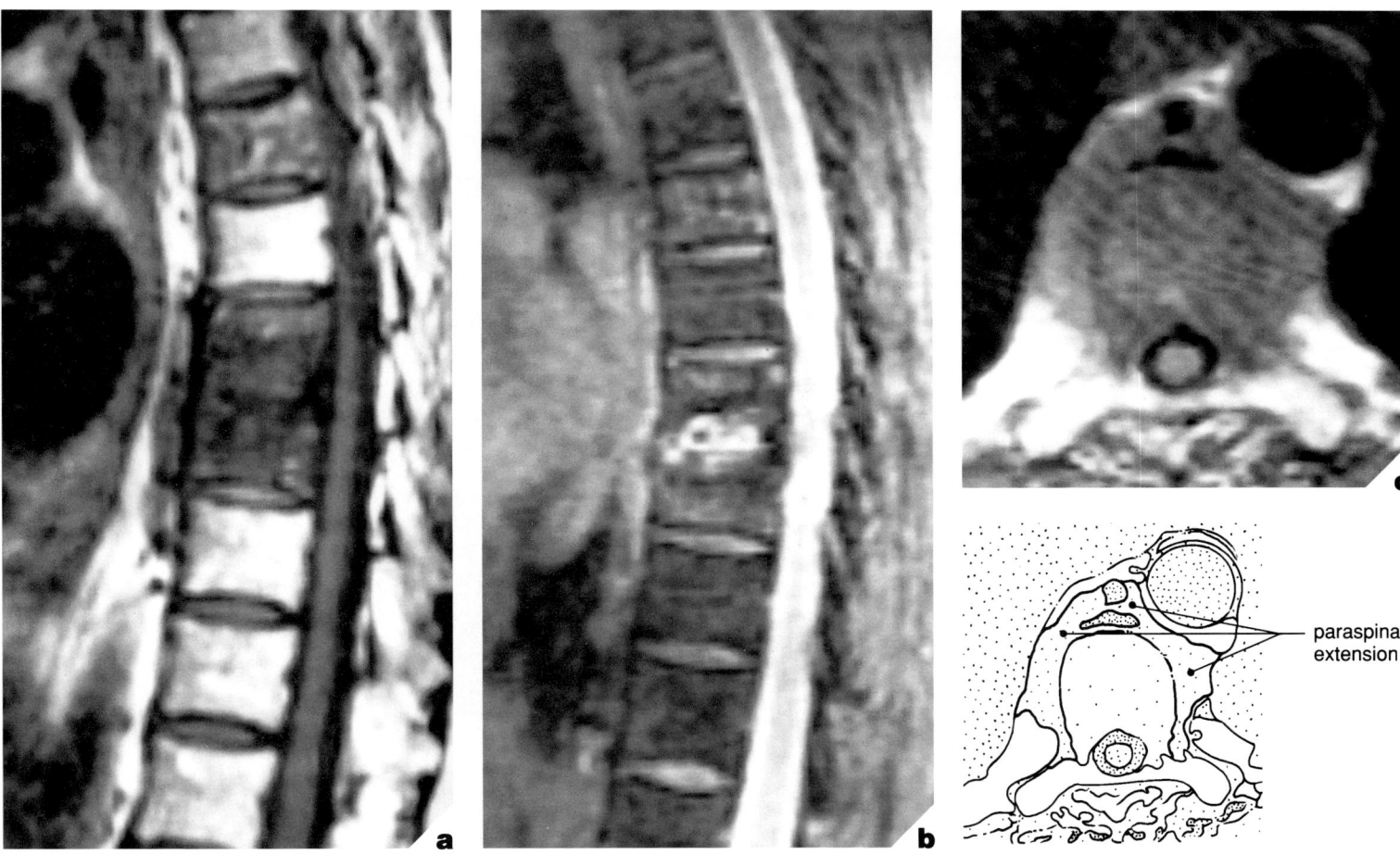

paraspinal
extension

Figure 9.4

Spinal tuberculosis. **a** *Sagittal T1 and* **b** *T2 and* **c** *axial T1-weighted images of the lower thoracic spine demonstrate signal abnormality within multiple adjacent and separated vertebral bodies. A paraspinal mass is demonstrated anteriorly* *which allows for extension of infectious material beneath the anterior longitudinal ligament to other levels. There is associated discitis; this is usually a late finding in tuberculosis of the spine.*

cobacteria extend beneath the anterior longitudinal ligament and often involve vertebral bodies above and/or below the primarily infected vertebrae. The most common site of involvement is the lower thoracic spine. There is often collapse of the anterior portions of one or more thoracic vertebral bodies, producing the characteristic gibbus deformity (Fig. 9.5). Unlike pyogenic infections, discitis is usually not a dominant feature of spinal tuberculosis and may only occur late in the disease.

MISCELLANEOUS SPINAL INFECTIONS

Nonbacterial infections of the spine are most common in immunocompromised individuals. These include fungi such as *Cryptococcus neoformans* and *Coccidioides immitis*, which commonly affect AIDS patients. Parasitic infection of the spine by *Echinococcus* or *Cysticercosis* is rare. The site of infection may be extradural, intradural/extramedullary or even intramedullary.

Spinal Meningitis

Spinal bacterial meningitis may produce the characteristic meningeal enhancement similar to that which occurs in the meninges overlying the brain (see Chapter 3). Viral meningitis usually produces no radiographic abnormalities and evaluation of CSF chemistry and viral studies is usually required for diagnosis. Noninfectious arachnoiditis may occur following instillation of certain types of contrast material into the subarachnoid space.

Sarcoidosis

Sarcoidosis may result in granulomatous invasion of the meninges or spinal cord. It is difficult to distinguish from infectious processes. Correlation with chest radiographs is usually helpful.

Transverse Myelitis

Acute transverse myelitis is an idiopathic disorder which may produce widening of the spinal cord on

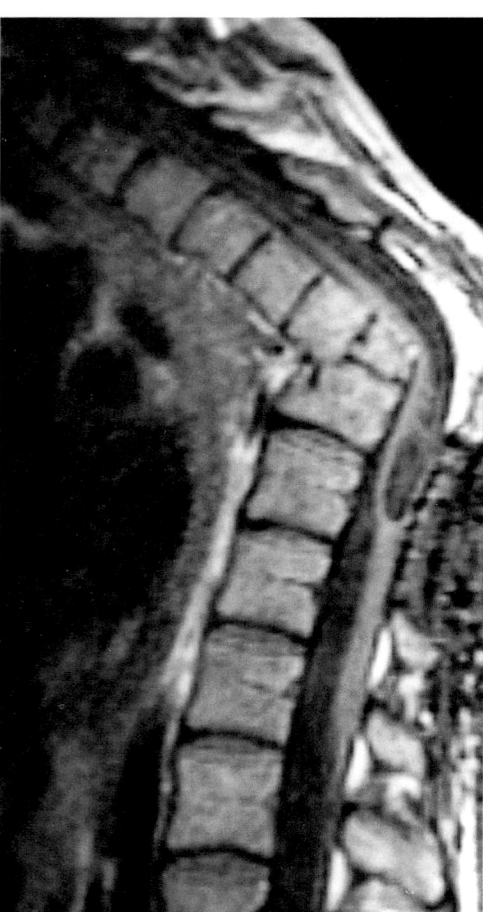

Figure 9.5
Spinal tuberculosis with gibbus deformity. Complete destruction of the anterior portion of a midthoracic vertebral body resulting in a sharply angled kyphosis (gibbus deformity) is shown on this T1-weighted sagittal MR image. The posterior vertebral body remnant is displaced into the spinal canal where it compresses an atrophic spinal cord. There is cystic change within the spinal cord at and distal to the site of involvement.

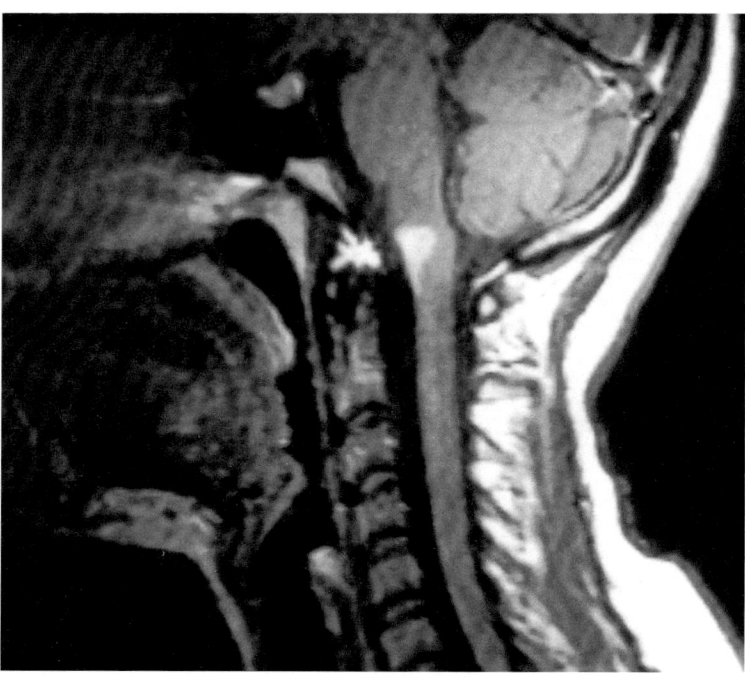

Figure 9.6
Multiple sclerosis plaque. Gadolinium-enhanced T1-weighted image demonstrates a large, intramedullary, active focus of demyelination at the cervical–medullary junction.

myelography or MRI. Typically, no focal signal abnormality is demonstrated. This disorder usually affects young adults.

MULTIPLE SCLEROSIS

Demyelinating lesions ("plaques") in the spinal cord are commonly demonstrated at autopsy in patients with multiple sclerosis. However, they remain somewhat elusive to MRI. Large, solitary (Fig. 9.6) or smaller, multifocal lesions (Fig. 9.7) may be demonstrated on high-field, T2-weighted MR images. Although these lesions might be difficult to distinguish from infectious or neoplastic disorders of the spinal cord, correlation with the patient's brain MRI usually reveals lesions in the characteristic locations of multiple sclerosis plaques.

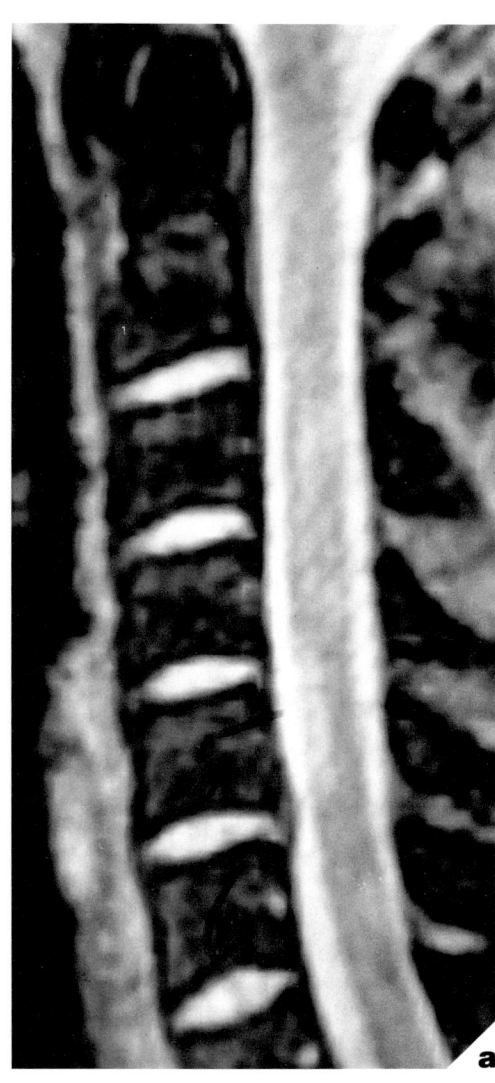

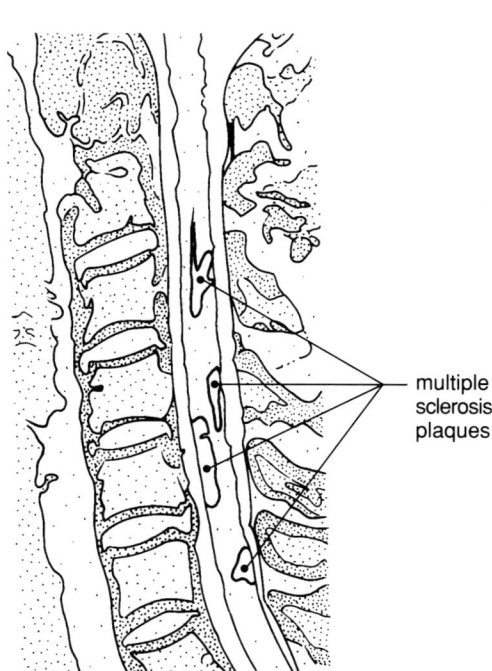

multiple
sclerosis
plaques

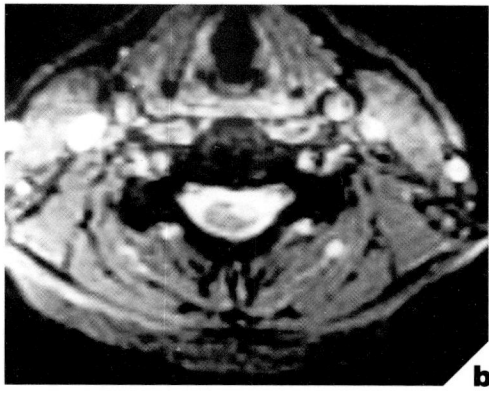

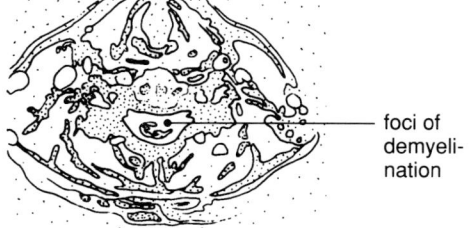

foci of
demyeli-
nation

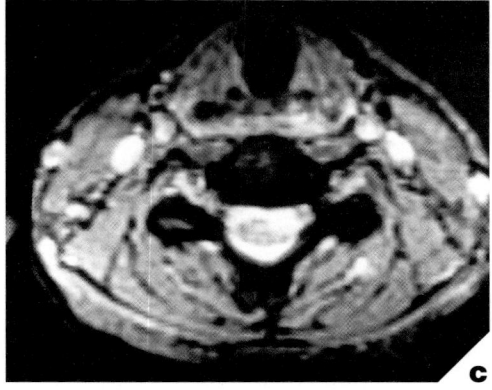

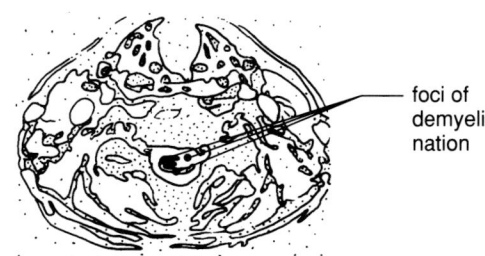

foci of
demyeli-
nation

Figure 9.7

*Numerous multiple sclerosis plaques in the cervical spinal cord. T2-weighted **a** sagittal and **b, c** axial MR images of the cervical spinal cord show numerous large and small intramedullary bright-T2 foci of signal abnormality in this patient with known multiple sclerosis. Incidentally demonstrated is a mild central disc bulge and associated posterior osteophyte formation at C5/6.*

Inflammatory Diseases of the Spine

10

Neoplastic Diseases of the Spine

eoplasms of the spine represent a diverse group of disorders ranging from primary malignancies of the spinal cord to benign bony tumors of the posterior elements. Statistically, metastases comprise the most important single category of spinal tumors. As with other types of spinal lesions, involvement of the central spinal canal or neural foramina is key in determining the presence and type of neurologic signs and symptoms.

Astrocytomas of the spinal cord are most common in the cervical region and progressively decrease in frequency caudally. In contrast, ependymomas are most common at the caudal end of the neural axis. Whatever the cell type, intramedullary gliomas demonstrate widening of the spinal cord, conus medullaris, or filum terminale. MRI usually demonstrates dark-T1, bright-T2 signal abnormality (Fig. 10.1).

Cyst formation or syringohydromyelia occurs in approximately one-third of astrocytomas. Ring or

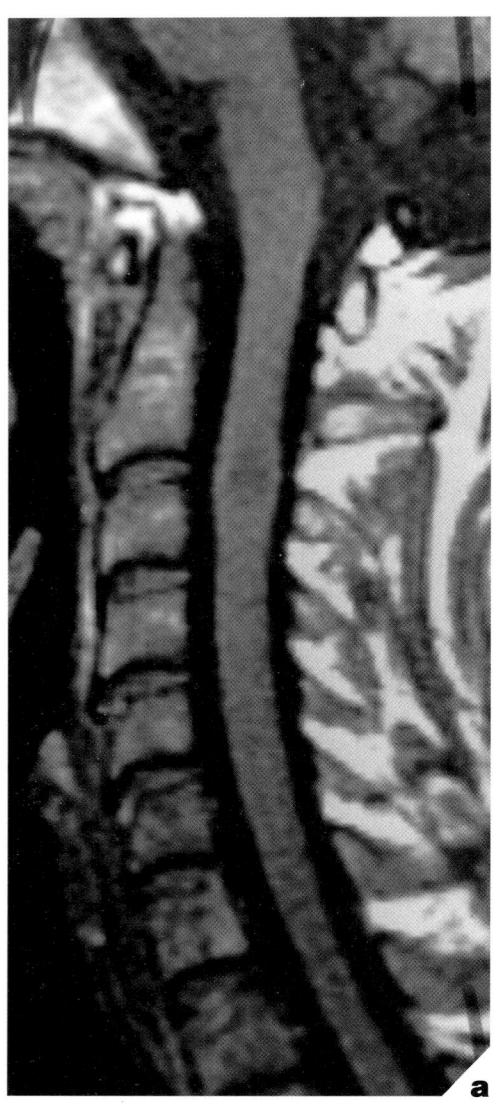
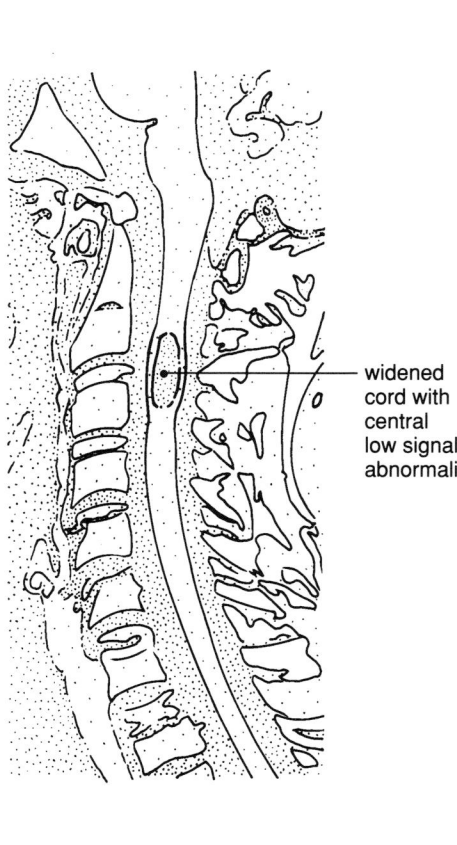

widened cord with central low signal abnormality

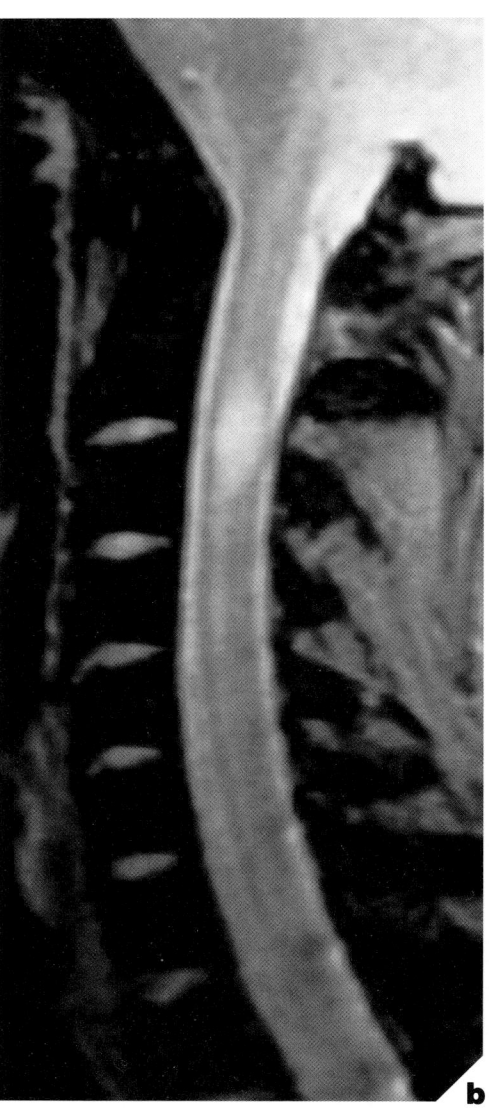

Figure 10.1

*Cervical spinal cord astrocytoma. **a** Sagittal T1- and **b** T2-weighted MR images show focal widening of the spinal cord at the level of C2/C3 and dark-T1, bright-T2 signal abnormality within the spinal cord at this level.*

nodular enhancement following intravenous administration of Gadolinium-DTPA may be seen with MR imaging. Myelography usually shows widening of the spinal cord which, when large, may result in a block of flow of intrathecal contrast medium (Fig. 10.2). Slow-growing infiltrative lesions may cause scalloping of the posterior margins of the vertebral bodies and thinning and lateral displacement of the pedicles and lamina.

Astrocytomas of the spinal cord are usually of the infiltrative type and therefore low-grade. Glioblastoma multiforme and oligodendroglioma of the spinal cord are very uncommon.

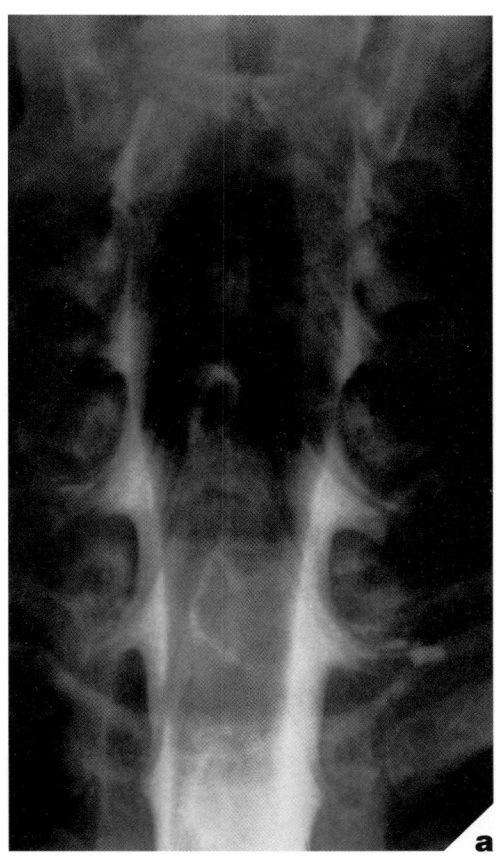
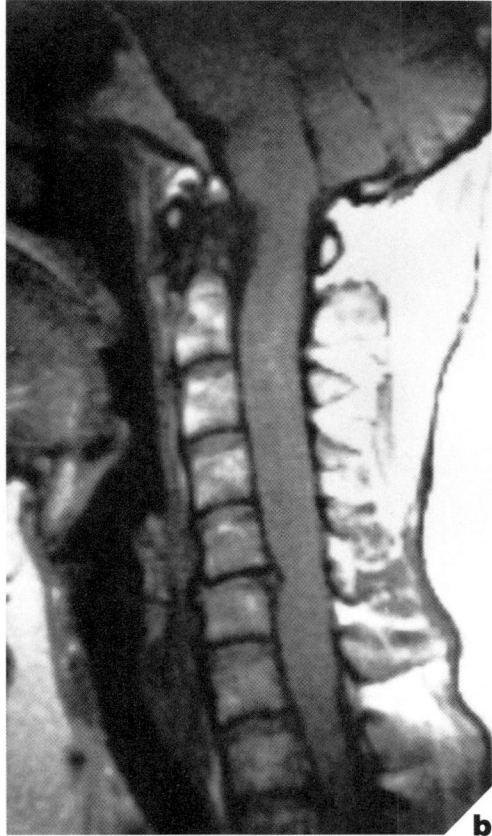
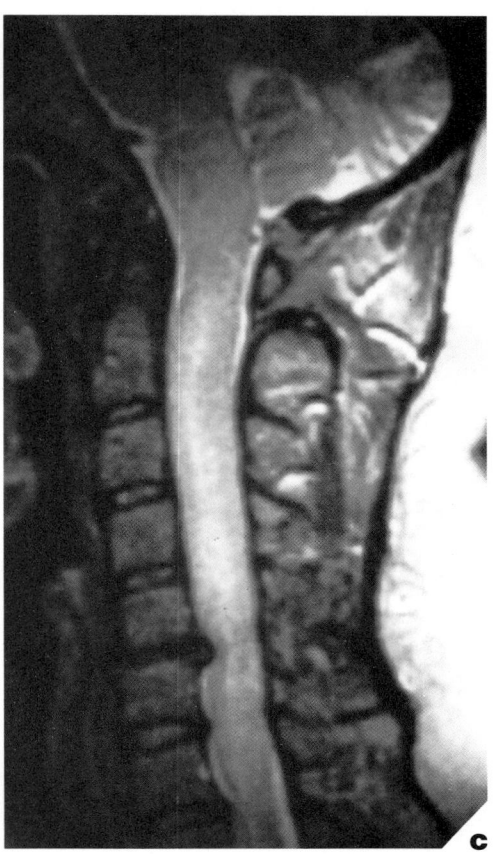

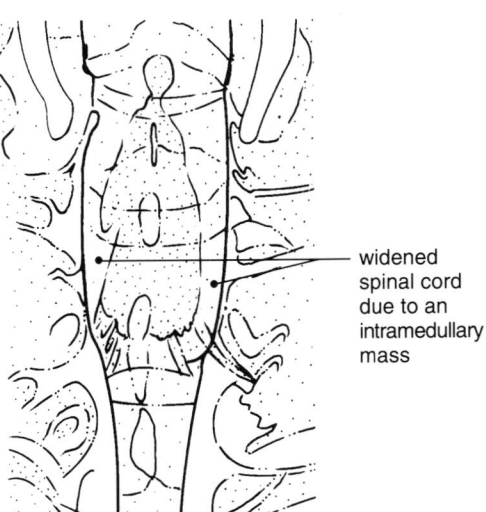

widened spinal cord due to an intramedullary mass

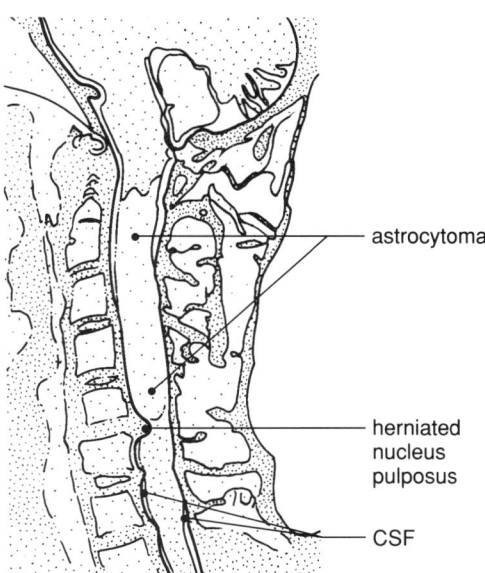

astrocytoma

herniated nucleus pulposus

CSF

Figure 10.2

Cervical spinal cord astrocytoma.
*a This cervical myelogram shows a large intramedullary mass and a complete block to flow of contrast medium at the level of C5. These findings are confirmed on sagittal **b** T1- and **c** T2- weighted MR images of the cervical spine. This infiltrative glioma extends from the cervical-medullary junction through the level of T1. There is no cerebral spinal fluid signal demonstrated between C2 and C6. Incidentally demonstrated is a large central disc herniation at the level of C5/C6 which compresses the tumor.*

Neoplastic Diseases of the Spine

Ependymomas are the most common type of spinal glioma. They are rare in the cervical cord and tend to predominate in the conus medullaris (Fig. 10.3) or filum terminale (Fig. 10.4), and are usually better demarcated from the surrounding normal neural tissue than infiltrating astrocytomas. Contrast enhancement on MRI is common. Ependymomas are usually hypervascular; they may bleed and cause spinal subarachnoid hemorrhage. Cyst formation and syringohydromyelia occur in approximately one-half of ependymomas. Metastatic spread to other levels of the spinal cord, or less frequently, to the brain may occur. Likewise, an ependymoma of the spinal cord may represent a metastatic implant from a primary brain lesion, particularly posterior fossa tumors.

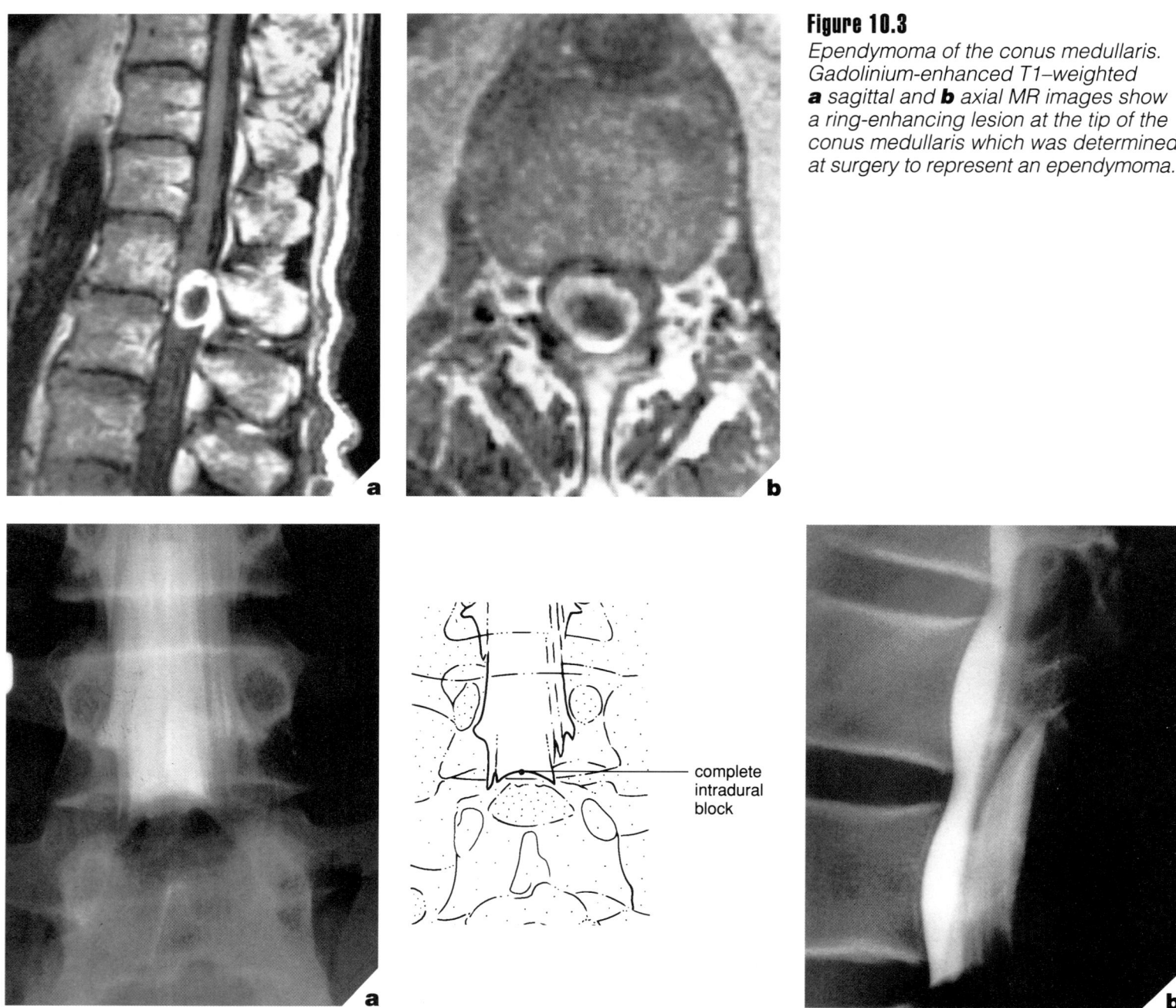

Figure 10.3

*Ependymoma of the conus medullaris. Gadolinium-enhanced T1–weighted **a** sagittal and **b** axial MR images show a ring-enhancing lesion at the tip of the conus medullaris which was determined at surgery to represent an ependymoma.*

complete
intradural
block

Figure 10.4

*Ependymoma of filum terminale. **a** AP and **b** lateral films from a myelogram show a complete block of flow of contrast medium at L4/L5 by an intradural mass. At surgery this was proven to be an ependymoma of the filum terminale.*

METASTATIC DISEASE

Metastatic disease represents the most common form of neoplastic disease of the spine. Most lesions involve the pedicles (Fig. 10.5) and vertebral bodies. Lesions may be grossly destructive (Fig. 10.6) or mostly infiltrative. Bony lesions which arise from malignancies of the lung, kidney, thyroid gland, and melanoma are usually lytic. Prostate and gastrointestinal tract metastases are usually blastic in nature. Breast metastases may be mixed or predominantly either lytic or blastic. MRI is the procedure of choice in evaluating spinal metastases.

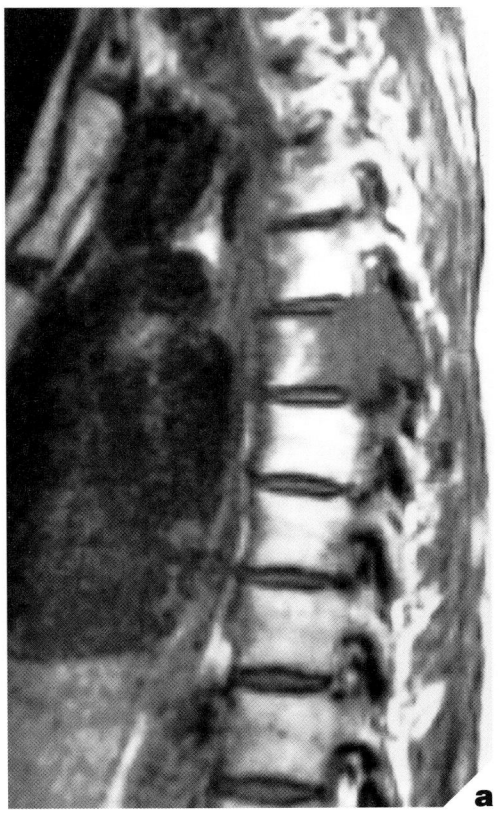

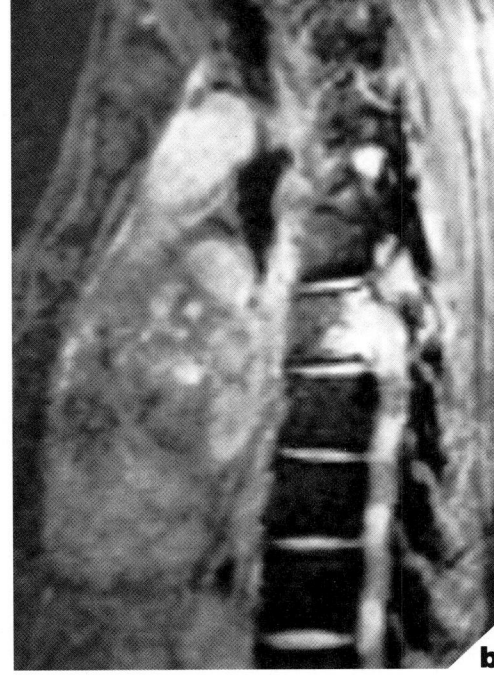

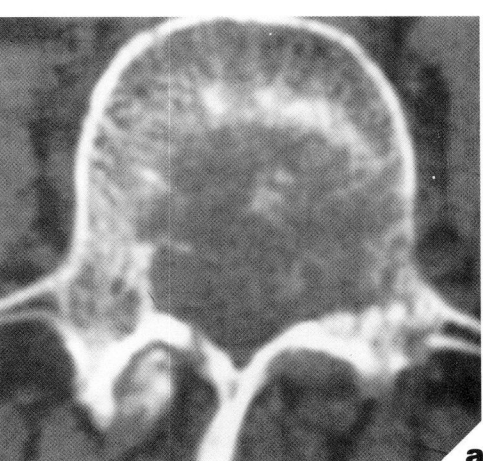

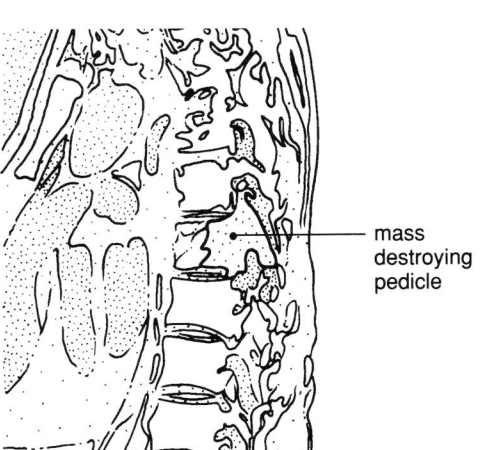

mass destroying pedicle

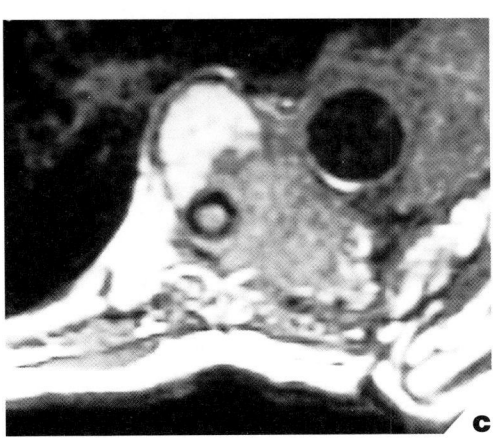

Figure 10.5

*Spinal metastases. Sagittal **a** T1 and **b** T2 and **c** axial T1-weighted images show metastatic disease to the spine from a bronchogenic carcinoma of the lung. There is predominantly involvement of the left pedicle of T5 with extension into the posterior portion of the left side of the T5 vertebral body and into the paraspinal soft tissues. Metastatic disease to the spine typically involves the pedicles first.*

Figure 10.6

*Spinal metastases. **a,b** CT scans through the L3 vertebral body demonstrate a grossly destructive lytic metastasis which has resulted in fracture of the posterior third of the vertebral body and left pedicle and posterior extension of bony and soft tissue material into the spinal canal.*

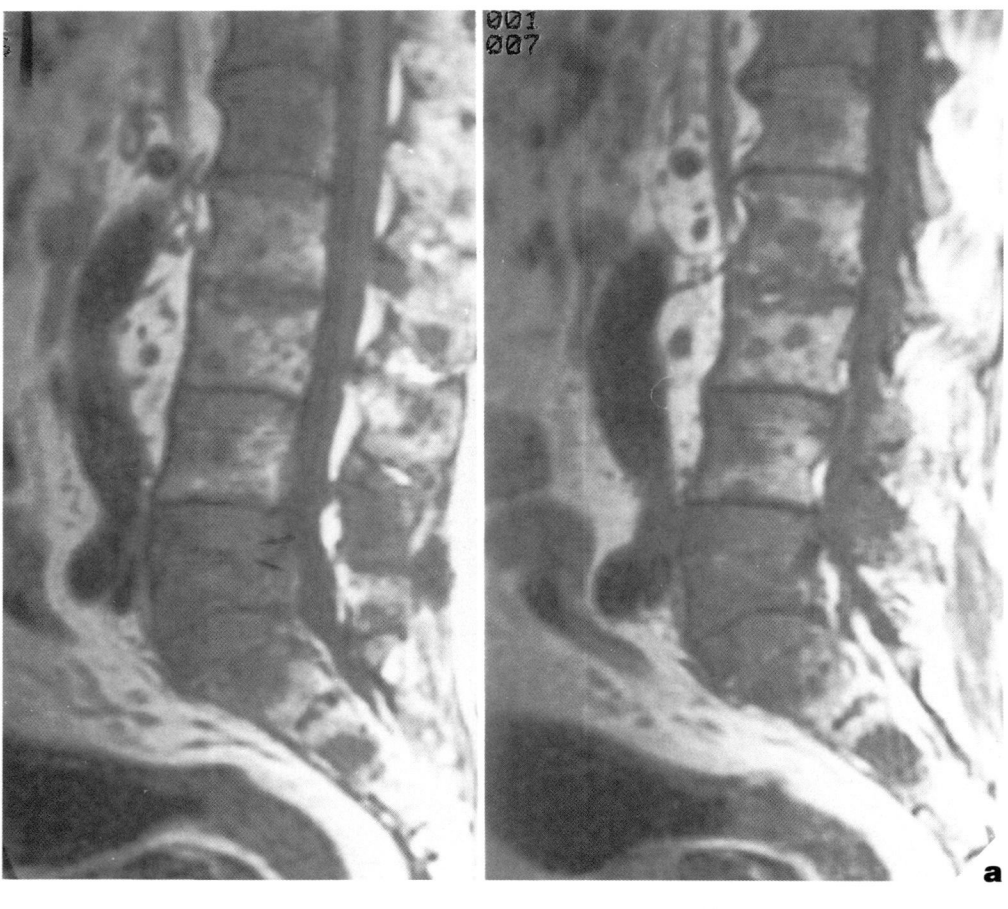

a

Figure 10.7

*Extensive metastases to the spine without spinal canal compression. Innumerable destructive lesions are demonstrated within the **a** lumbar spine, sacrum, and **b** thoracic spine which are represented by areas of hypointensity on these T1-weighted images. There is no invasion of the spinal canal and the patient had no neurologic signs or symptoms.*

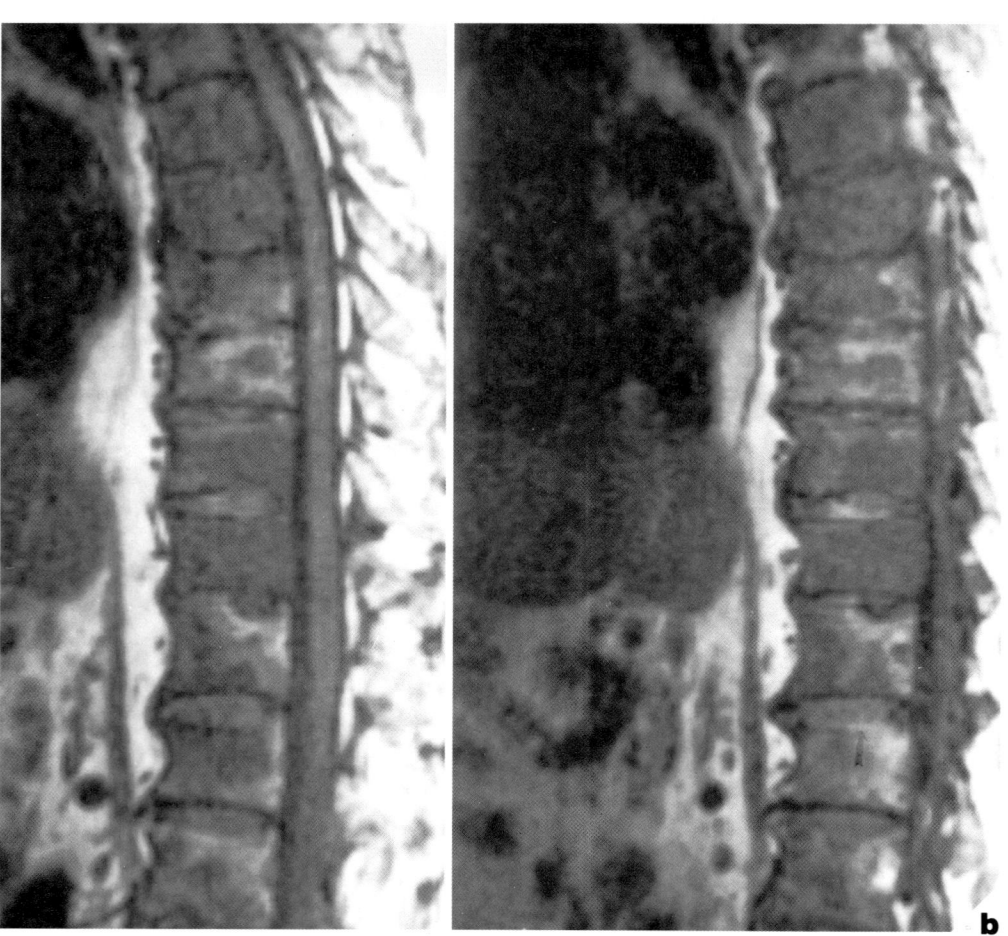

b

Metastatic disease of the spine may be quite extensive (Fig. 10.7) but only result in neurologic symptoms if there is invasion into the spinal canal. Paraspinal masses from metastatic disease are common and may develop rapidly (Fig. 10.8). Vertebral body compression (Fig. 10.9) frequently occurs and must be distinguished from compression fractures related to osteoporosis or trauma. Compression fractures due to osteoporosis are frequently wedge shaped and often only affect the anterior portion of the vertebral body. Neoplastic compression tends to predominate in the posterior portion of the vertebral body but there are many exceptions to this rule and considerable overlap exists.

Metastatic neuroblastoma frequently involves the spine (Fig. 10.10). Lesions arising in the sympathetic

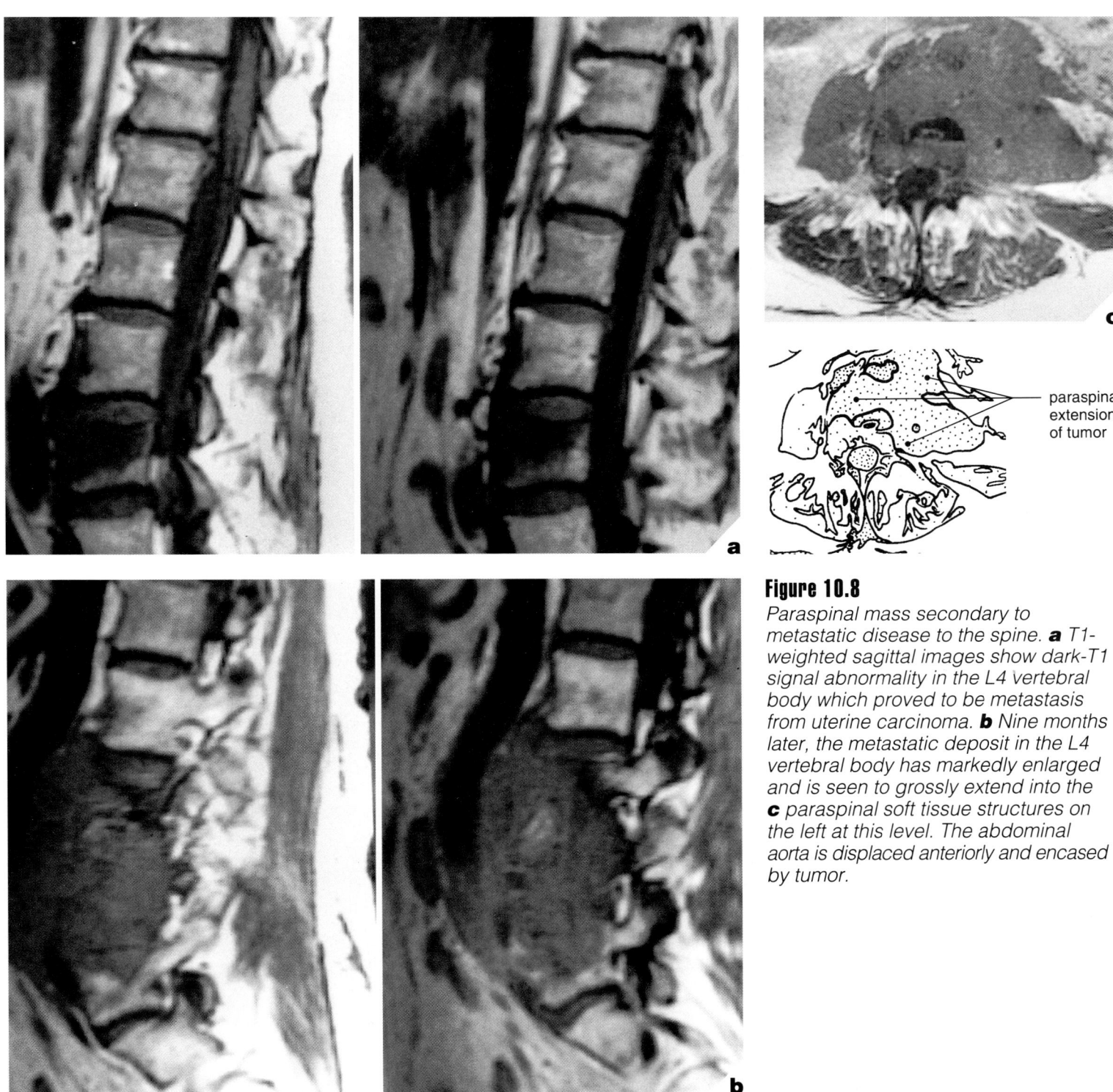

paraspinal extension of tumor

Figure 10.8

Paraspinal mass secondary to metastatic disease to the spine. **a** *T1-weighted sagittal images show dark-T1 signal abnormality in the L4 vertebral body which proved to be metastasis from uterine carcinoma.* **b** *Nine months later, the metastatic deposit in the L4 vertebral body has markedly enlarged and is seen to grossly extend into the* **c** *paraspinal soft tissue structures on the left at this level. The abdominal aorta is displaced anteriorly and encased by tumor.*

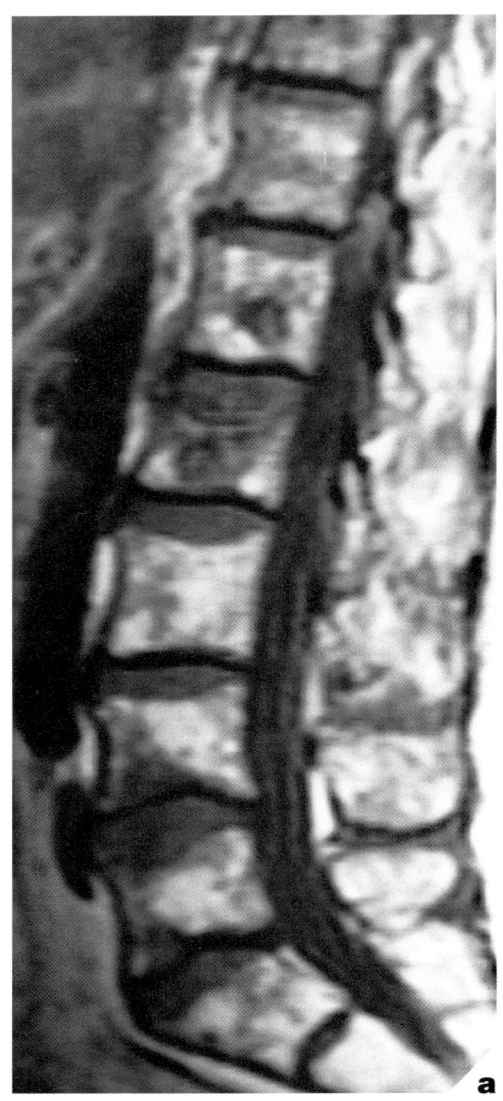
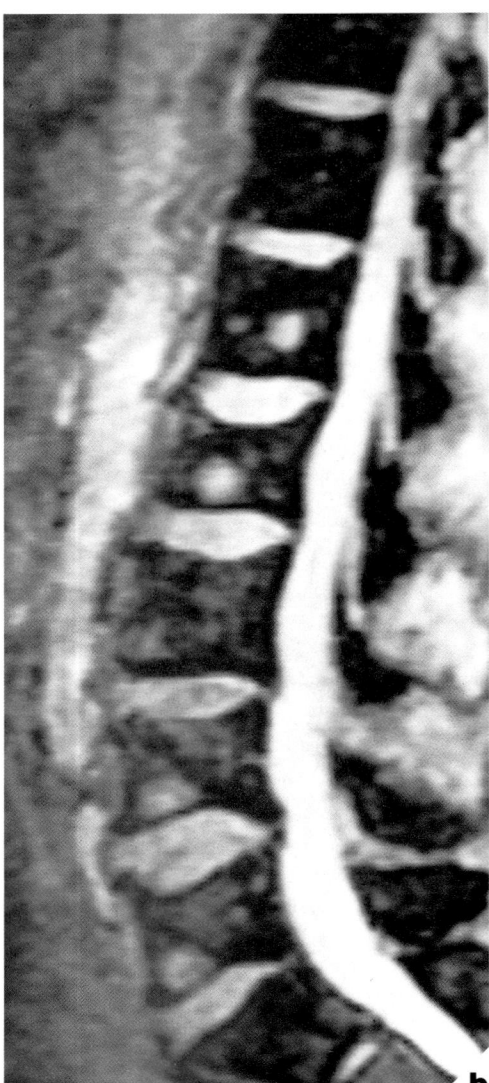
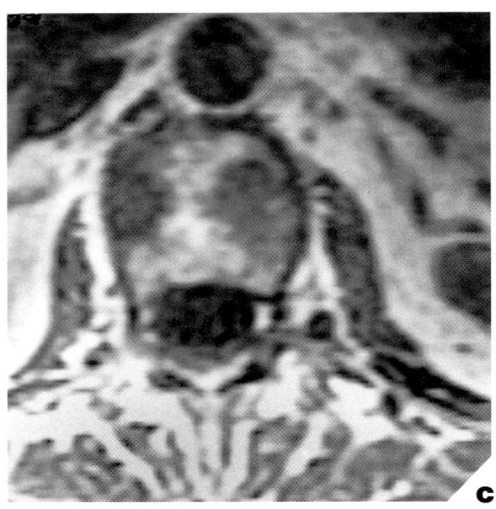
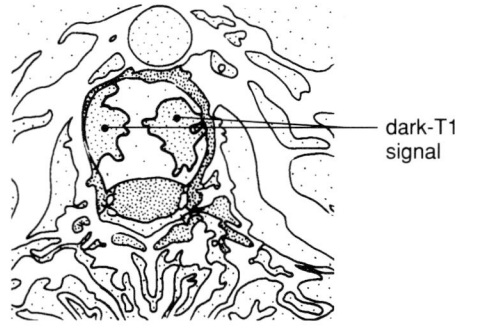

c

dark-T1 signal

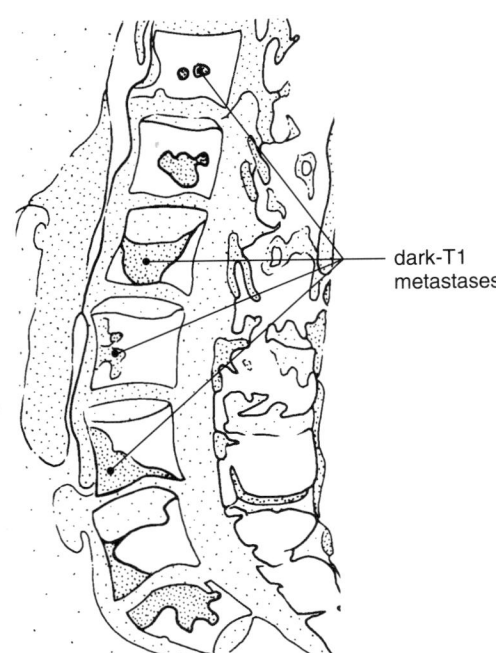

dark-T1 metastases

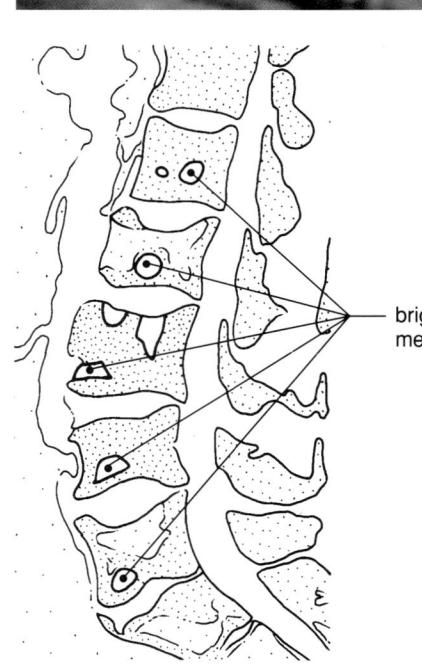

bright-T2 metastases

Figure 10.9

Metastatic disease to the spine with compression deformities. Sagittal a T1 and b T2 and c axial T1-weighted MR images of the lumbar spine show extensive metastatic disease manifested by characteristic hypointense-T1 and hyperintense-T2 signal abnormalities. Endplate compression deformities are noted at L2, L4, and L5. No intraspinal extension of tumor tissue is demonstrated.

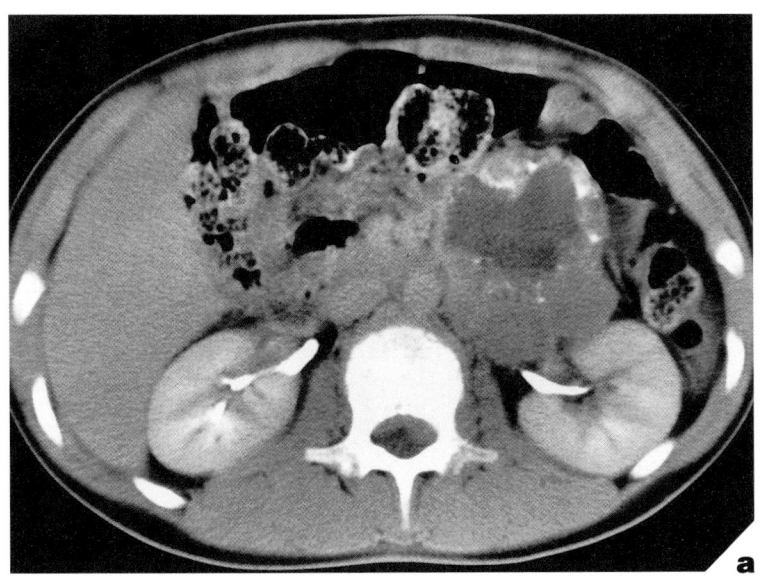

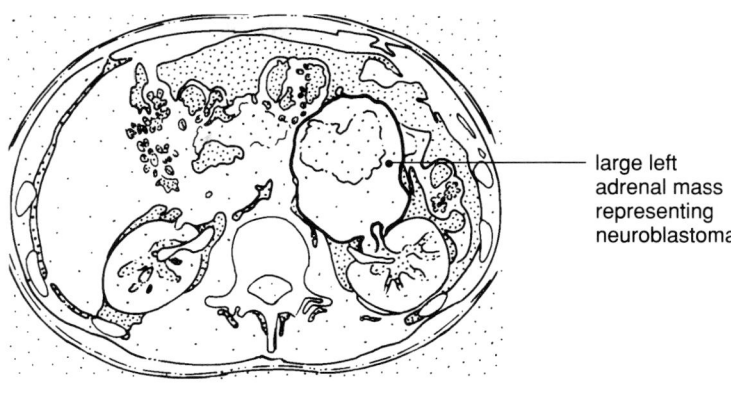

large left
adrenal mass
representing
neuroblastoma

a

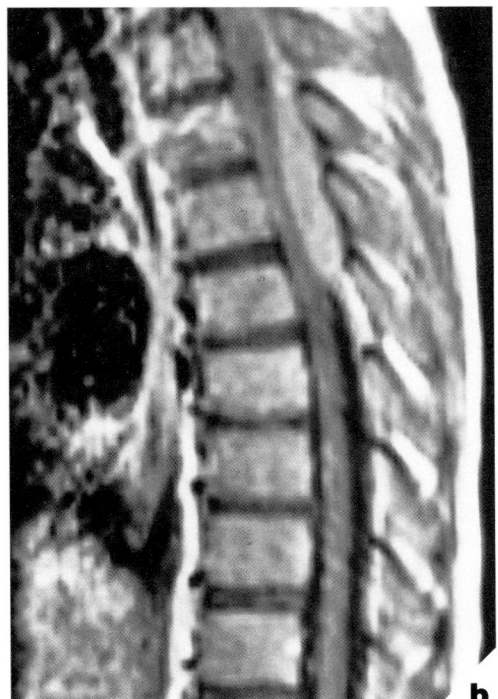

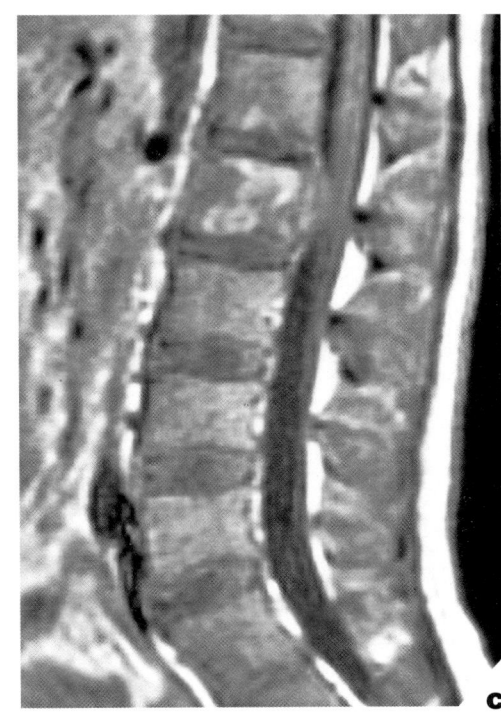

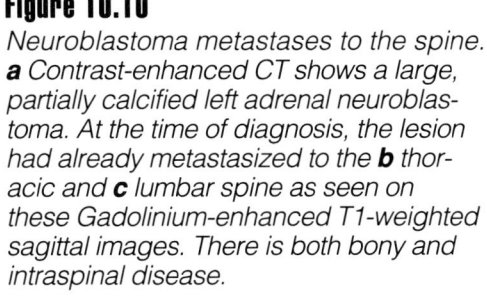

Figure 10.10

Neuroblastoma metastases to the spine.
a *Contrast-enhanced CT shows a large,
partially calcified left adrenal neuroblastoma. At the time of diagnosis, the lesion
had already metastasized to the **b** thoracic and **c** lumbar spine as seen on
these Gadolinium-enhanced T1-weighted
sagittal images. There is both bony and
intraspinal disease.*

b

c

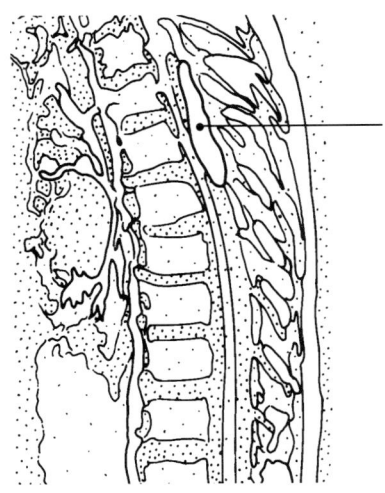

enhancing
intraspinal
neuro-
blastoma
metastasis

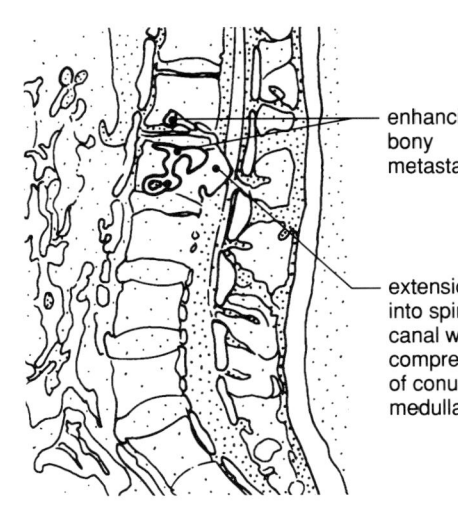

enhancing
bony
metastases

extension
into spinal
canal with
compression
of conus
medullaris

chain usually demonstrate a paraspinal mass. Neuroblastoma may spread into the spinal canal through a neural foramen. Such intraspinal extension (Fig. 10.11) usually produces scalloping of the posterior margins of nearby vertebral bodies. Leukemia (Fig. 10.12) results in diffuse vertebral demineralization which weakens the bone. This can result in compression fractures.

Radiation therapy changes in the spine usually create bright-T1 signal within the vertebrae. Following irradiation, active red marrow undergoes fatty degeneration and the marrow signal becomes increas-

ingly hyperintense on T1-weighted images. The involved areas are sharply demarcated from nonradiated areas (Fig. 10.13).

Although most metastatic disease of the spine involves the extradural tissue, subarachnoid and intramedullary metastases may also occur. Subarachnoid metastases are most commonly "drop" metastases from a posterior fossa medulloblastoma. Medulloblastoma metastases may be diffuse and plaque-like (Fig. 10.14) or they may be multiple, seed-like nodules (Fig 10.15) implanted within the subarachnoid space. There may be associated blastic

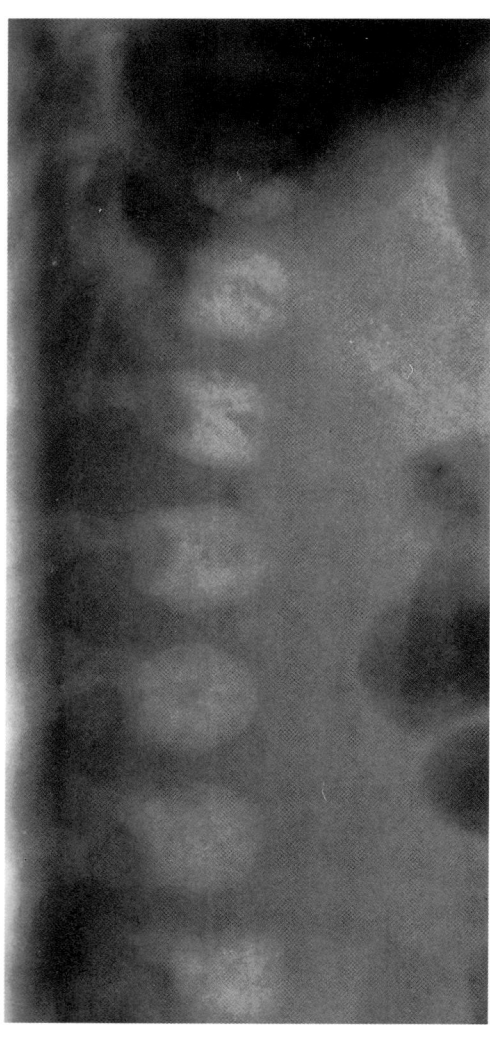

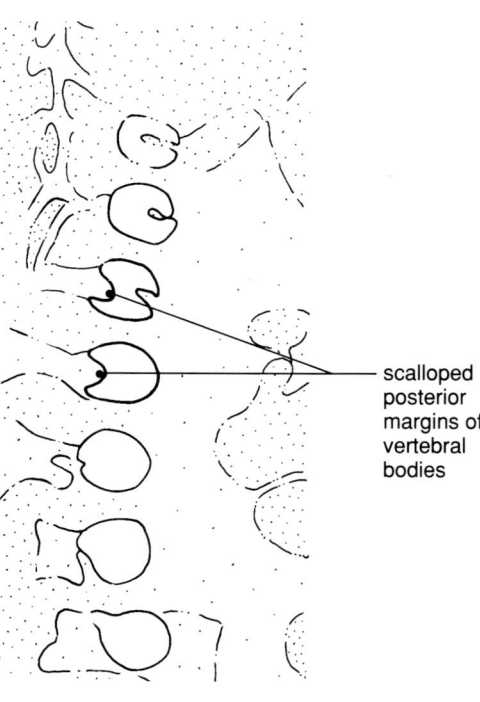

scalloped posterior margins of vertebral bodies

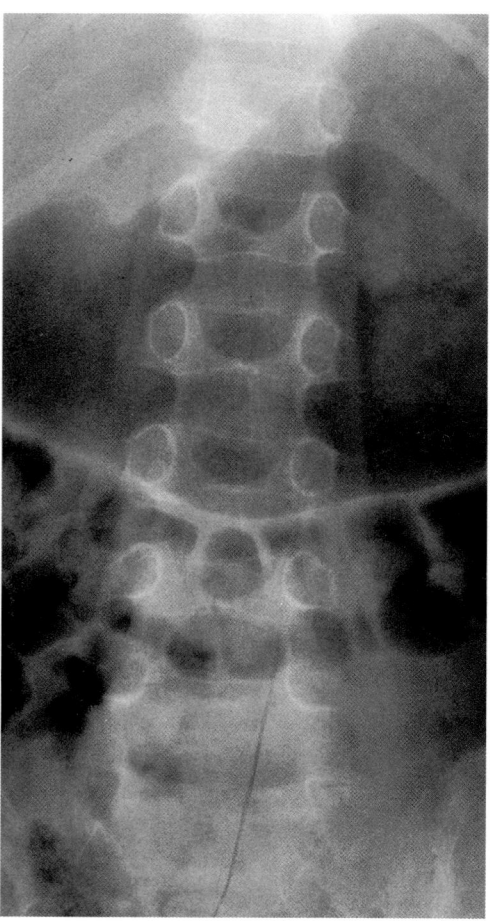

Figure 10.12

Acute lymphocytic leukemia. Lumbar spine film shows and diffuse bony demineralization and diminished height of most vertebral bodies.

Figure 10.11

Intraspinal neuroblastoma. Lateral plain film of the thoracolumbar spine shows posterior scalloping of several vertebral bodies caused by pressure erosion from metastatic neuroblastoma, which has invaded the central spinal canal.

bony medulloblastoma metastases. Drop metastases also result from ependymomas, choroid plexus papillomas, pineal tumors, meningiosarcomas, gliosarcomas, and glioblastoma multiforme. Intradural metastases may result from lung and breast carcinoma and melanoma. No matter what the cell type is, Gadolinium-enhanced MRI is essential for accurate evaluation of intradural metastases.

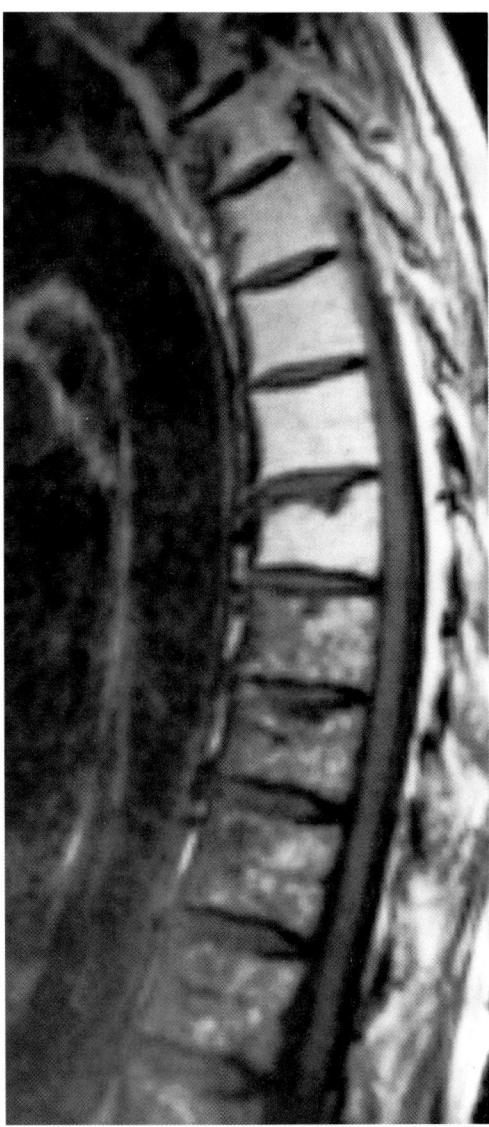

Figure 10.13

Radiation therapy changes to the spine. The thoracic vertebra to the level of T7 show hyperintensity on this T1-weighted image due to changes following radiation therapy. Below T7 there is extensive hypointense-T1 signal abnormality within the vertebral bodies due to metastatic disease. There is a mild anterior wedge-shaped compression deformity of T7. No intraspinal extension of tumor is demonstrated.

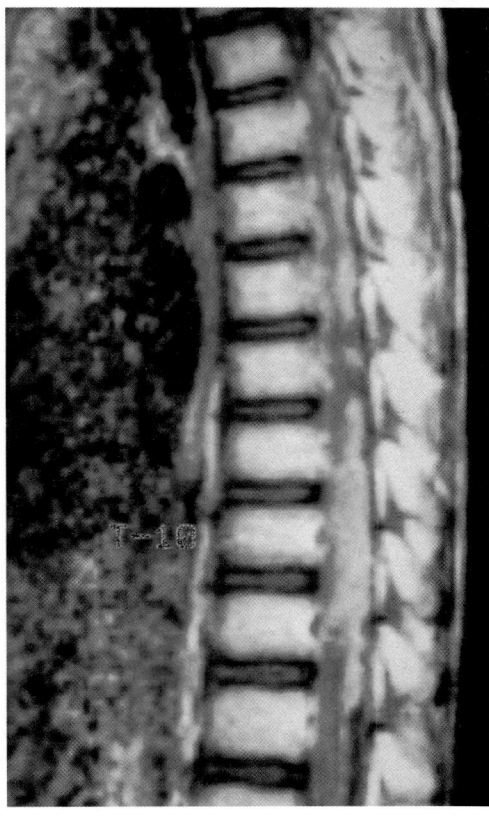

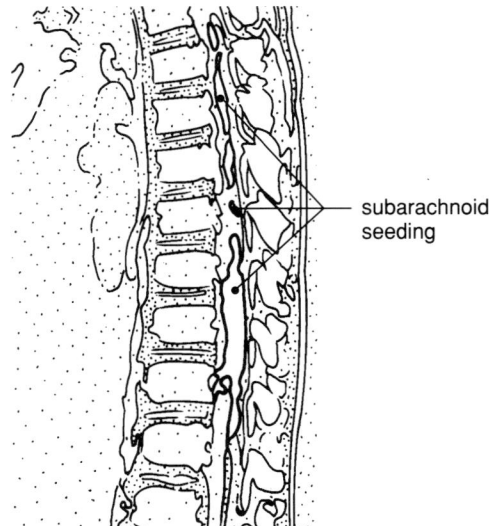

Figure 10.14

Subarachnoid metastases from medulloblastoma. Plaque-like areas of Gadolinium enhancement are demonstrated along the meninges in this patient with a posterior fossa medulloblastoma.

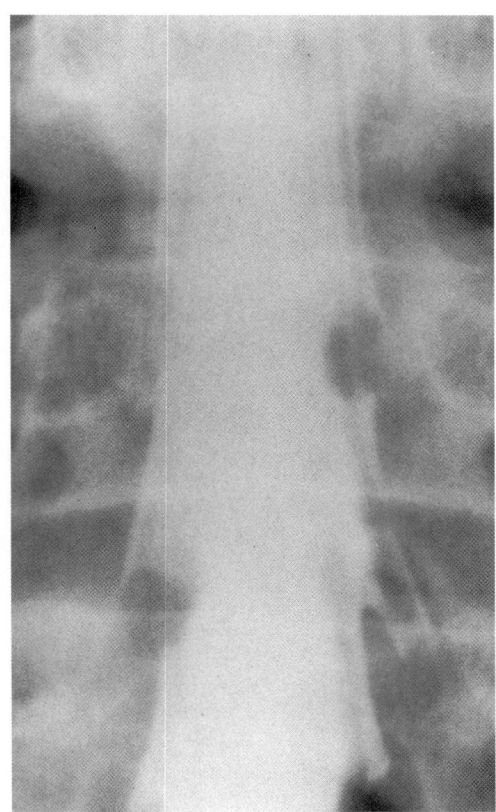

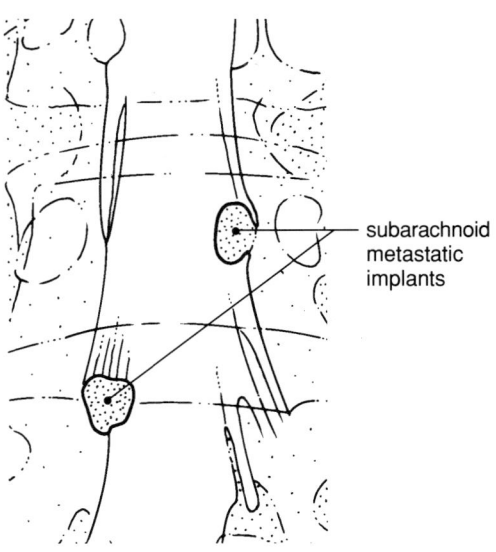

Figure 10.15

Metastatic implants from medulloblastoma. Several intradural, extramedullary nodular-shaped mass lesions are demonstrated along the course of nerve roots in the lumbar spine in this patient with medulloblastoma.

MULTIPLE MYELOMA

Multiple myeloma commonly involves the spine. Unlike metastatic disease, myeloma tends to primarily invade the vertebral bodies rather than the pedicles. Myeloma often results in osteopenia and compression fractures. Typically, there is a permeative type of bony demineralization (Fig 10.16). Blastic changes from myeloma occur in 1.5% of patients. Unlike spinal metastases, nuclear medicine bone scans may be normal in patients with multiple myeloma due to the lack of a significant reparative response.

LYMPHOMA

Lymphoma may involve the vertebra (Fig. 10.17), spinal extradural space, or rarely, the spinal cord. It is often associated with systemic lymphoma, particularly involving the retroperitoneal space. It has a greater propensity for the lumbar spine than other regions and may affect one or multiple levels. Dark-T1, bright-T2 signal abnormality is seen on MRI. There usually is enhancement following Gadolinium-DTPA administration.

MENINGIOMA

Spinal meningiomas occur most commonly in middle age: there is a 4:1 female:male predominance. They are most common in the thoracic spine, followed by the cranio-cervical junction and the cervical spine. The lesions frequently show calcification on CT but MRI is the ideal method of examination, particularly following Gadolinium-DTPA administration. Even without contrast, spinal meningiomas are easier to identify than their intracranial counterparts. Like intracranial meningiomas, spinal meningiomas may be represented by a nodular mass (Fig. 10.18) or

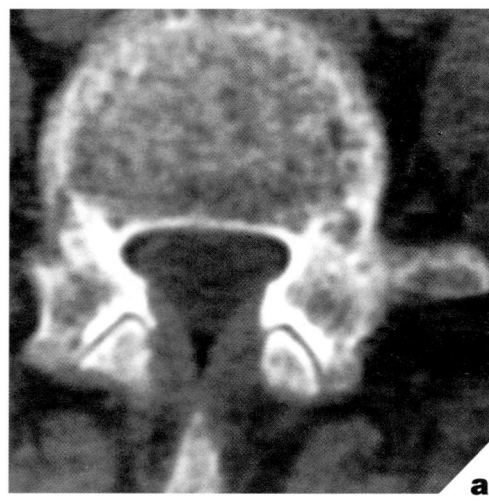
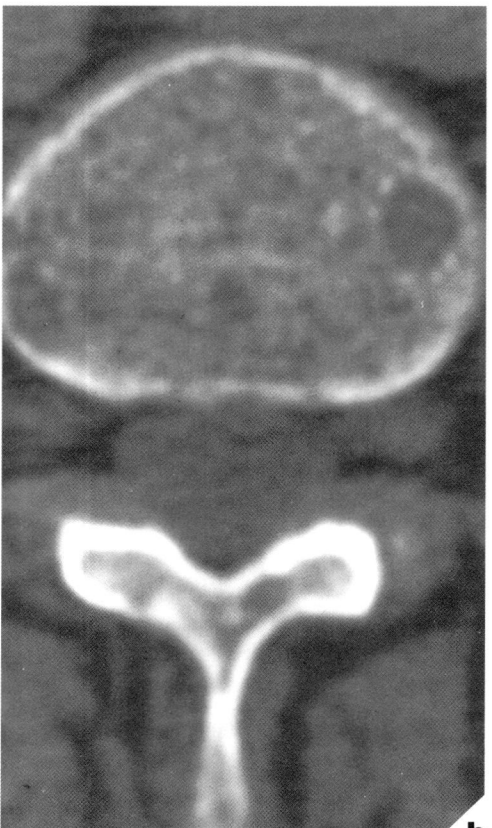
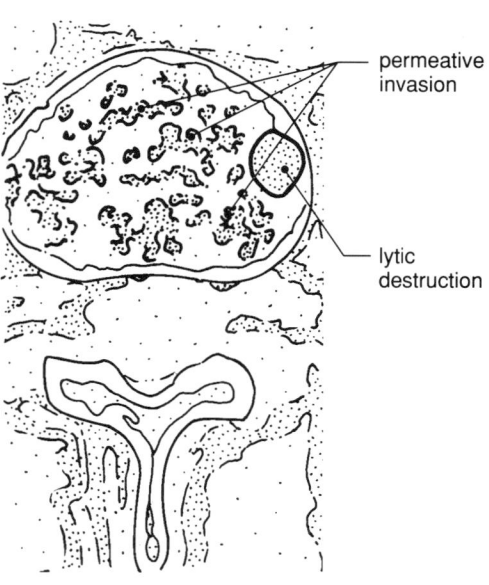

permeative invasion

lytic destruction

Figure 10.16

Multiple myeloma involving the spine.
a *CT section shows a permeative, infiltrative pattern of tumor invasion of the vertebral body, pedicles, and left transverse process.* ***b*** *A section at a higher level shows several focal areas of lytic destruction as well as generalized demineralization and infiltration of the vertebral body.*

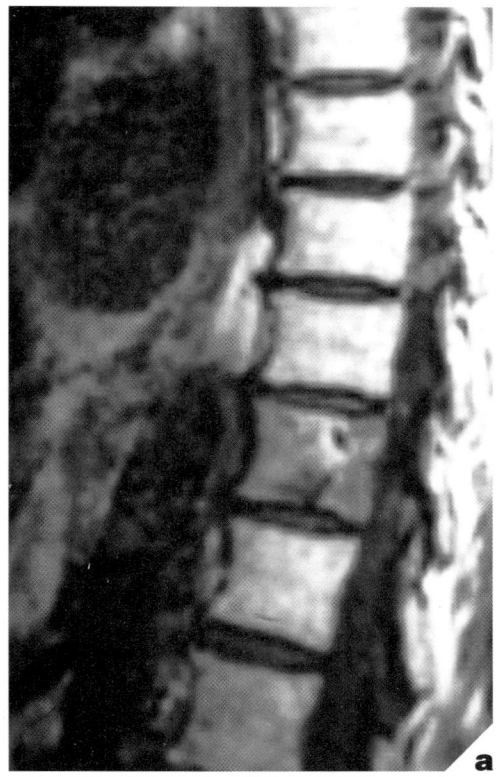

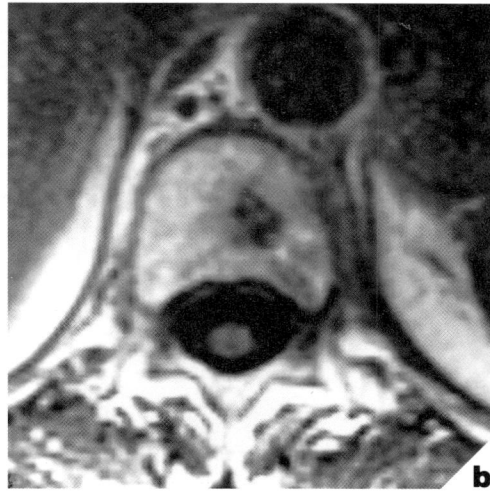

Figure 10.17
Lymphoma of the spine. **a** Sagittal and **b** axial T1-weighted images reveal T1 hypointensity in a lower thoracic vertebral body. This was proven at surgery to represent lymphoma.

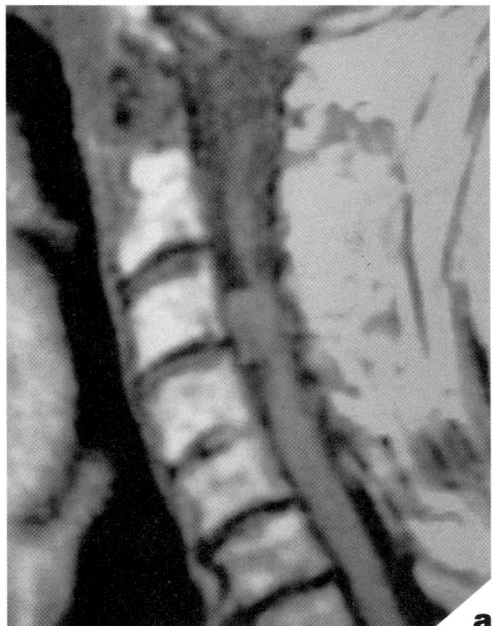

meningioma

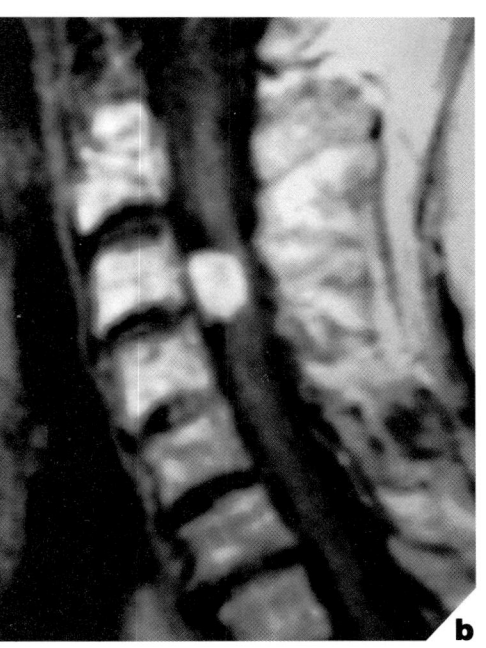

Figure 10.18
Extradural spinal meningioma. **a** Unenhanced and **b** Gadolinium-DTPA-enhanced T1-weighted images of the cervical spine show an isointense, intensely enhancing nodular, extradural mass at the level of C3–4 which compresses the spinal cord.

plaque-like sheets (Fig. 10.19) of tumor. Most meningiomas are extradural in nature and compress the spinal cord extrinsically. However, some lesions are primarily intradural (Fig. 10.20). Unlike schwannomas, meningiomas only rarely extend outside the spinal canal.

SCHWANNOMAS

Schwannomas of spinal nerves frequently have a "dumbbell" configuration due to their tendency to have both intraspinal and extraspinal components (Fig. 10.21). The lesions usually arise from glial cells of posterior nerve roots in an intradural, extramedullary location. Approximately one-third of schwannomas tend to grow through the dura and develop extradural components as well. The tumor becomes narrowed as it passes through the bony margins of a neural foramen. Pressure erosion often results in widening of the involved foramen (Fig. 10.22). These lesions are benign but may become quite large and present as a posterior mediastinal mass. Cyst formation and hemorrhage are rare.

Schwannomas are usually isodense to extradural soft tissues on unenhanced CT (Fig. 10.23) and there-

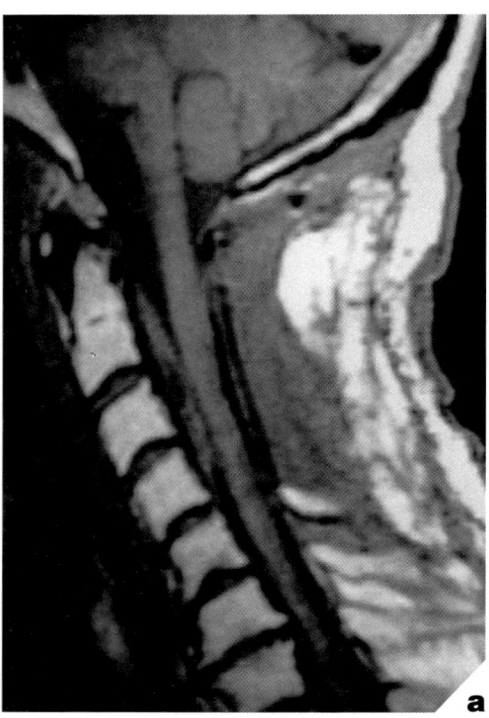 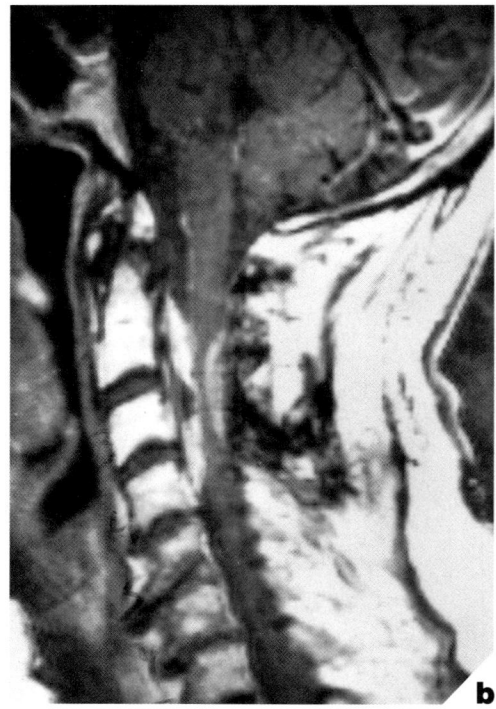 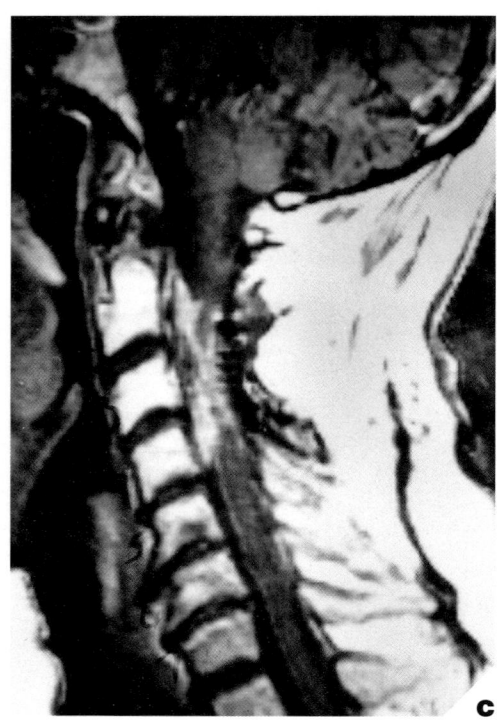

a   b   c

Figure 10.19

*Meningioma en plaque. **a** Unenhanced and **b,c** Gadolinium-DTPA-enhanced T1-weighted images of the cervical spine show circumferential thickening of the dura with a sheet-like configuration around the cervical spinal cord. As is characteristic of meningiomas, there is intense contrast enhancement.*

sheets of meningioma

fore MRI is the preferred method of diagnosis. When compared to the spinal cord, schwannomas usually are hypointense on T1- and hyperintense on T2-weighted images. They typically enhance intensely following Gadolinium-DTPA administration.

When associated with type-1 neurofibromatosis (NF-1), true neurofibromas frequently are demonstrated in the spine (Fig. 10.24). These lesions differ from schwannomas in that they contain neural as well as glial elements. In addition, neurofibromas may undergo malignant degeneration into neurofibrosarcomas. Patients with NF-1 frequently have a sharply angled scoliosis deformity. There may be scalloping of the posterior margins of the vertebral bodies due to dural ectasia (Fig. 10.25). Spinal meningiomas and gliomas are also more common in patients with NF-1 than the general population.

ARTERIOVENOUS MALFORMATIONS

Arteriovenous malformations may affect the spinal meninges, the spinal cord (Fig. 10.26), or both. Detection is often made incidentally on myelography or MRI. Rarely, spinal AVMs bleed and cause subarachnoid hemorrhage. Serpentine filling defects are

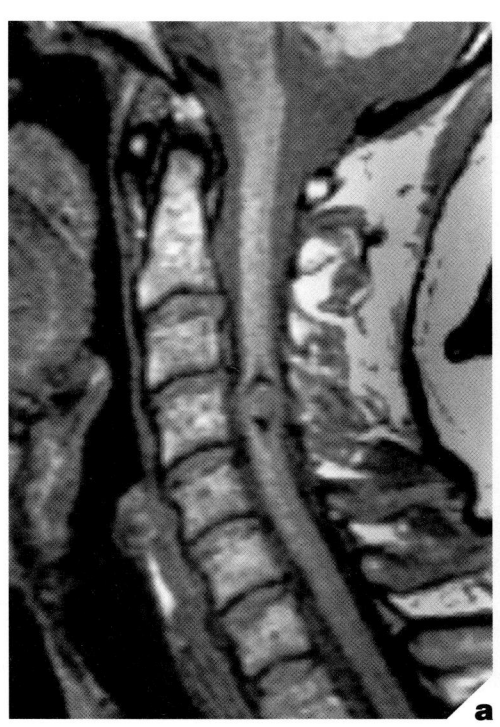
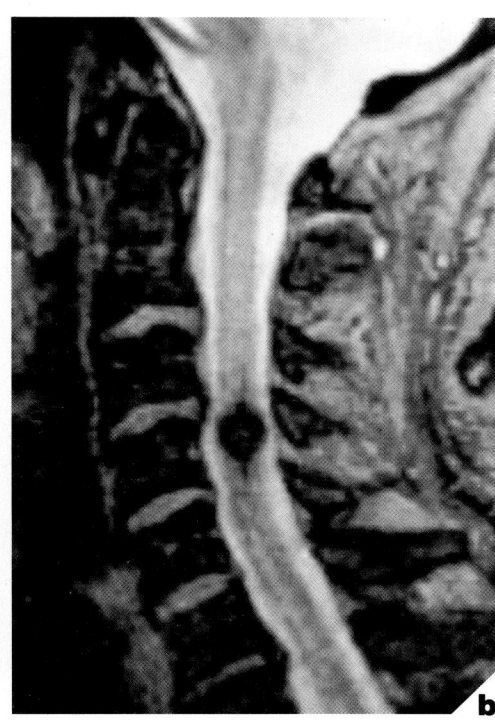
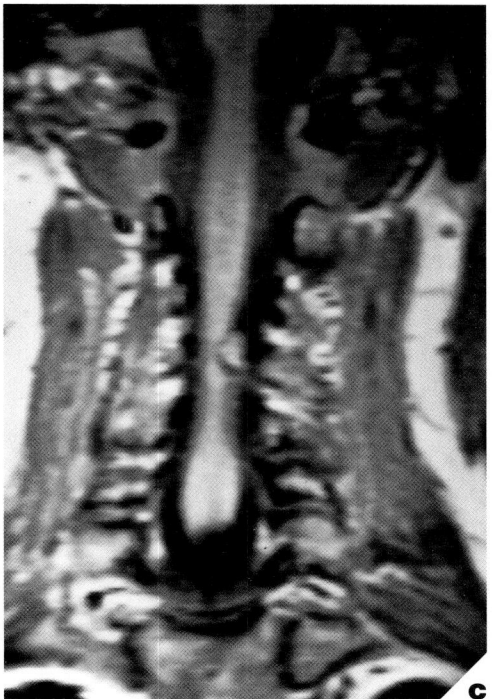

Figure 10.20

*Intradural spinal meningioma. Sagittal **a** T1, **b** T2, and **c** coronal T1-weighted images demonstrate a nodular, intradural mass compressing the spinal cord on the left at the level of C4. The mass has dark-T2 signal characteristics which represent calcification.*

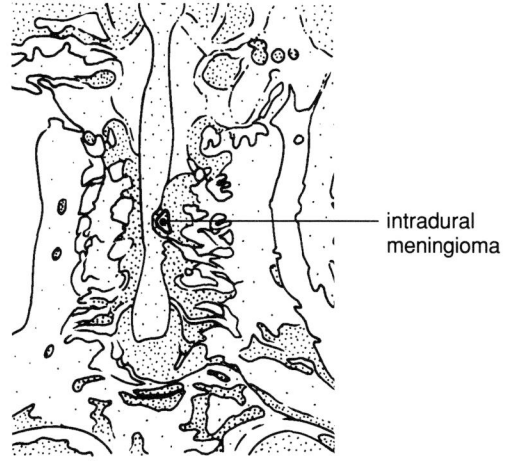

intradural meningioma

Neoplastic Diseases of the Spine

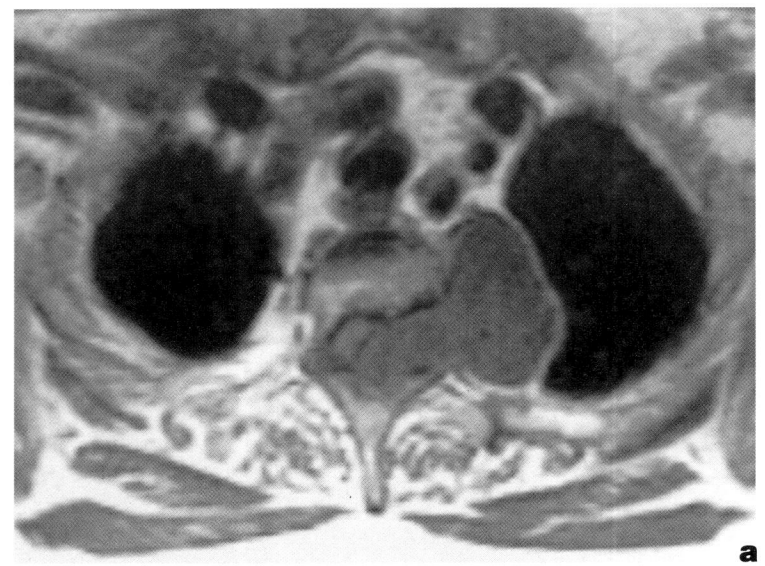

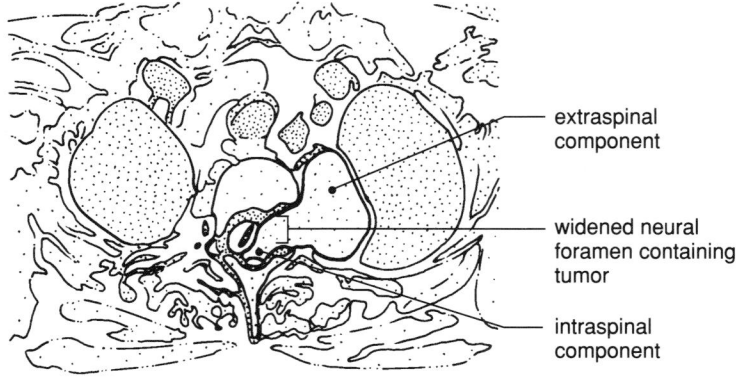

extraspinal component

widened neural foramen containing tumor

intraspinal component

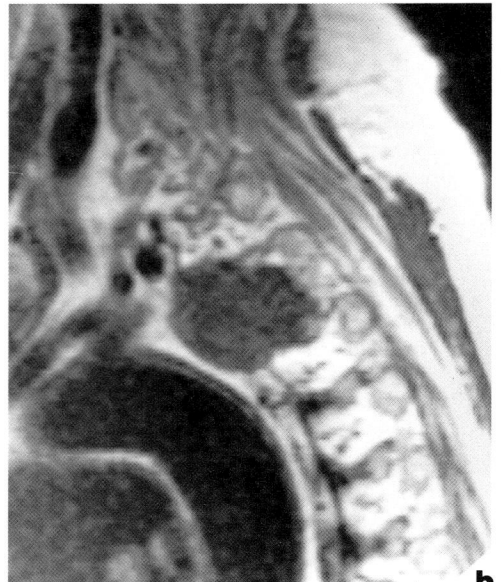

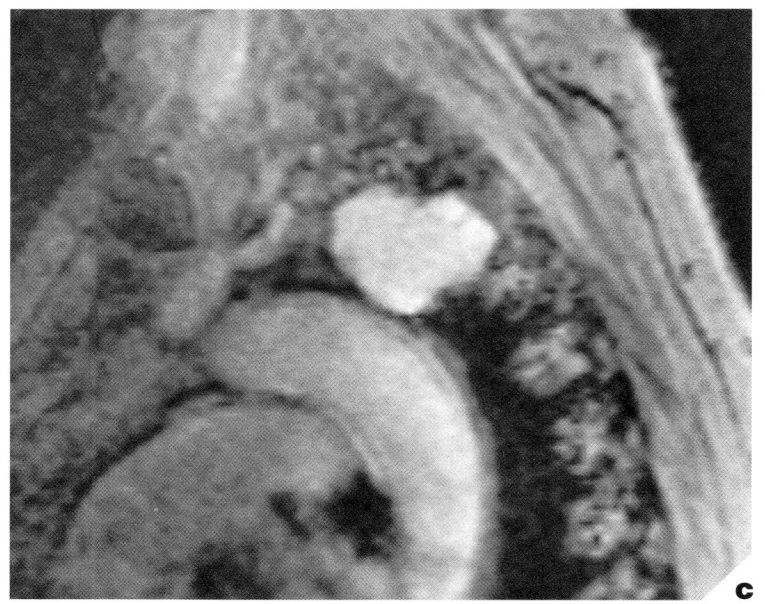

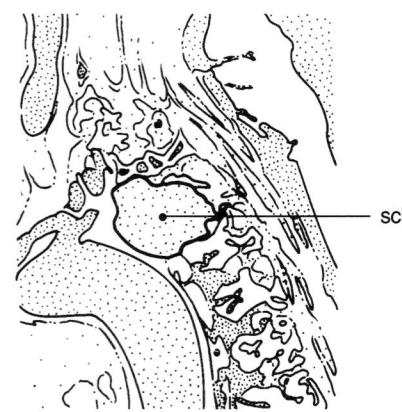

schwannoma

Figure 10.21

*Dumbbell schwannoma. **a** Axial T1-weighted image shows a large, left-sided paraspinal mass extending through a widened neural foramen into the spinal canal. There is spinal cord compression. Sagittal **b** T1- and **c** T2-weighted images show dark-T1, bright-T2 signal characteristics. This lesion presented as a posterior mediastinal mass on a chest radiograph.*

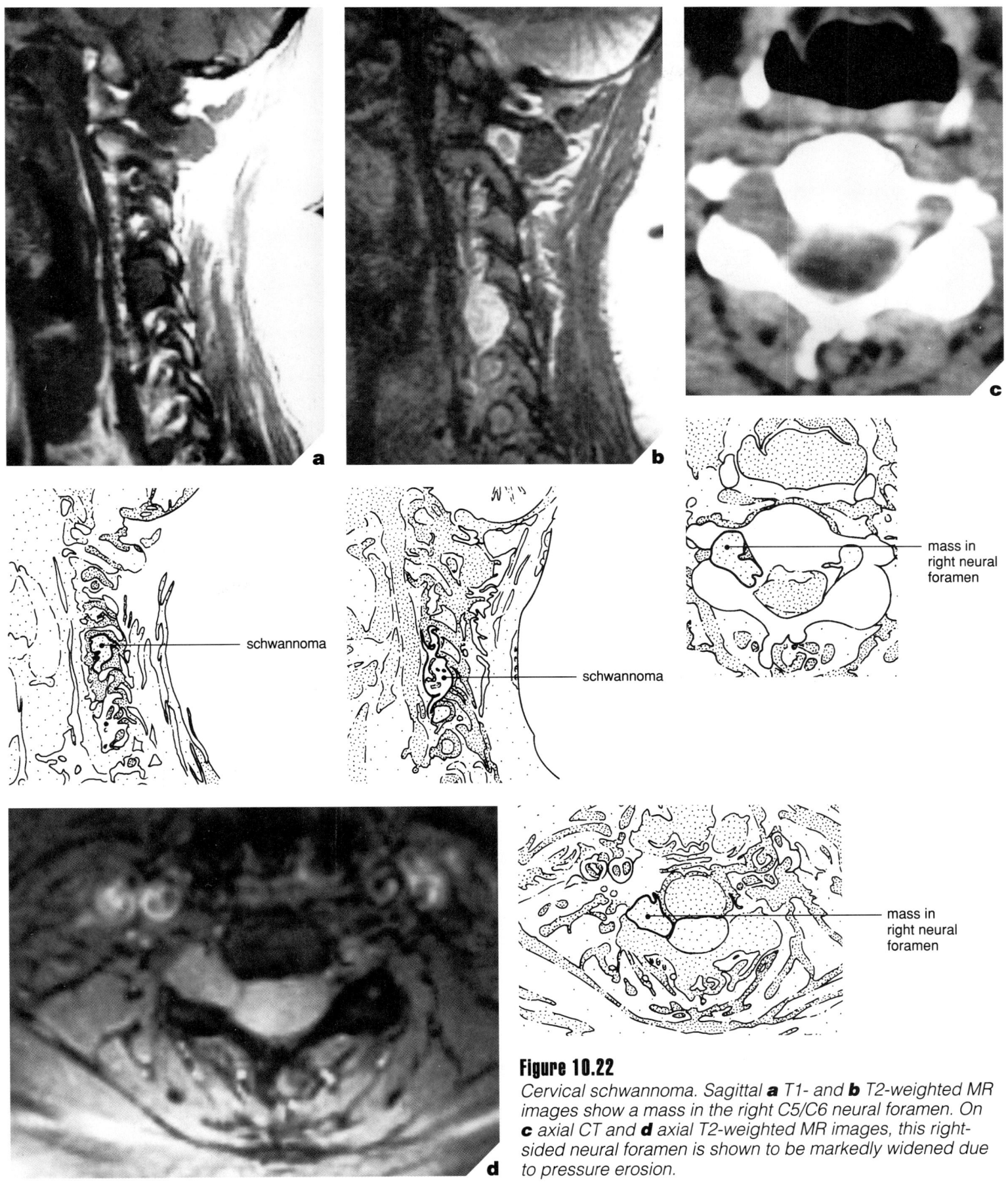

schwannoma

schwannoma

mass in right neural foramen

mass in right neural foramen

Figure 10.22

*Cervical schwannoma. Sagittal **a** T1- and **b** T2-weighted MR images show a mass in the right C5/C6 neural foramen. On **c** axial CT and **d** axial T2-weighted MR images, this right-sided neural foramen is shown to be markedly widened due to pressure erosion.*

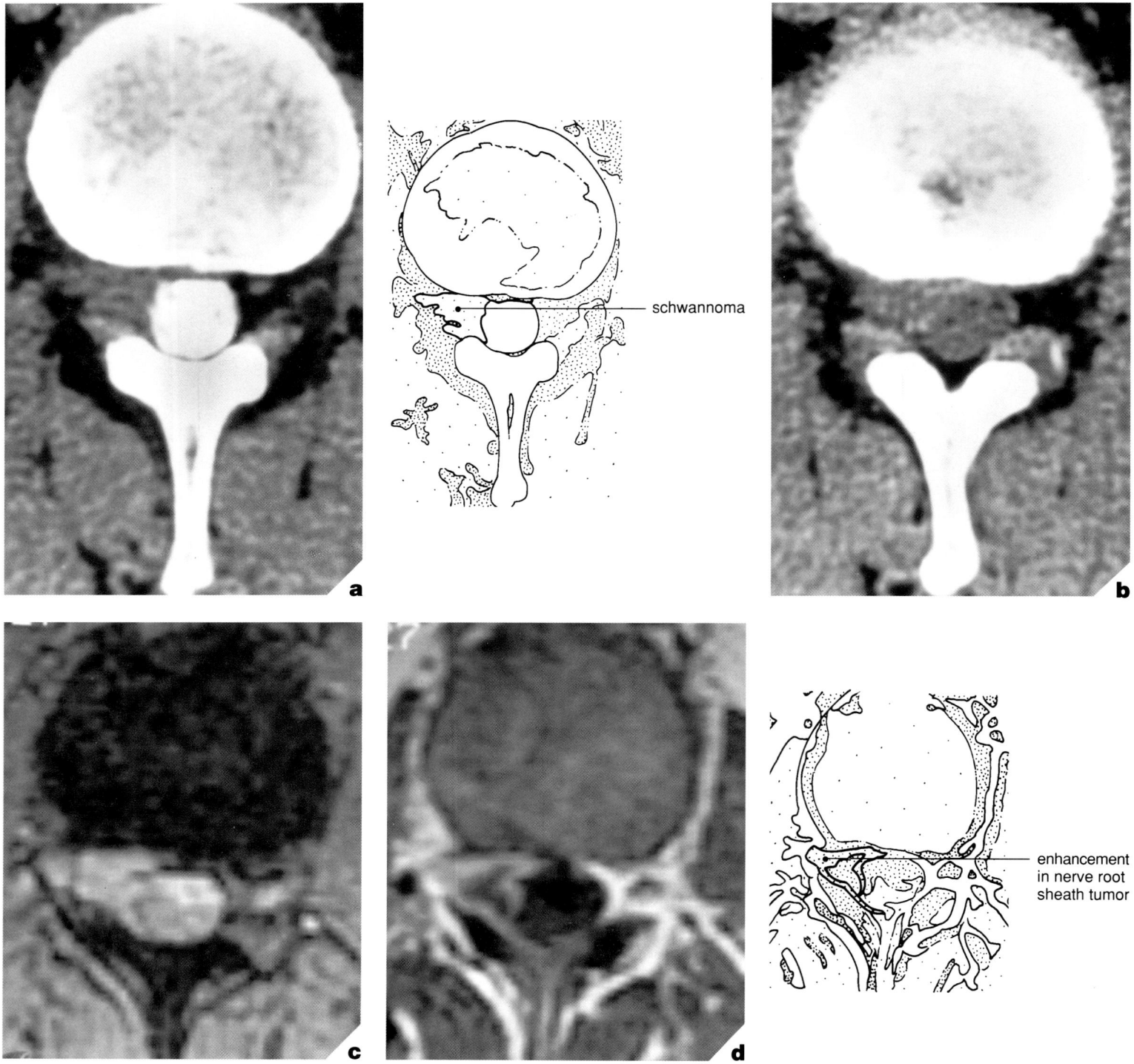

Figure 10.23

*Schwannoma. **a,b** Axial CT images show a soft tissue mass attached to the right L5 nerve root sleeve extending into a nonwidened neural foramen. **c** This mass has bright-T2 signal characteristics and **d** its margins enhance with Gadolinium-DTPA.*

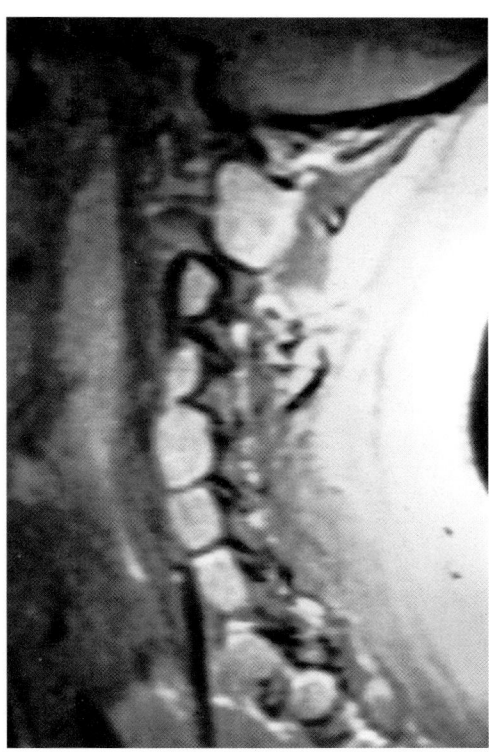

Figure 10.24
Neurofibromas. MRI shows neurofibromas at virtually all levels of the cervical spine. This patient had typical skin lesions of neurofibromatosis.

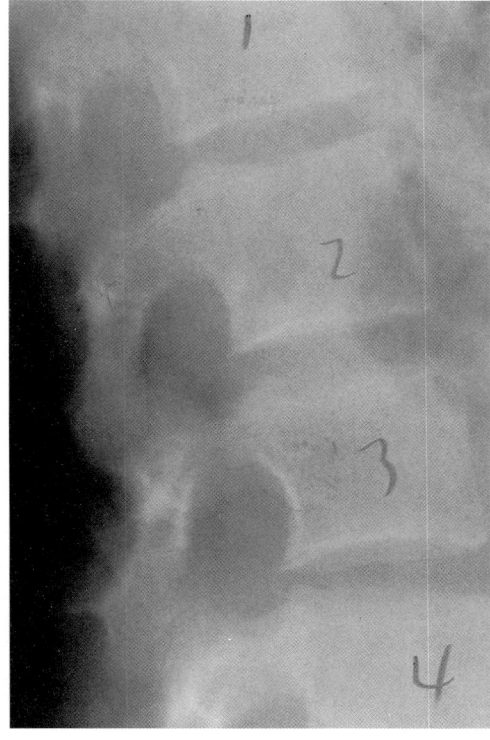

Figure 10.25
Dural ectasia. Lateral plain film shows posterior scalloping of all of the lumbar vertebral bodies in this patient with neurofibromatosis.

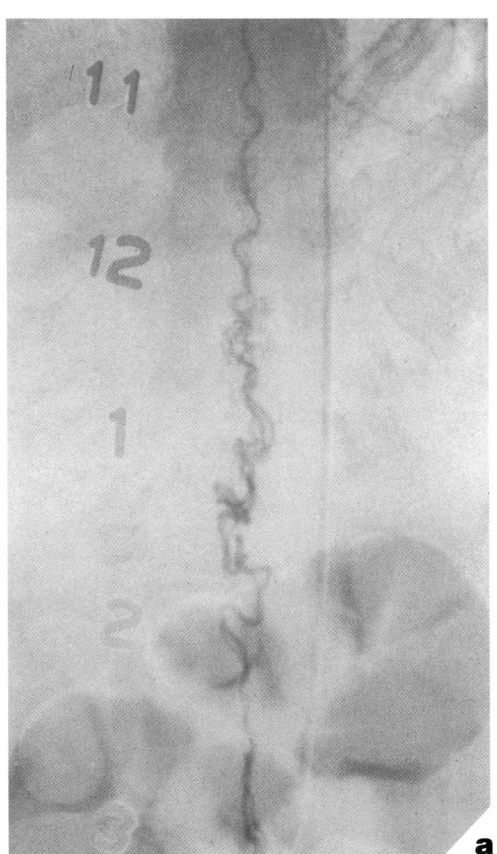

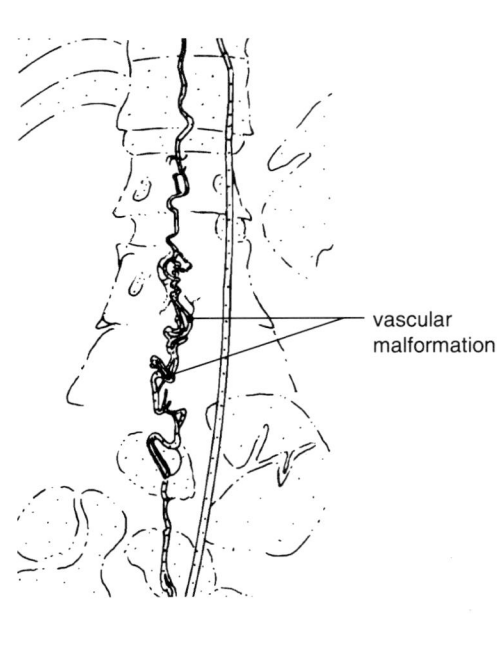

vascular malformation

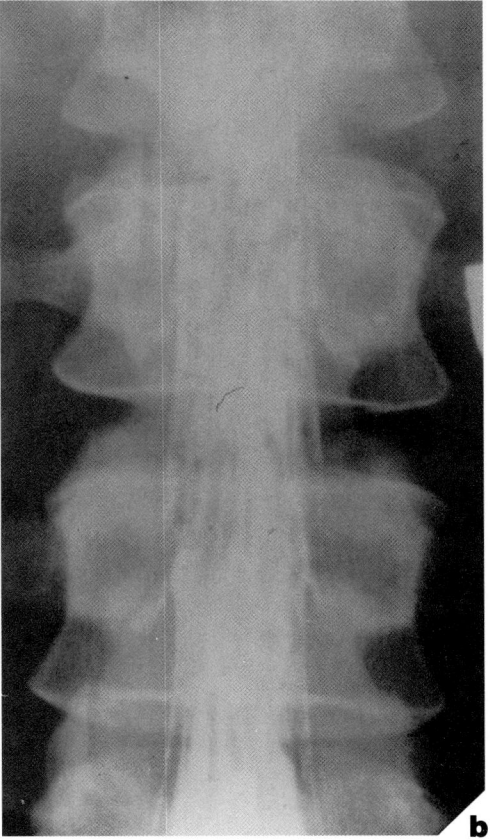

Figure 10.26
*Spinal arteriovenous malformation (AVM). **a** Film from a spinal angiogram demonstrates abnormal, prominent, and tortuous feeding arteries extending from T12 through L2. **b** These are demonstrated on myelography as serpentine filling defects.*

demonstrated at myelography which need to be distinguished from the more common dilatation and tortuosity of epidural veins and nerve roots caused by spinal stenosis (Fig. 10.27).

Angiographic confirmation and demonstration of arteriovenous malformations require extensive catheterization of numerous spinal and systemic arteries. All of the feeding vessels need to be identified for proper embolization or neurosurgical planning.

MISCELLANEOUS BONY NEOPLASMS

Numerous benign and malignant primary bone tumors which occur throughout the skeleton may also affect the spine. These lesions include aneurysmal bone cyst (Fig. 10.28), giant cell tumor, hemangioma (Fig. 10.29), osteoid osteoma, osteoblastoma (Fig. 10.30), osteosarcoma, sacral teratoma (Fig. 10.31), nonossifying fibroma (Fig. 10.32), chordoma, chondrosarcoma (Fig. 10.33), and Ewing's sarcoma

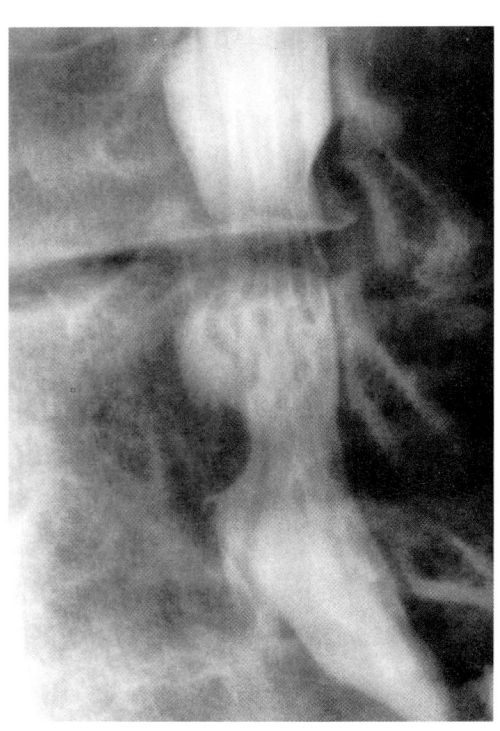

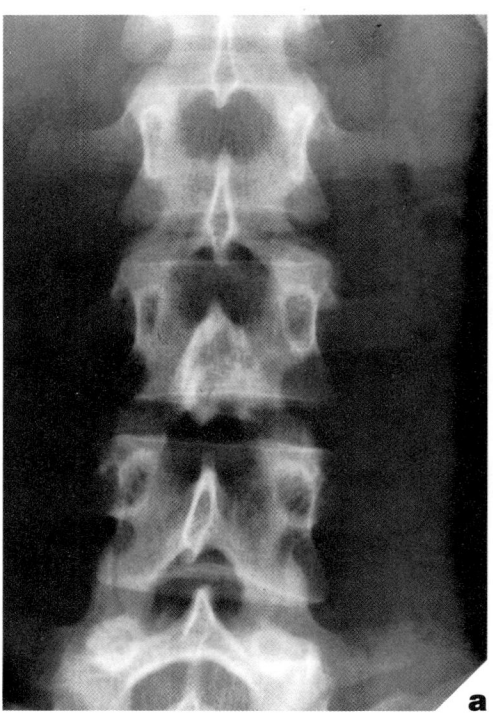

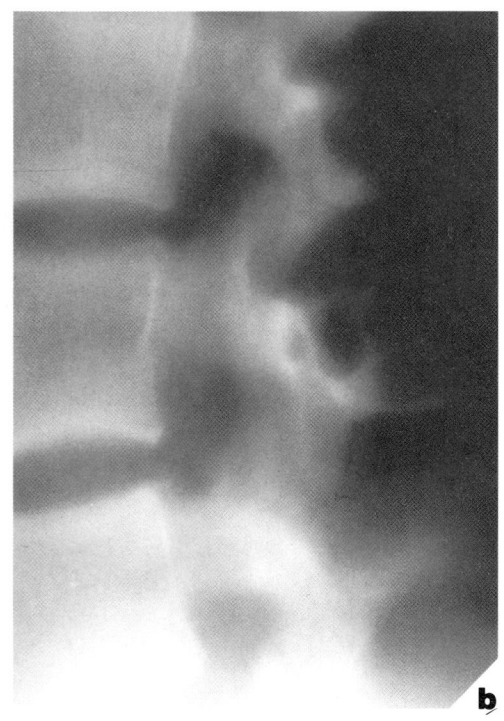

a

b

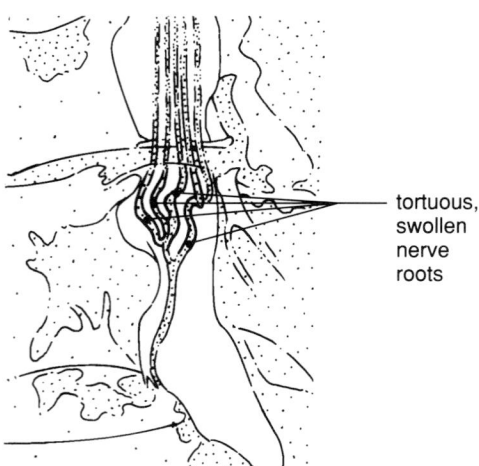

tortuous, swollen nerve roots

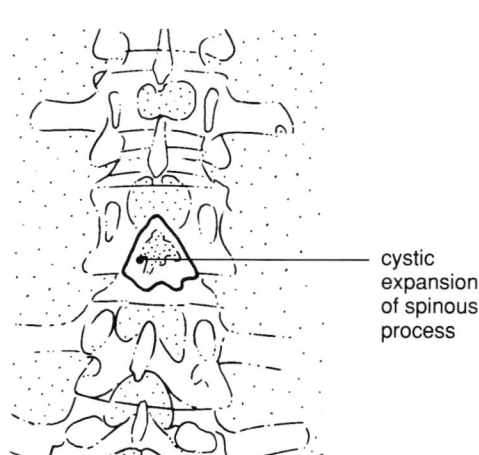

cystic expansion of spinous process

Figure 10.28

*Aneurysmal bone cyst. **a** Plain radiograph of the lumbar spine shows a bubbly expansion of the L3 spinous process. **b** Lateral tomogram shows multiseptated expansion of the spinous process with thinning of its cortex.*

Figure 10.27

Spinal stenosis mimicking spinal AVM. Redundant, swollen spinal nerve roots caused by spinal stenosis produce filling defects which might be mistaken for the serpentine defects seen with arteriovenous malformations.

(Fig. 10.34). Eosinophilic granuloma (Fig. 10.35), the most benign form of Histiocytosis X, is the most common cause of platyspondyly in pediatric patients. All of these bony lesions may invade or compress the spinal canal and/or neural foramina and result in neurologic signs and symptoms. Differentiation may be difficult since many of these tumors are expansile, multicystic, and grossly destructive. Patient's age, symptomatology, and the precise location of the lesion are helpful distinguishing criteria.

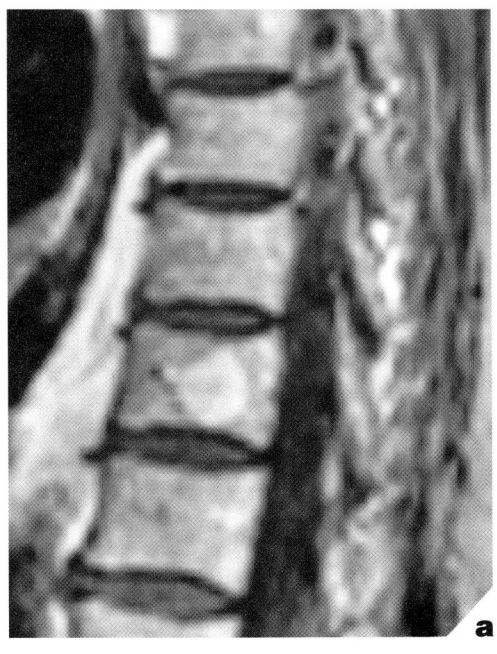
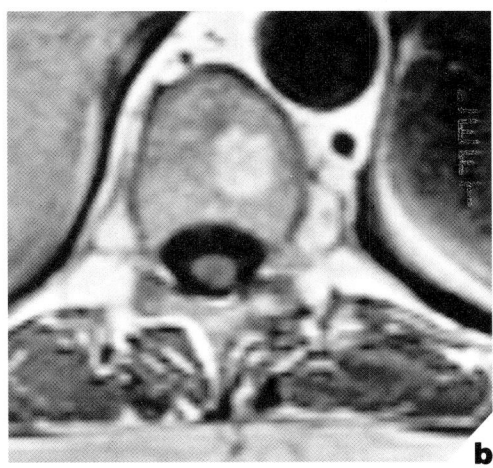

Figure 10.29

*Spinal hemangioma. T1-weighted **a** sagittal and **b** axial MR images show a rounded area of bright signal abnormality in the left side of the L1 vertebral body characteristic of a hemangioma. Plain films showed a characteristic "corduroy" trabecular pattern.*

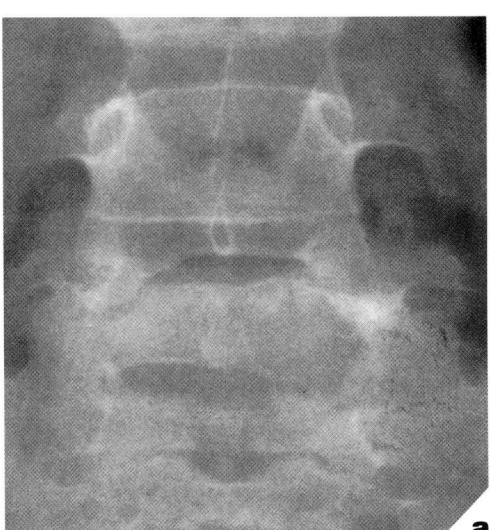
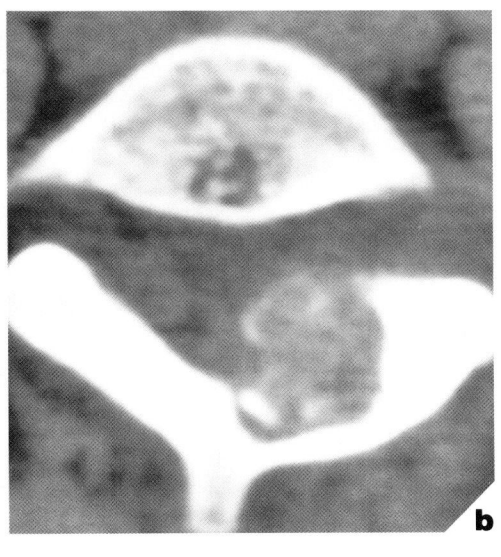
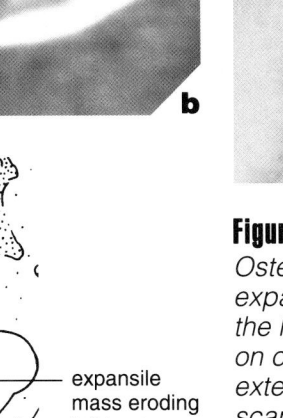

expansile mass eroding left lamina

expansile mass eroding left lamina

Figure 10.30

*Osteoblastoma. **a** Plain film shows an expansile, erosive process destroying the left lamina of L5. **b** This is confirmed on computed tomography which shows extension into the spinal canal. **c** Bone scan shows intense uptake on the left at L5. At surgery this was confirmed to represent an osteoblastoma.*

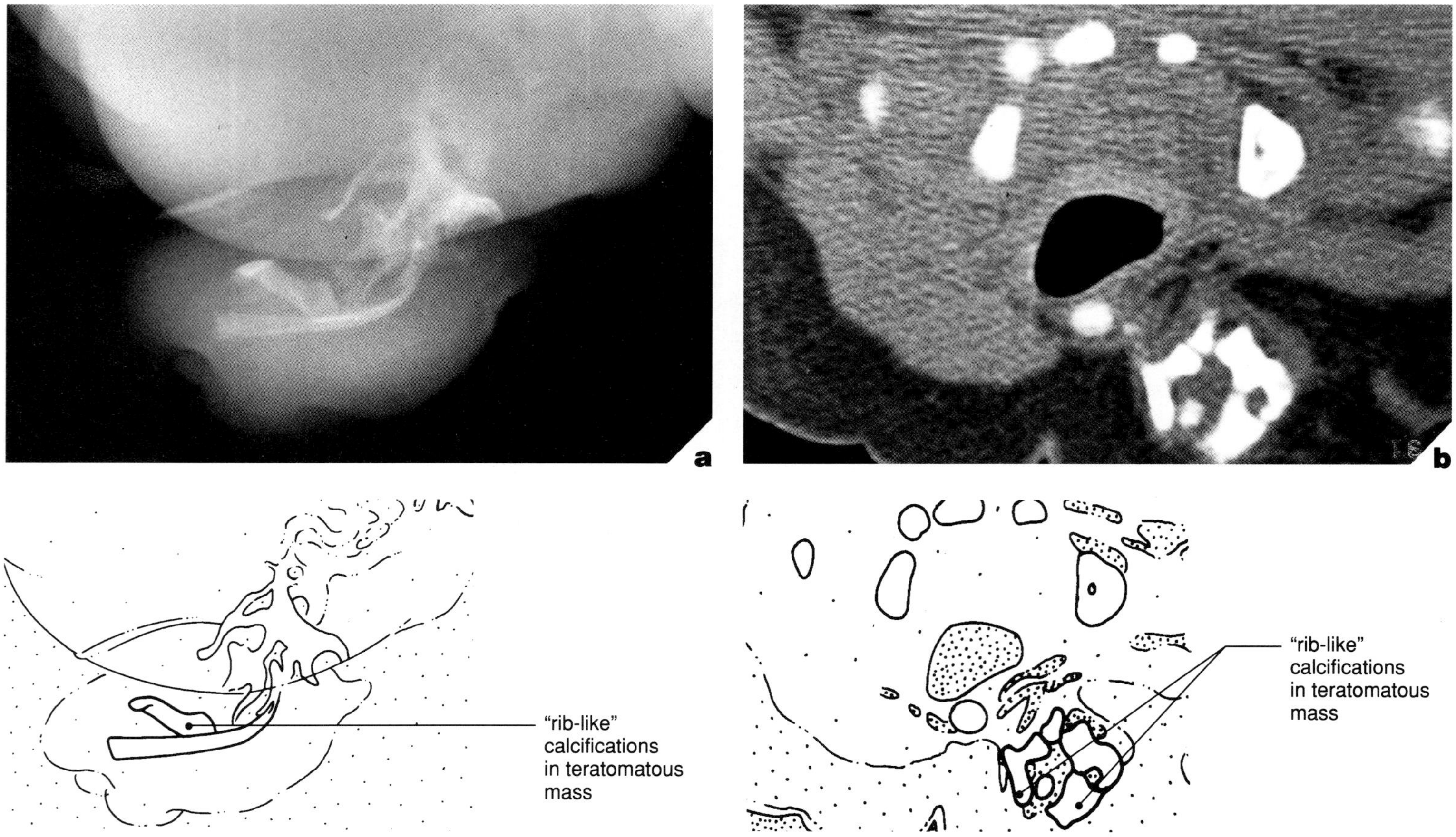

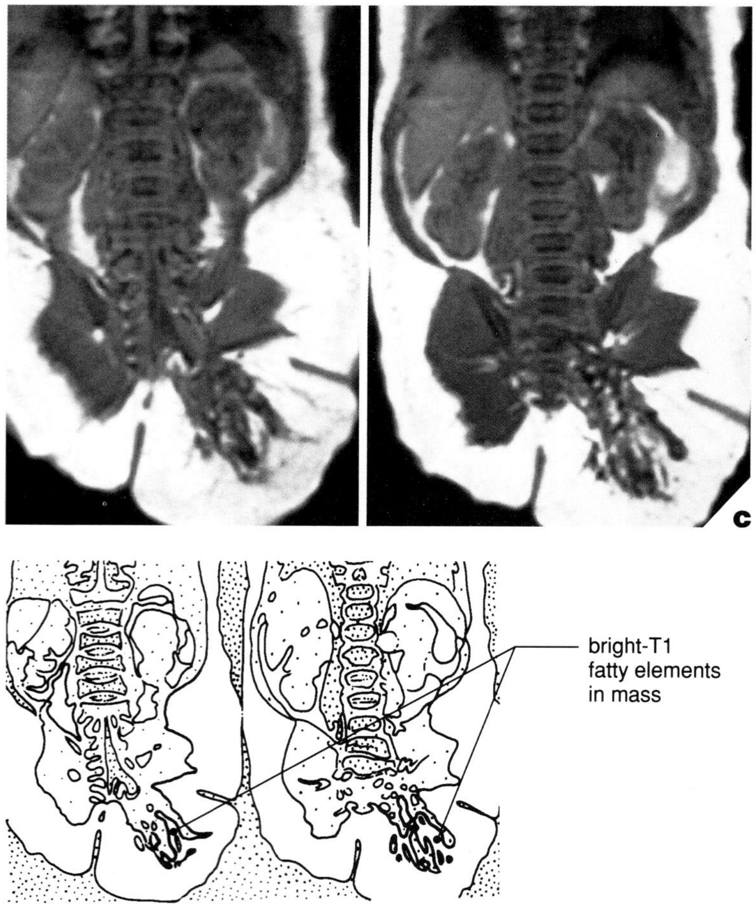

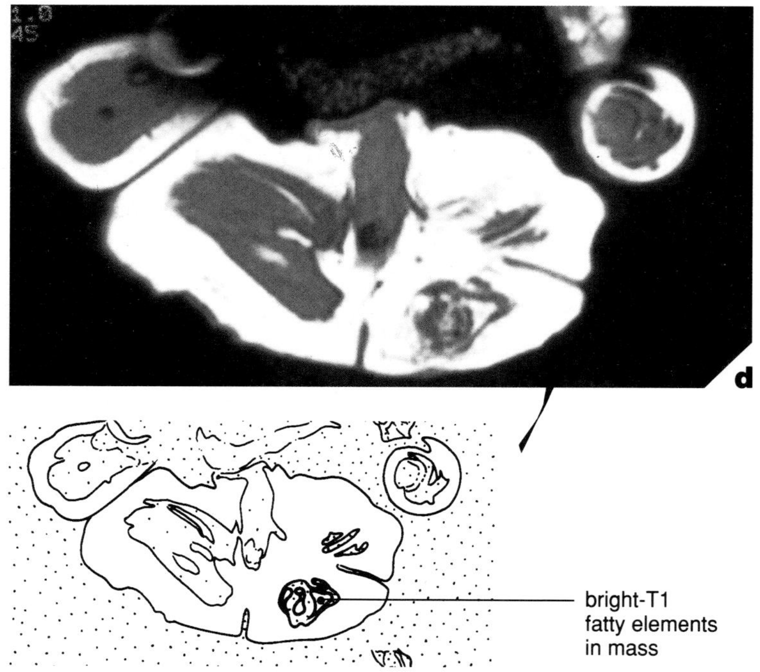

"rib-like" calcifications in teratomatous mass

"rib-like" calcifications in teratomatous mass

bright-T1 fatty elements in mass

bright-T1 fatty elements in mass

Figure 10.31

Sacral teratoma. *a* Plain film and *b* CT show a large mass containing rib-like calcifications extending posteriorly from the sacrum and left buttock. The mass contains fatty elements which are best seen as bright-T1 signal on the *c* coronal and *d* axial MR images.

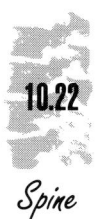

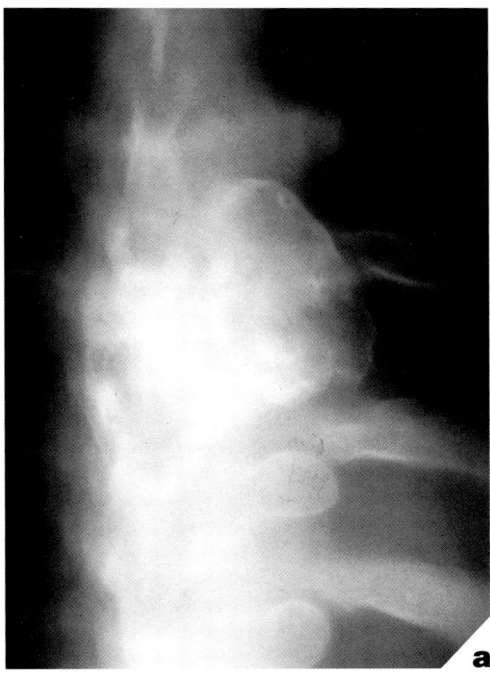

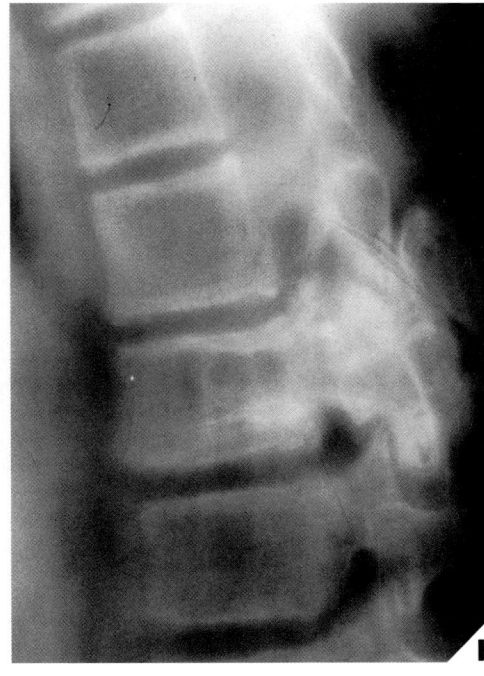

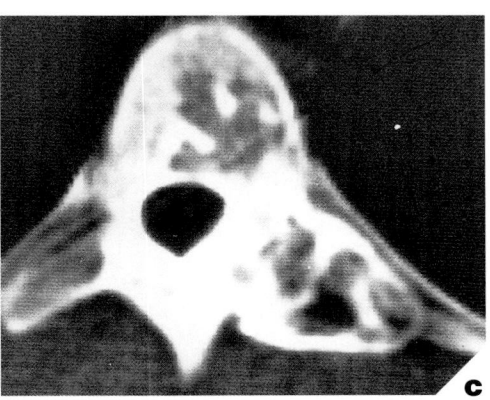

Figure 10.32

*Nonossifying fibroma. **a** AP and **b** lateral tomograms show a sclerotic, well-defined expansile mass in the left pedicle, lamina and transverse process of T7. **c** This is demonstrated to better advantage on computed tomography. There is some compression of the spinal canal.*

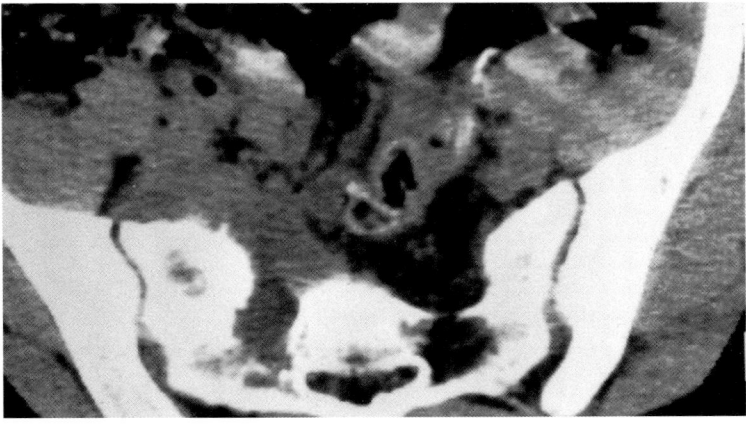

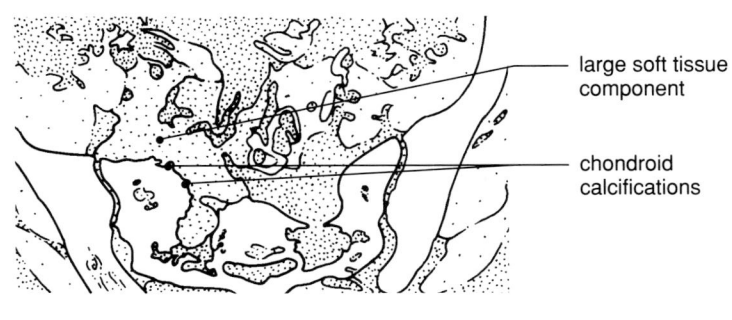

large soft tissue component

chondroid calcifications

Figure 10.33

Chondrosarcoma. There is a destructive mass in the right side of the sacrum with a large soft tissue component extending anteriorly which displaces the right psoas muscle. A portion of this mass contains hyperdense streaks representing calcification of chondroid material.

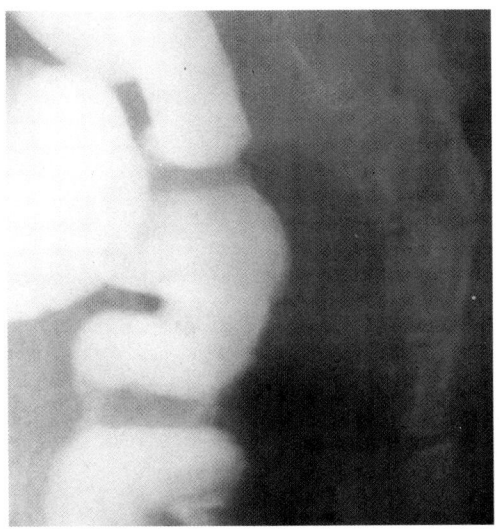

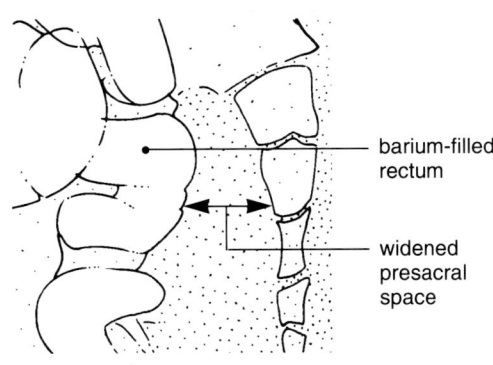

barium-filled rectum

widened presacral space

Figure 10.34

Ewing's sarcoma. Lateral film from a barium enema demonstrates destructive changes and demineralization within the sacrum and coccyx. There is a very large presacral soft tissue mass displacing the contrast-filled rectum anteriorly.

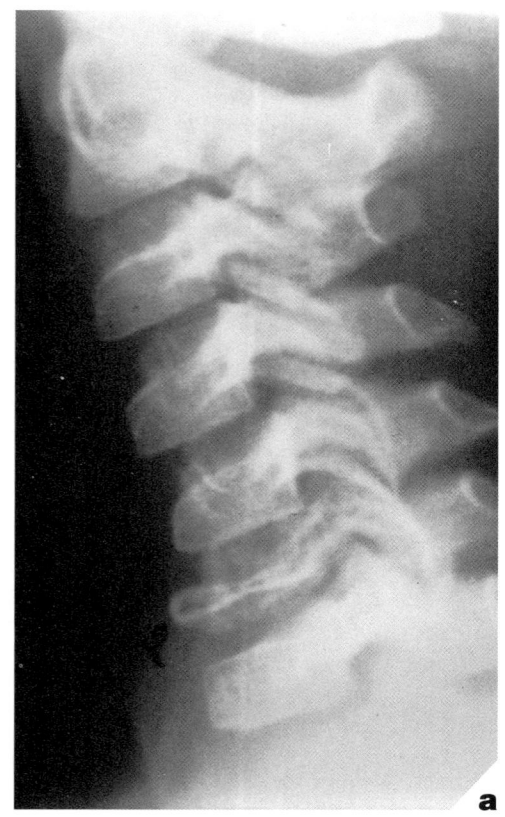

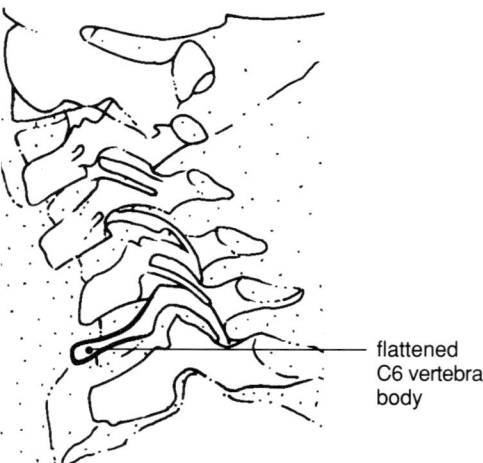

flattened
C6 vertebral
body

Figure 10.35

*Eosinophilic granuloma. **a** Lateral plain film of the cervical spine shows flattening of the C6 vertebral body. **b** MR performed the following day shows considerable posterior extension of soft tissue material into the spinal canal. **c** A follow-up MR performed two years later shows resorption of the hemorrhage and other intraspinal soft tissue components but persistent platyspondyly at C6.*

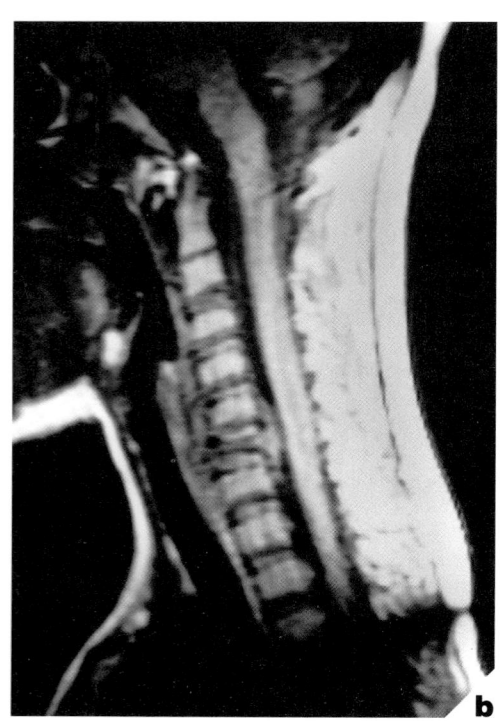

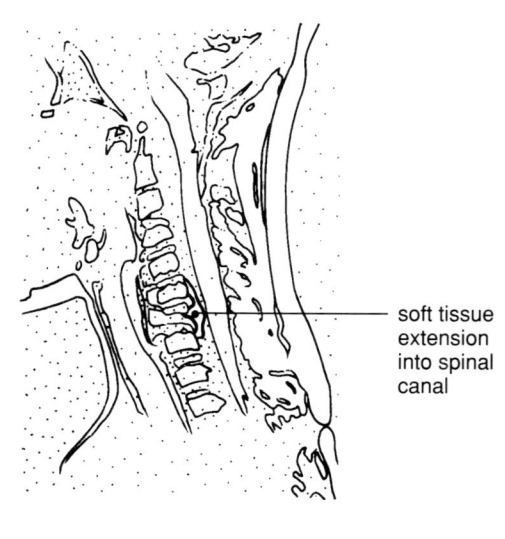

soft tissue
extension
into spinal
canal

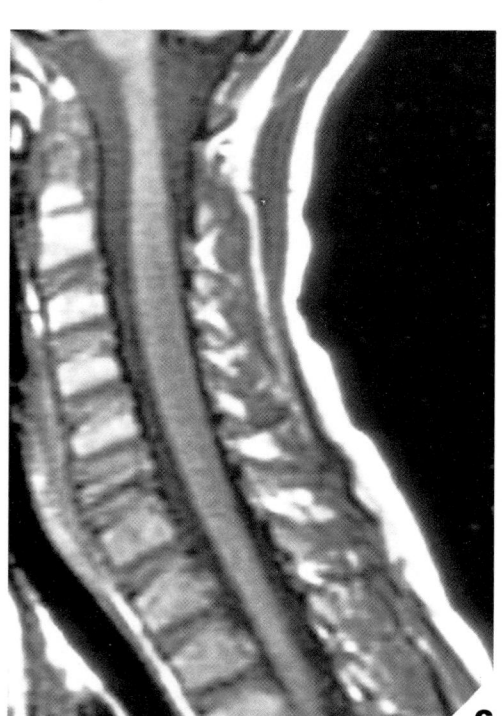

11

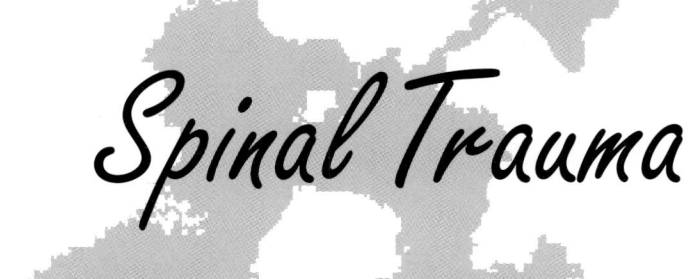

Spinal Trauma

*e*valuation of spinal trauma is a vital function of the neuroradiologist. Precise diagnosis of bony and soft tissue injury is necessary for proper patient care. This requires knowledge of the causes and mechanisms of spinal trauma as well as familiarity with the types of fractures and soft tissue disruptions that occur.

Spinal trauma usually involves the cervical or lumbar spine. Thoracic fractures and soft tissue injuries are much less common. Most cervical spinal trauma is due to a blow to the head rather than direct injury to the neck itself. The cervical spine acts a fulcrum or pivot point between the head and the rest of the body. Like the middle of a "wishbone," it is this center of the fulcrum which "cracks" or undergoes disruption. In a similar fashion, the lumbar spine acts as a fulcrum between the pelvis and lower extremities with the upper body. Motor vehicle accidents, sports-related injuries, and falls are the most common causes of spinal injuries.

When evaluating spinal trauma, the vertebrae should be thought of in terms of vertical columns. The most useful model is to consider the vertebral bodies and intervertebral discs as the "anterior column" and the posterior elements as the "posterior column." An alternative model distinguishes the posterior one-third of the vertebral body, anulus fibrosus and the posterior longitudinal ligament as a separate, "middle column." These approaches help to categorize areas of injury which may be confined to a particular column or extend to other areas; this has particular prognostic and stability implications. The mechanisms of spinal injury can often be deduced by separating the columns into a compression vector and a distraction vector; thus flexion injuries cause compression of the anterior column and distraction of the posterior column while extension injuries result in the reverse.

Although invisible on plain films, the ligaments of the spine are of paramount importance in maintaining stability and normal motion. Ligamentous injury frequently accompanies spinal trauma; its presence must be determined indirectly. The anterior longitudinal ligament is attached to the anterior margins of the vertebral bodies. Its fibers become intertwined with the outer layer of the anulus fibrosus at the level of the intervertebral discs. Tearing of the anterior longitudinal ligament frequently occurs with extension injuries of the cervical spine. The posterior longitudinal ligament is attached to the posterior margin of the vertebral bodies and anulus fibrosus. Located near the center of the spinal axis, it is prone to injury by many different mechanisms. The ligamenta flava connect lamina at different levels. Along with the intervertebral discs, they permit much of the movement of the spine. The ligamenta flava are prone to rupture during flexion or rotation-type injuries. The transverse ligament of the atlanto-axial joint connects the odontoid process (dens) with the arch of C1. This ligament may be torn resulting in atlanto-axial subluxation. Interspinous and supraspinous ligaments connect spinous processes at multiple levels.

It is helpful, although frequently impossible, to determine whether an injury of the spine is stable or unstable. Such evaluation needs to consider clinical as well as radiological criteria and requires determination of present and future range-of-motion capabilities, the potential for further injury or neurologic impairment, the effect of subsequent minor trauma and a cumulative assessment of all of the bony and soft tissue injuries. In general, there are certain types of fractures (e.g., Jefferson fracture) or types of ligamentous injury (e.g., rupture of the anterior longitudinal ligament secondary to hyperextension of the neck) which are known to be unstable. A fracture or disruption of either the anterior or posterior column alone is usually stable but fractures which involve both the vertebral body and the posterior elements are usually unstable. Any dislocation of the spine is potentially unstable. Deformity, including changes in alignment, scoliosis, and kyphosis, may be indicators of instability.

The portable, lateral view of the cervical spine is usually the first radiographic image obtained in acutely traumatized individuals. This film must include the entire cervical spine, including the C7/T1 interspace. It is extremely useful in identifying most types of unstable fractures of the cervical spine. Exceptions include the Jefferson fracture and fractures of the odontoid process. Unstable injuries, especially those due to sudden extension of the neck, often show no bony abnormalities and indirect findings such as pre-vertebral soft tissue swelling or subtle widening or narrowing of intervertebral disc spaces or interspinous spaces need to be carefully identified. If an unstable injury is discovered, the patient's neck should not be moved. Further films should only be obtained with the patient in a cervical collar. Although flexion/extension films may dramatically confirm a ligamentous disruption, these views must be deferred in patients with a known or suspected unstable injury.

Classification of spinal fractures is made difficult by the wide diversity of fractures which occur. This is underscored by the large number of individual vertebra and the central location of the spine in the body making it susceptible to a multitude of injuries. Except for a few fractures with generally accepted eponyms (e.g., "hangman's fracture"), spinal trauma is best categorized by the mechanism of injury which produced it. This often has to be deduced on the basis of the radiologic findings, since highly detailed clinical histories are seldom obtainable.

NORMAL CONDITIONS THAT MIMIC SPINAL TRAUMA

There are several normal conditions that may mimic fractures or dislocations. These are most common in the cervical spine. The os odontoideum (Fig. 11.1) represents an accessory ossification center located at the tip of the dens. It should not be confused with a type I odontoid fracture. Generally, its margins are smooth and well corticated, and the os odontoideum is smaller than a normal odontoid tip.

There are numerous variations in the normal development of the arch of C1 (Fig. 11.2) that should not be confused with a fracture. The pre-odontoid space represents the distance between the anterior margin of the dens and the posterior margin of the

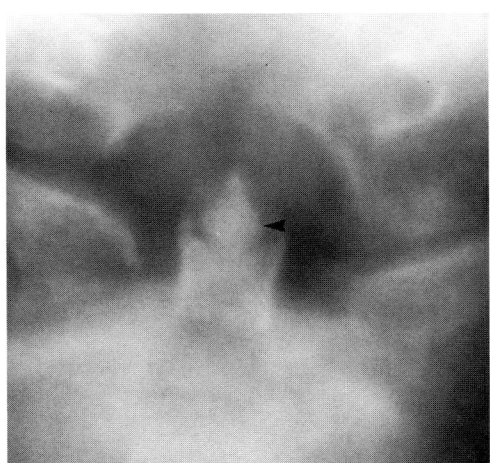

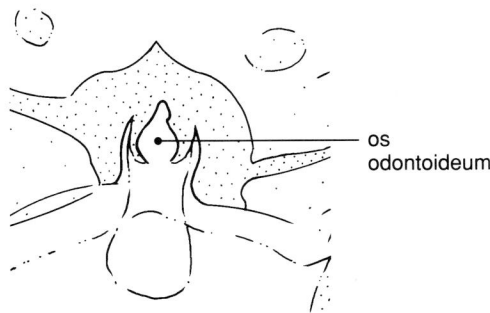

os odontoideum

Figure 11.1

Os odontoideum. Tomogram shows a well-corticated oval-shaped bony density at the tip of the odontoid process (arrow) which is separated from the rest of the dens. This represents a variation in development.

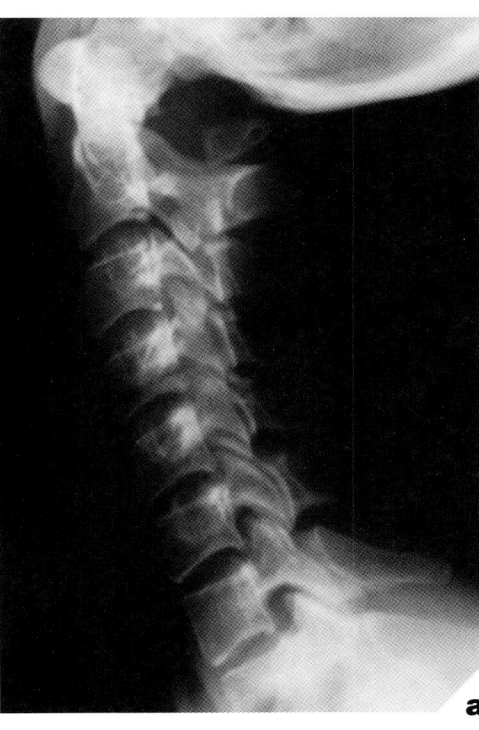

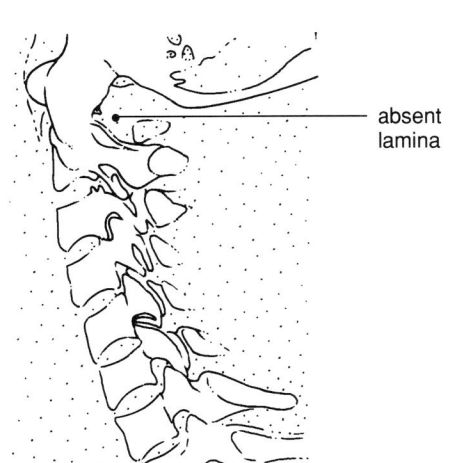

absent lamina

a

b

Figure 11.2

*Congenital absence of lamina of C1. **a** Lateral and **b** oblique films of the cervical spine show absence of the lamina of the atlas. This represents a developmental variation.*

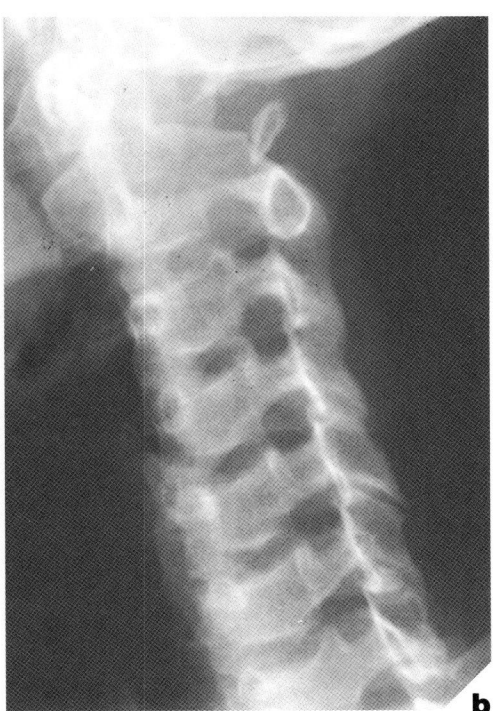

11.3

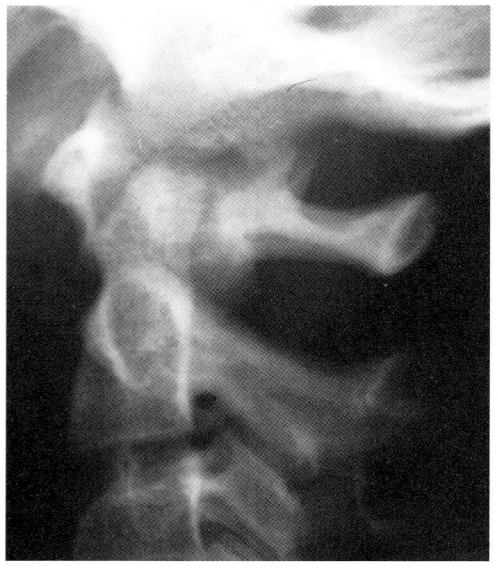

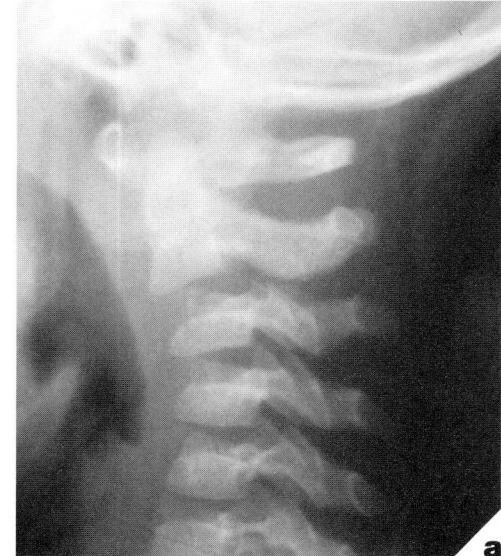

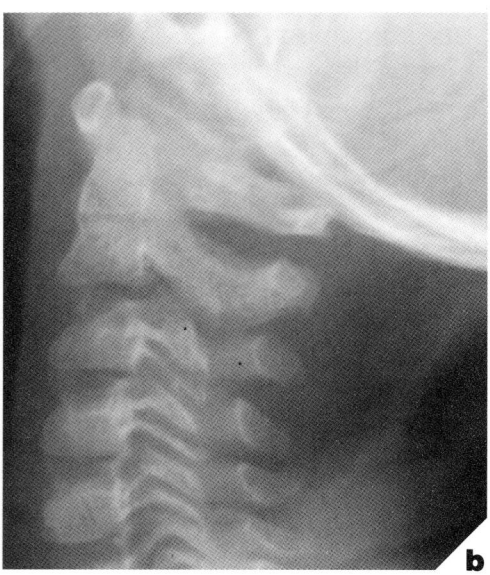

pre-odontoid space

pseudo-subluxation

normal alignment

Figure 11.3

Wide preodontoid space. The space between the posterior margin of the anterior arch of C1 and the anterior margin of the odontoid process measures 5 mm in this 11 year old. This is the upper limit of normal for children. Atlanto-axial subluxation should be considered if this distance is more than 3 mm in adults.

Figure 11.4

Pseudosubluxation of C2 upon C3.
a Flexion view shows 2-mm anterior subluxation of C2 on C3 which should

be considered a normal variation in children. **b** This displacement is reduced on the extension view.

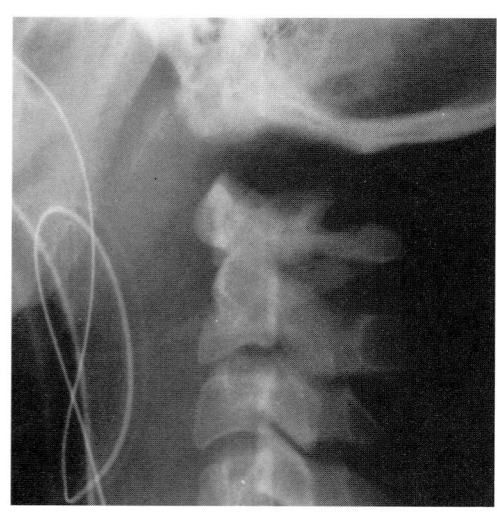

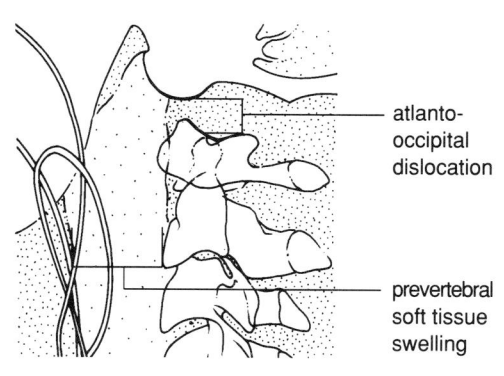

atlanto-occipital dislocation

prevertebral soft tissue swelling

Figure 11.5

Cranio-vertebral dissociation. Lateral view of the cervical spine shows 1.5 cm separation of the occiput from the arch of C1 and odontoid process. The cervical spine is displaced posteriorly in relation to the foramen magnum. There is marked prevertebral soft tissue swelling.

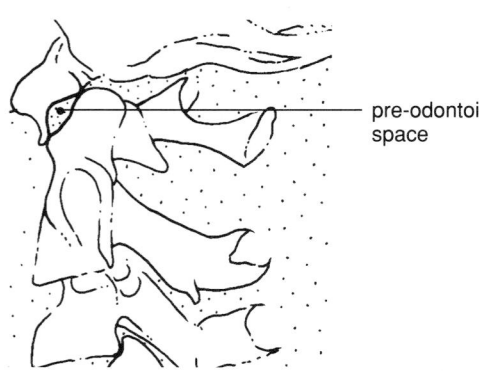

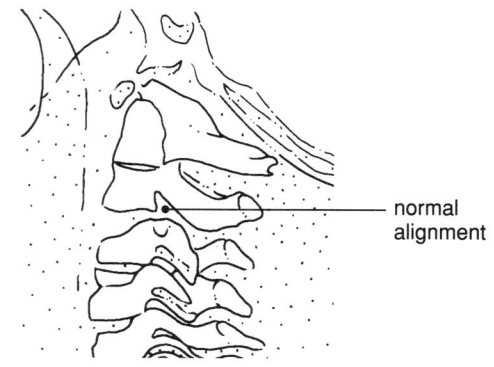

anterior arch of C1. Generally, this space is less than 1 mm. On flexion films, it may normally widen to up to 3 mm in adults and, presumably due to greater ligamentous laxity, 5 mm separation may be considered normal in children (Fig. 11.3). If extension films do not show appropriate re-alignment, atlanto-axial subluxation should be suspected. Children and infants may also have a physiologic subluxation of C2 on C3 during flexion (Fig 11.4). This is generally no greater than 2 mm and reduces completely on films obtained with the neck in extension.

CRANIO-VERTEBRAL DISSOCIATION

Atlanto-occipital dislocation (Fig. 11.5) usually occurs as a result of motor vehicle trauma in which there is a severe twisting force of the head. These injuries result in tearing of the synovial joint and the many ligaments which connect C1 to the occiput including the anterior longitudinal ligament, the tectorial membrane, the apical odontoid ligament, and the alar ligaments. Associated fractures of the arch of C1 and the occipital condyles are frequently present and there is usually marked prevertebral soft tissue swelling. Cranio-vertebral dissociations are usually fatal.

ATLANTO-AXIAL TRAUMA

Pure atlanto-axial subluxation (Fig. 11.6) or instability may be related to Down's syndrome, rheumatoid arthritis, ankylosing spondylitis, or destruction of the transverse ligament by tumor or infection. Rarely, Morquio's disease, spondyloepiphyseal dysplasia, and metatropic dwarfism are causes of atlantoaxial dislocation. Down's syndrome is often associated with a hypoplastic dens (Fig. 11.7) which predisposes these individuals to atlanto-axial subluxation. Much more commonly, bony malalignment and fractures are related to trauma.

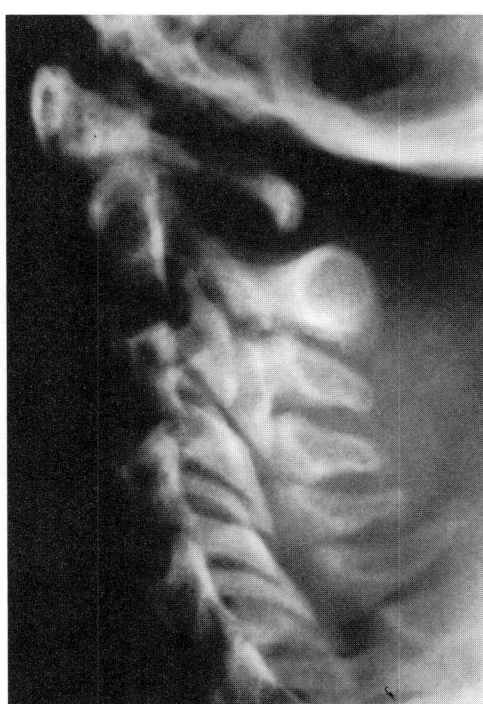

Figure 11.7
Hypoplastic dens. The odontoid process is small and does not extend fully behind the anterior arch of C1. This patient has Down's syndrome, a known association with hypoplasia of the dens.

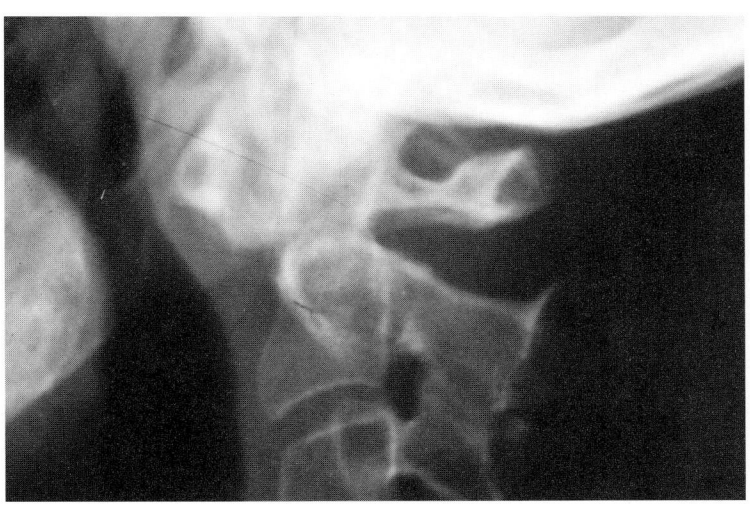

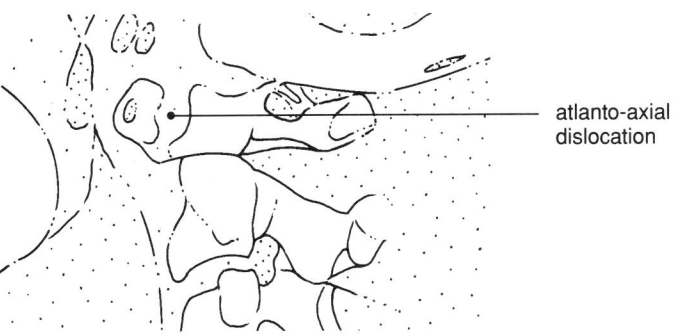

atlanto-axial dislocation

Figure 11.6
Atlanto-axial subluxation. There is a 6-mm anterior subluxation of C1 on C2.

In the craniovertebral junction, the most common fracture is that of the odontoid process. Fractures of the odontoid process are usually associated with an anterior or posterior dislocation of the arch of C1. Although mechanisms of injury vary considerably, fractures of the dens associated with an anterior dislocation (Fig. 11.8) usually result from a flexion injury whereas extension injuries produce posterior dislocations or subluxations of C1.

Fractures of the odontoid process have been categorized into three types, depending upon the level of the fracture line. These may not be visualized on the standard lateral plain film of the cervical spine and often require an "open-mouth view," computed tomography or plain tomography for accurate evaluation.

Type I fractures are uncommon. They are a result of a fracture at the tip of the dens, probably representing an avulsion fracture due to rupture of the alar ligaments which attach the tip of the dens to the medial edge of the occipital condyles.

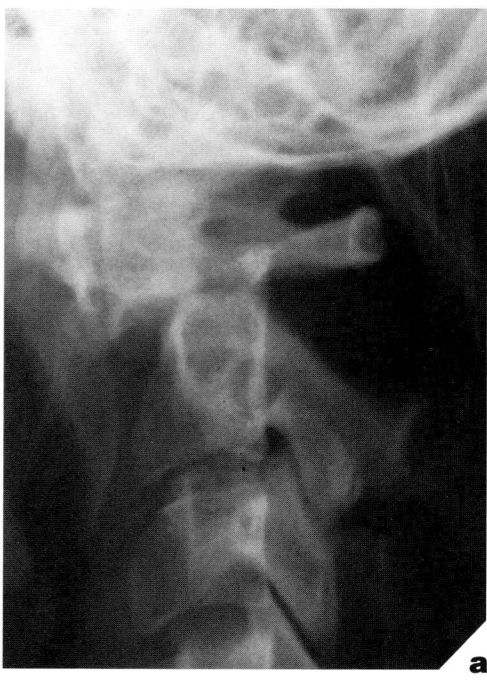

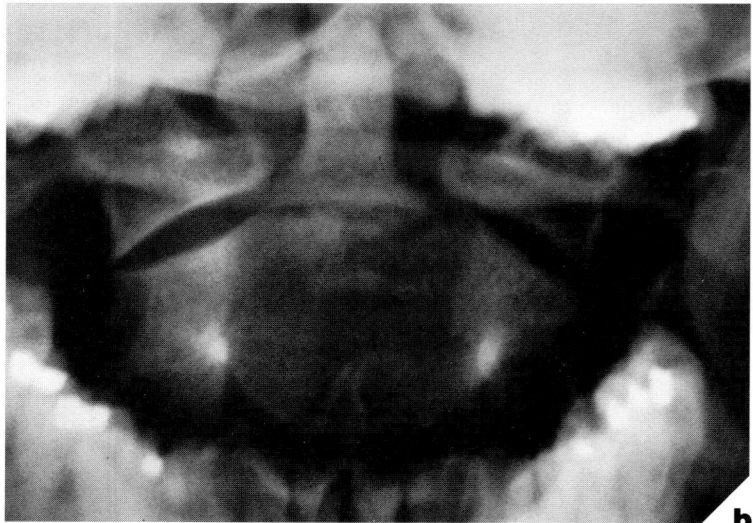

Figure 11.8

*Fracture dislocation of odontoid process. **a** There is anterior dislocation of the odontoid process which is fractured at its base. **b** Open-mouth view shows a horizontal fracture at the base of the odontoid process.*

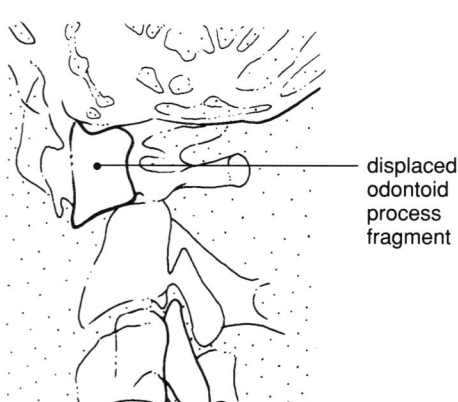

displaced odontoid process fragment

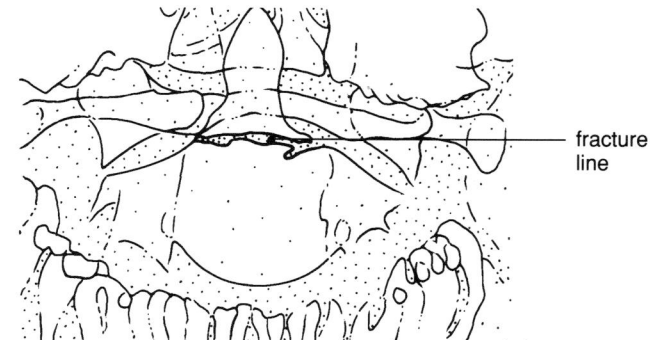

fracture line

Spine

Type II odontoid fractures occur at the base of the odontoid process just above the body of the axis (Fig. 11.9). There may be displacement or angulation of fracture fragments. This is the most frequent type of odontoid fracture.

Type III fractures occur through the body of the axis (Fig. 11.10). These fractures tend to be more sta-

ble than type II odontoid fractures, which frequently lead to nonunion.

Atlanto-axial rotatory dislocation and fixation is an idiopathic disorder in which the atlas and axis are displaced during rotation. This is well demonstrated by fluoroscopy. The atlas begins to turn without accompanying rotation of the axis. Ultimately, this may

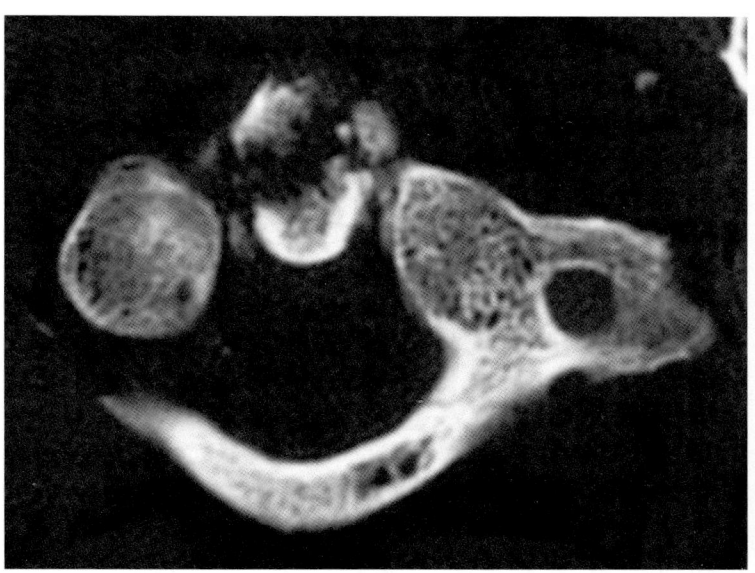

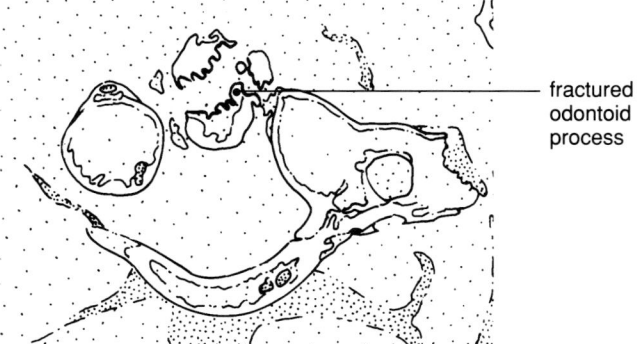

Figure 11.9

Type II odontoid fracture. There is a comminuted fracture through the odontoid process with fracture fragments extending anteriorly.

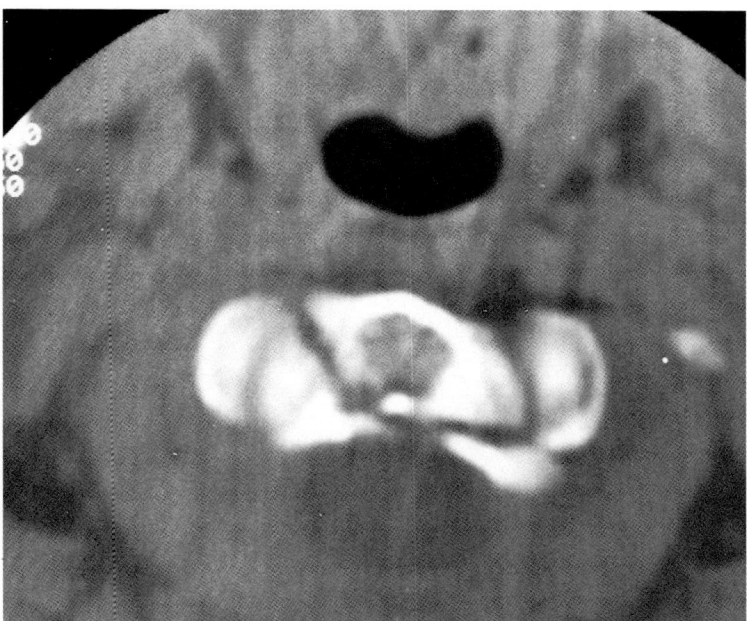

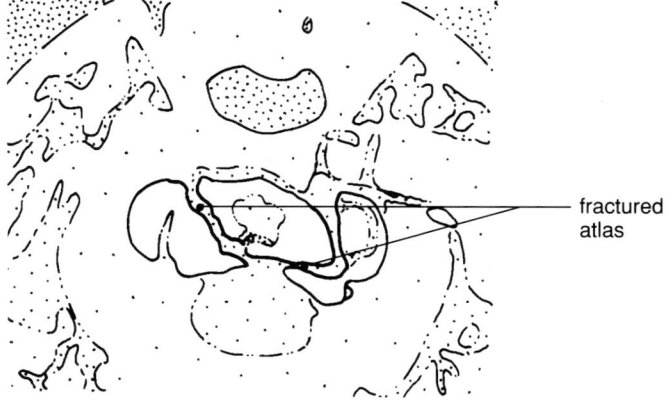

Figure 11.10

Type III odontoid fracture. CT scan demonstrates a comminuted fracture through the base of the odontoid extending into the body of C2.

become nonreducible (fixation) (Fig. 11.11). Clinically, this disorder usually occurs in childhood and presents with torticollis. It is occasionally associated with a recent upper respiratory tract infection or minor trauma. Atlanto-axial rotatory subluxation is usually self limiting and reversible. This disorder needs to be distinguished from congenital muscular torticollis, a disorder of infancy in which a short sternocleiodomastoid results in tilting of the head but the cervical spine itself is usually structurally normal.

A Jefferson fracture results from an axial compressive load to the head, usually from a motor vehicle accident or a diving injury. The ring of C1 is fractured, classically in four places. The lateral masses of C1 are shown to be displaced laterally from the odontoid process on the open-mouth view. In practice, however, there are many variations in the number and location of C1 fractures (Fig. 11.12). CT is frequently helpful for exact delineation of the location of the fracture fragments. C1 fractures are unstable if they are associated with rupture of the transverse ligament.

The so-called hangman's fracture (Fig. 11.13) represents bilateral fractures of the pedicles of C2 which may be associated with subluxation of the body of the axis. It is associated with sudden hyperextension

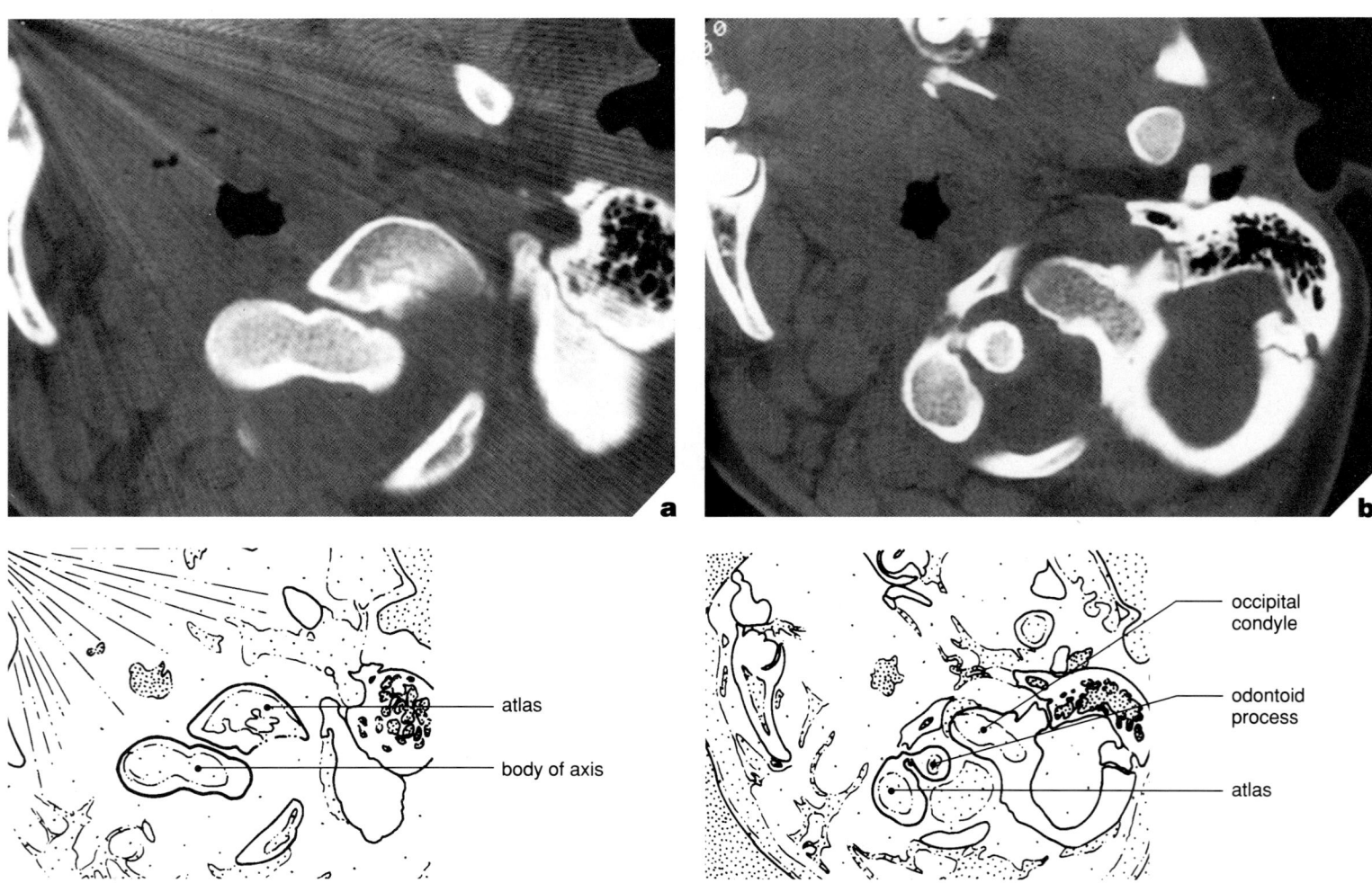

Figure 11.11

*Atlanto-axial rotatory fixation. **a,b** CT images show marked rotation of the atlas on the axis. The atlas is properly aligned with the foramen magnum and head. This results in torticollis.*

of the neck, usually related to motor vehicle accidents. It had previously been associated with victims of judicial hanging, although the term "hangee's fracture" would be more appropriate. A hangman's fracture with associated spondylolisthesis is usually diagnosed by the lateral plain film. When nondisplaced, CT may be essential for diagnosis. Prevertebral soft tissue hematomas are usually present.

HYPERFLEXION INJURIES OF THE CERVICAL SPINE

Flexion injuries of the cervical spine may result in hyperflexion sprain, bilateral facet dislocation, unilateral facet dislocation, compression fractures of the vertebral body (flexion teardrop fracture), and odontoid process fractures. Any associated rotational or compressive component will tend to favor one particular pattern of injury over another. As a general rule for flexion injuries, the area of the posterior longitudinal ligament acts as the fulcrum; structures anterior to it tend to be compressed while structures behind it tend to be splayed apart.

Hyperflexion sprain results from injury to the ligamenta flava and interspinous ligaments. This may result in widening of the interspinous distance, especially at C5/C6 or C6/C7. There may be narrowing of the anterior intervertebral disc space height due to compressive forces. However, often there is no definite abnormality seen on the routine portable lateral view.

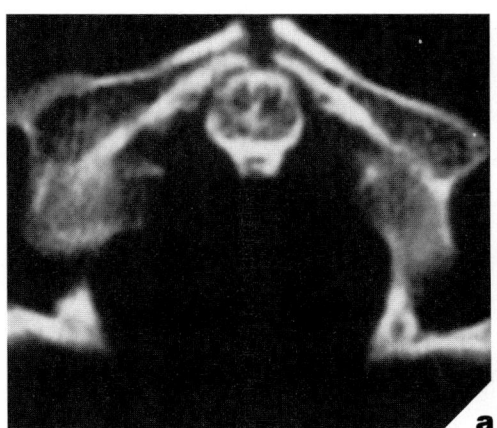 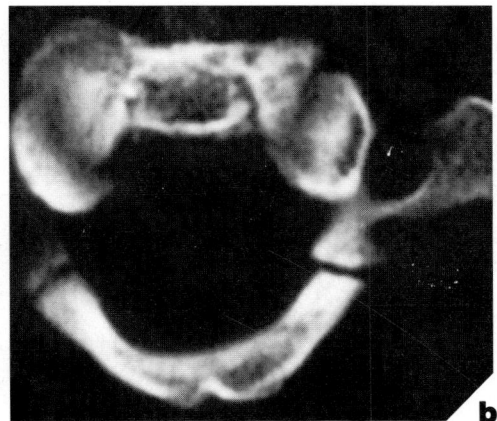

Figure 11.12

*Jefferson fracture. **a,b** CT images at the level of C1 show three fractures: a single fracture at the anterior aspect of the ring of C1 and fractures along both lateral aspects of C1. The classic Jefferson fracture consists of four fractures involving the arch of C1.*

Figure 11.13

Hangman's fracture. A lateral plain film of the cervical spine shows bilateral fractures of the pedicles of C2.

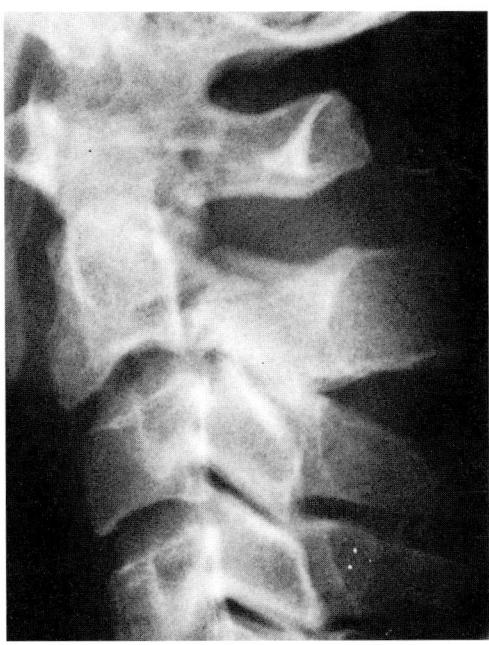 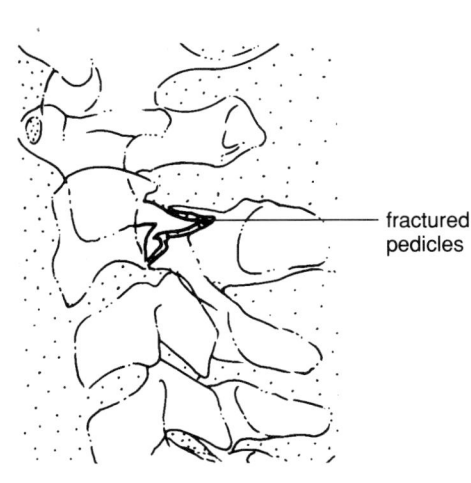

fractured pedicles

Bilateral facet joint dislocation (Figs. 11.14, 11.15) results from a more severe hyperflexion injury, usually resulting from a direct blow to the occipit. There is disruption of the anterior and posterior ligamentous structures, usually associated with a soft tissue hematoma. The facet joints become malaligned and completely dislocated, with the superior pillars locking anterior to the inferior pillars. Commonly, there are associated fractures of the posterior elements.

Unilateral facet dislocation may result when a hyperflexion-type injury occurs while the head is rotated. This may produce a "unilateral locked facet joint," in which a superior pillar is displaced anteriorly to an inferior pillar. Oblique views of the cervi-

cal spine or CT reconstructions show the dislocated facet to best advantage. C4/C5 and C5/C6 are the most commonly affected levels.

If a superior pillar does not quite dislocate anterior to the inferior pillar, it may come to lie "perched" on top of the inferior pillar. Such perched facets (Fig. 11.16) do not articulate properly. CT demonstrates the "naked" facet sign.

Compression fractures of cervical vertebra produced by flexion injuries may result in simple wedge compression fractures or the "teardrop" hyperflexion fracture dislocation. Simple wedge compression fractures result from a moderate flexion injury, which compresses the anterior aspect of the vertebra, partic-

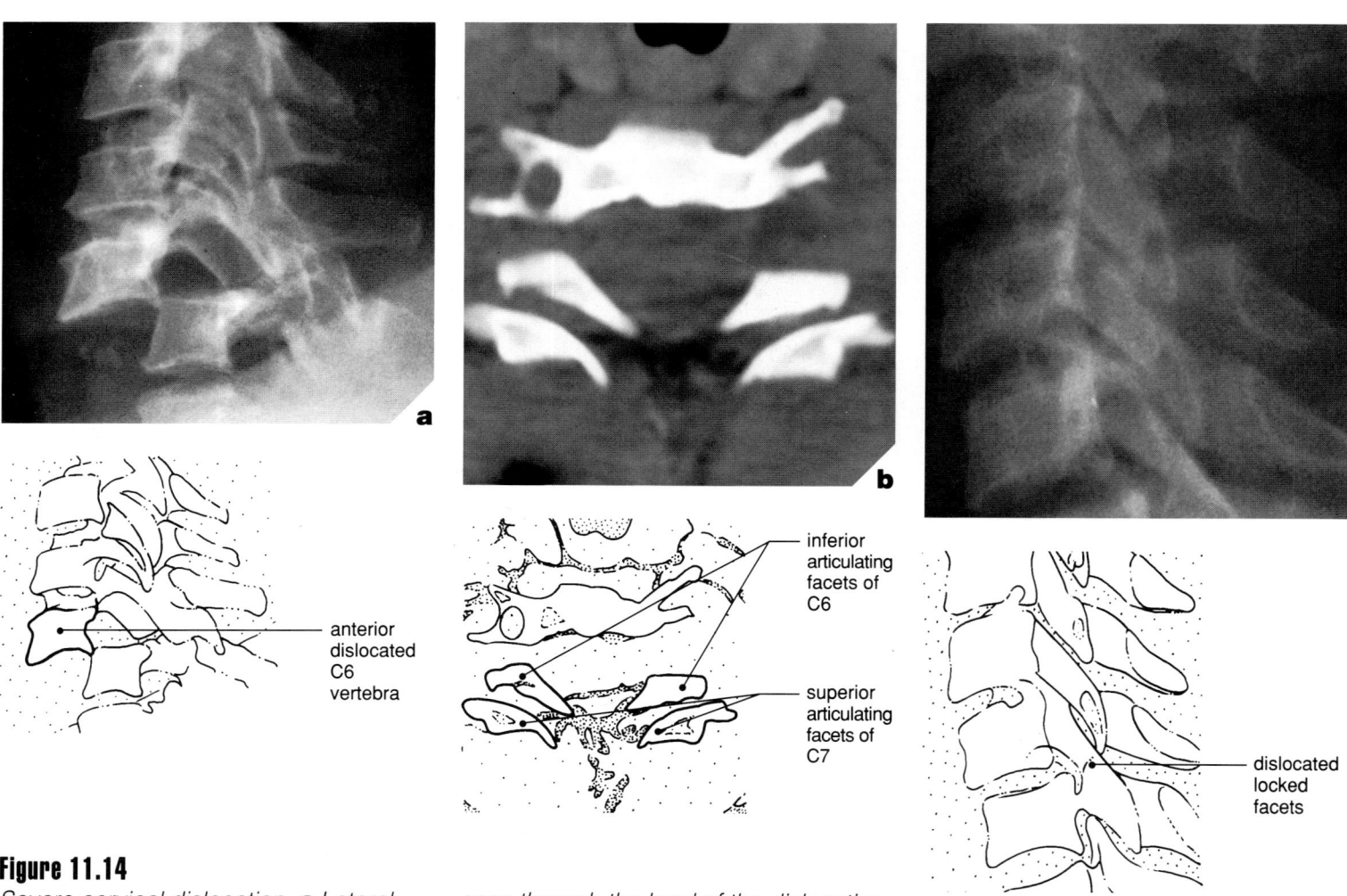

Figure 11.14

*Severe cervical dislocation. **a** Lateral plain film shows severe dislocation of the C6 vertebra anterior to C7 with bilateral dislocated and locked facets. **b** CT scan through the level of the dislocation shows the inferior articulating facets of C6 anterior to the superior articulating facets of C7.*

Figure 11.15

Bilateral facet joint dislocation. There is anterior dislocation of the C5 vertebral body and facet joints. The inferior articulating facets of C5 are "jumped and locked" in front of the superior articulating facets of C6.

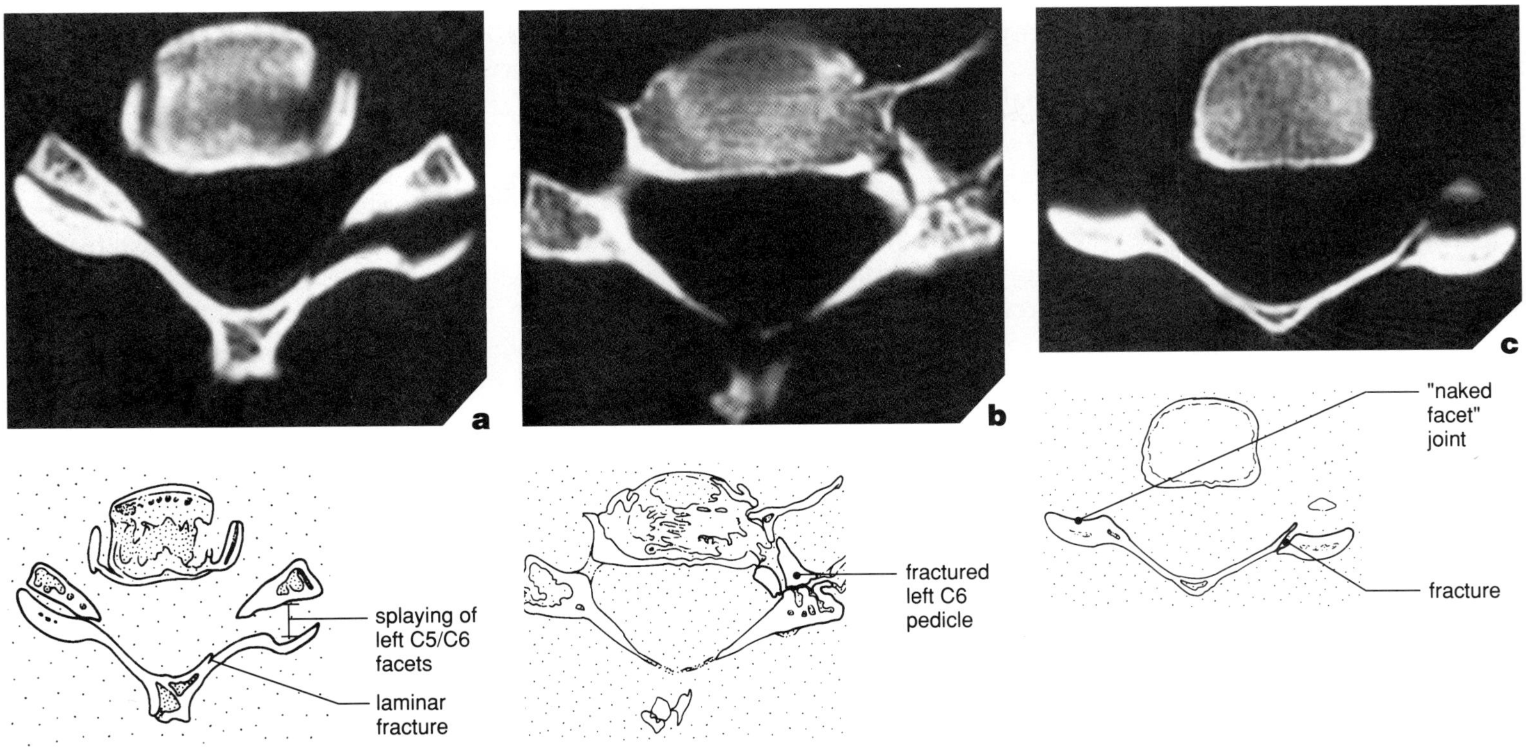

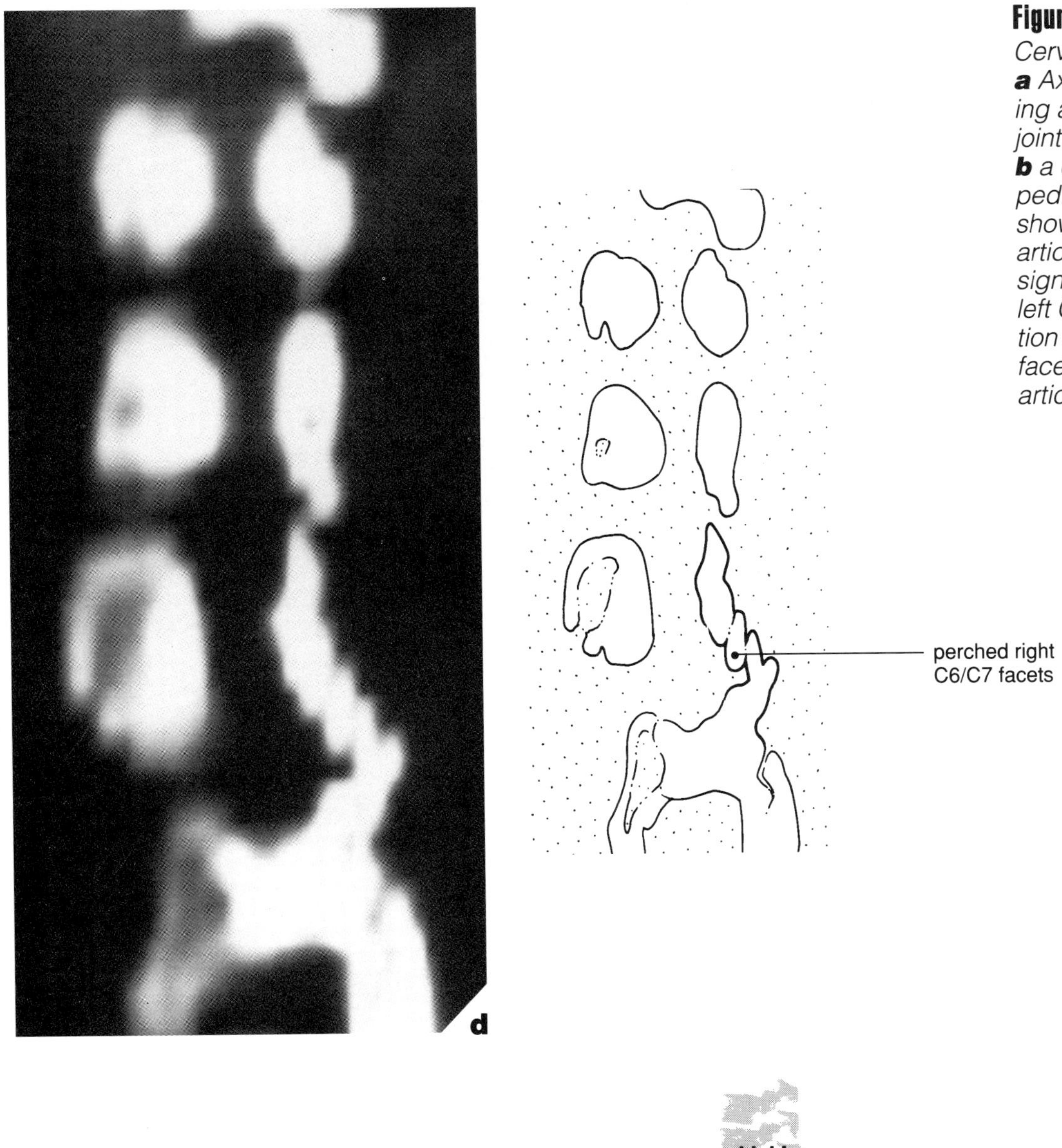

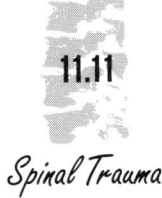

"naked facet" joint

splaying of left C5/C6 facets

laminar fracture

fractured left C6 pedicle

fracture

perched right C6/C7 facets

Figure 11.16

Cervical fractures and perched facets.
a *Axial CT image shows abnormal splaying and separation of the left C5/C6 facet joint, a left laminar fracture of C5, and* ***b*** *a comminuted fracture of the left C6 pedicle.* ***c*** *Axial CT at the C6/C7 level shows no articulation of the right superior articulating facet of C6 (the "naked facet sign") and separation and fracture of the left C6/C7 facets.* ***d*** *Sagittal reconstruction shows the right inferior articulating facet of C6 perched on top of the superior articulating facet of C7.*

a

b

c

d

ularly at C5 and/or C6. It is identified as loss of height of the anterior portion of a vertebral body. The vertebral body fracture is usually stable but it may be associated with other, more severe fractures or soft tissue injuries.

The teardrop hyperflexion fracture dislocation (Fig. 11.17) results from a severe flexion injury associated with a significant compressive force. Typically, the C5 or C6 vertebral body is fractured and compressed anteriorly, with retropulsion of fragments from the posterior portion of the vertebral body into the spinal canal. There is often an associated sagittal cleft fracture of the vertebral body (Fig. 11.18), posterior element fractures, narrowing of the adjacent intervertebral disc space and pillar fractures. This injury is commonly associated with diving accidents, falls, and motor vehicle accidents. Bony and soft tissue ex-

tension into the spinal canal often results in cervical spinal cord compression and quadriplegia.

EXTENSION INJURIES OF THE CERVICAL SPINE

Extension injuries of the cervical spine are notoriously difficult to diagnose. In the case of hyperextension strain, there are often no demonstrable radiologic abnormalities. Extension injuries usually result from an upward or backward striking injury to the jaw, face or forehead, most often as a result of a motor vehicle accident. Most serious hyperextension injuries are unstable and the patients should not undergo flexion/extension positioning.

Hyperextension fracture dislocation injuries occur most commonly in middle-aged or elderly patients

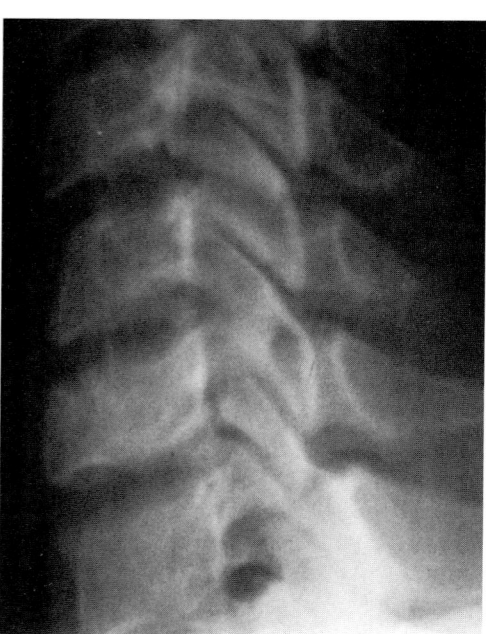

Figure 11.17
Teardrop hyperflexion fracture. Lateral plain film shows a compression fracture of the C6 vertebral body with a free fragment extending from its anterior/inferior margin.

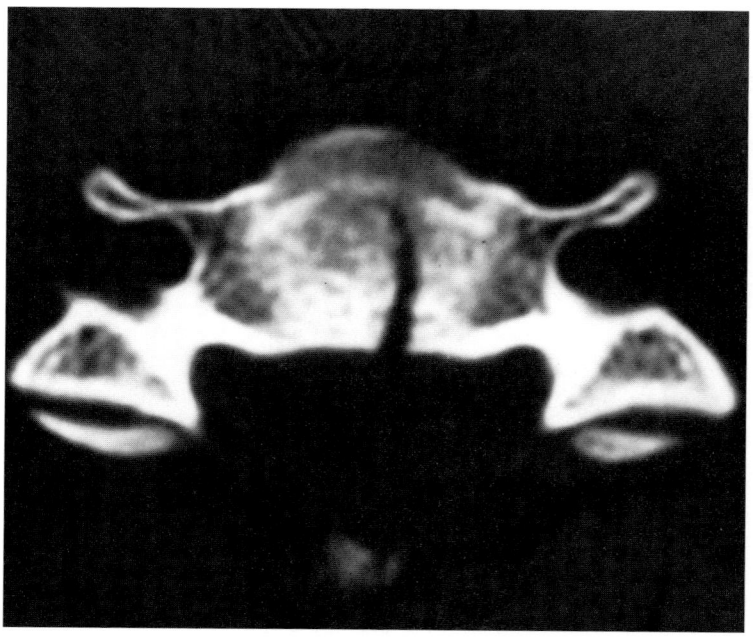

Figure 11.18
Sagittal cleft fracture of C4. CT shows a slightly displaced sagittally oriented incomplete fracture through the C4 vertebral body.

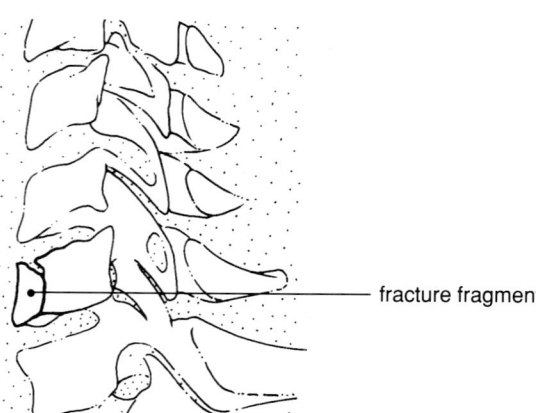

fracture fragment

with pre-existing degenerative disease of the cervical spine. The hyperextension fracture dislocation (Fig. 11.19) typically results from a combined extension and compressive force. This results in compression and fractures of the posterior elements (particularly the pillar), splaying of the vertebral bodies and intervertebral discs, rupture of the anterior longitudinal ligament with an associated prevertebral soft tissue hematoma and anterior dislocation of upper cervical vertebral bodies. Vacuum phenomenon may be demonstrated within the stretched intervertebral disc or behind a stretched (but not torn) anterior longitudinal ligament. There is often an associated avulsion fracture of the anterior–inferior portion of an inferior vertebral body endplate, particularly at C2 (Fig. 11.20). This is termed the *extension teardrop fracture*.

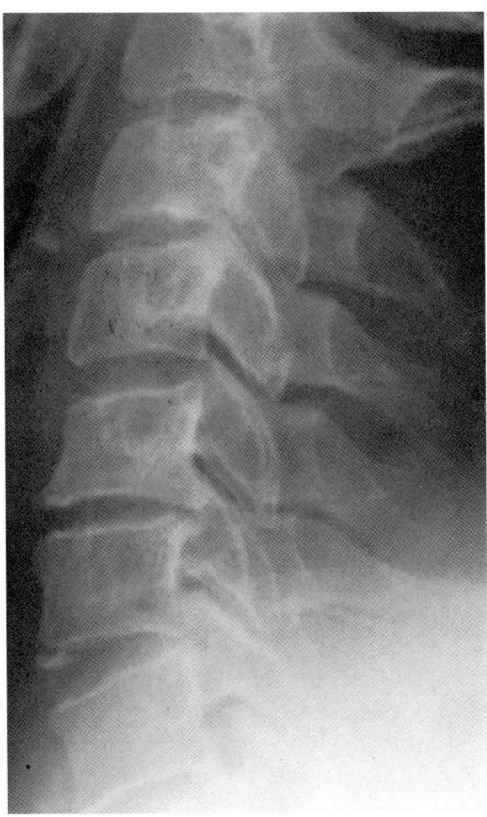

Figure 11.19
Hyperextension injury. There is an avulsion fracture involving the anterior/inferior endplate of C6 and widening of the C5/C6 intervertebral disc space. Incidentally noted are degenerative changes at C5/C6.

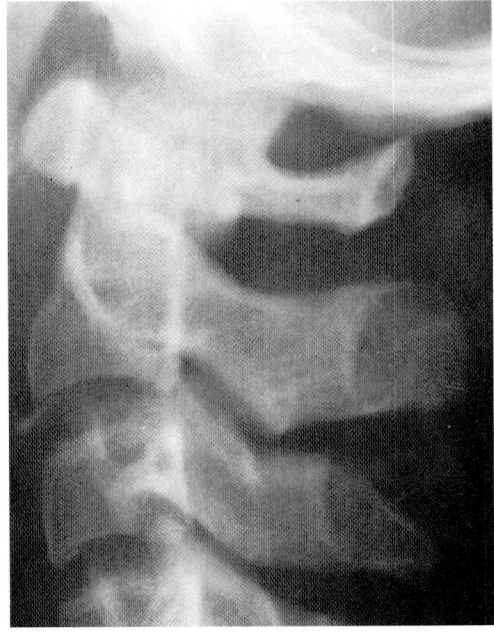

Figure 11.20
Extension teardrop fracture. There is a small avulsion fracture of the inferior endplate of the C2 vertebral body. This patient was a victim of a diving accident.

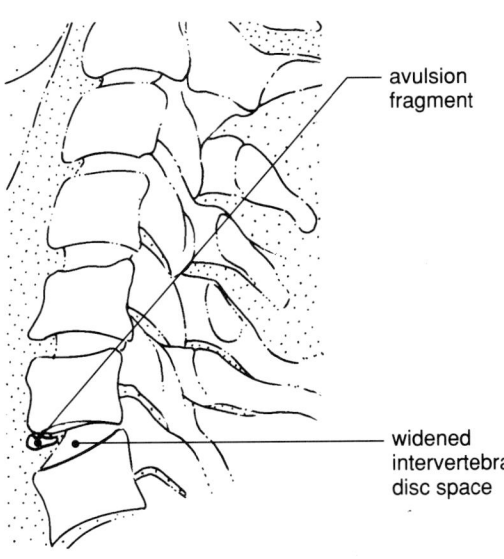

— avulsion fragment

— widened intervertebral disc space

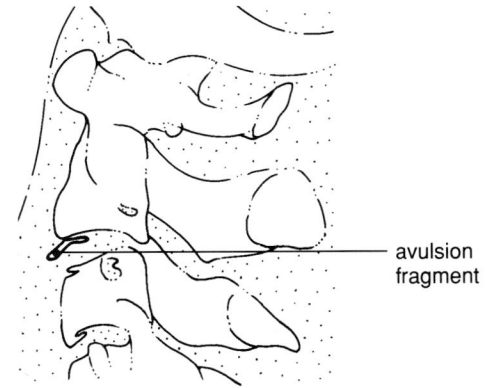

— avulsion fragment

Pillar fractures may be associated with hyperextension fracture dislocations or they may be the result of an isolated injury (Fig. 11.21). When there are no additional abnormalities, pillar fractures are usu- ally caused by lateral flexion or a mostly rotational component combined with a hyperextension vector. "Pillar view" plain radiographs, conventional tomography, or CT demonstrate these fractures best.

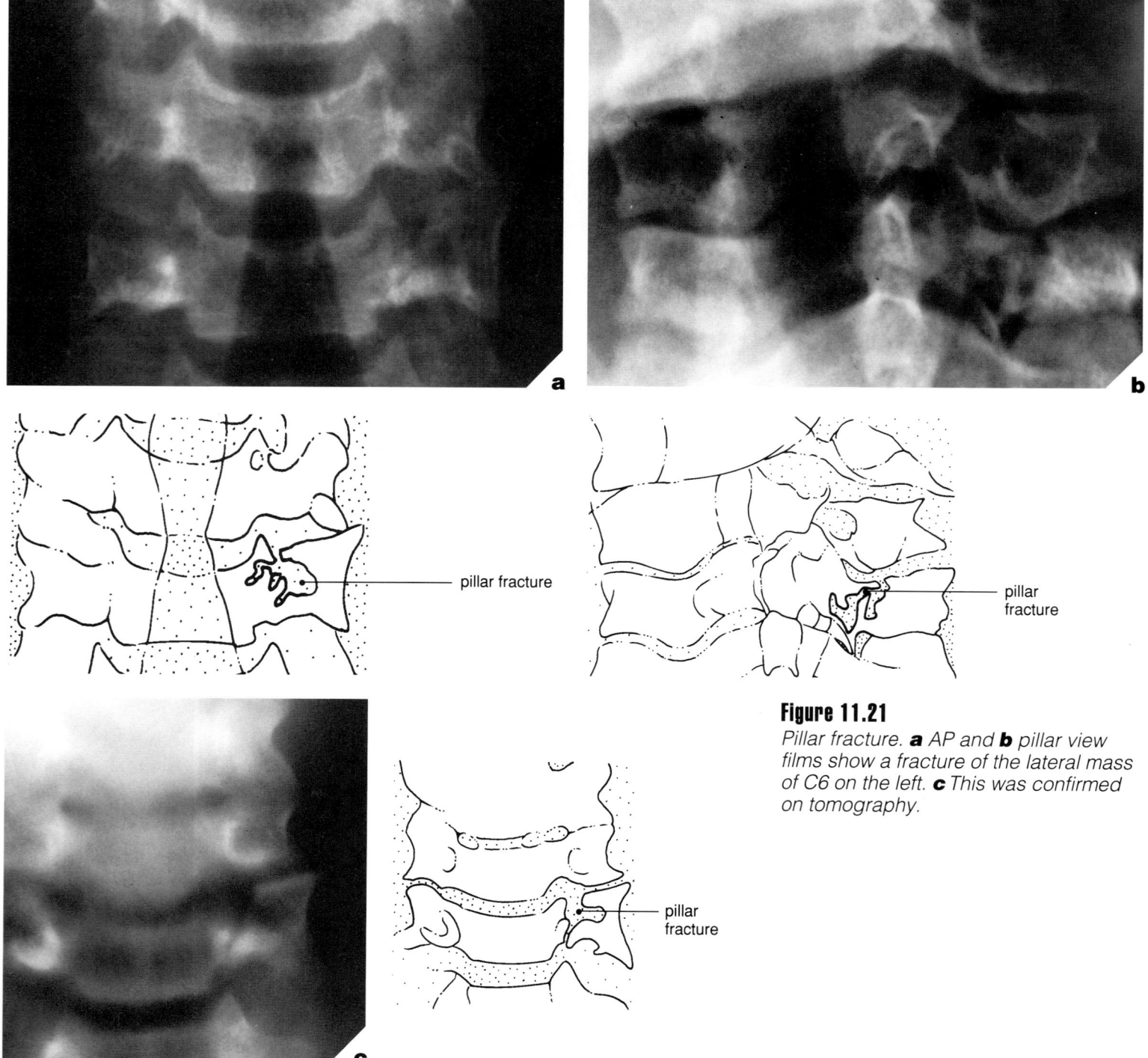

pillar fracture

pillar fracture

pillar fracture

Figure 11.21

*Pillar fracture. **a** AP and **b** pillar view films show a fracture of the lateral mass of C6 on the left. **c** This was confirmed on tomography.*

THORACIC AND LUMBAR SPINAL TRAUMA

Injuries of the thoracic and lumbar spine are less diverse than cervical injuries. For the most part, they can be divided into compression fractures, burst injuries, slice fractures, and spondylolysis/spondylolisthesis. The vertebra at the thoraco–lumbar junction are frequently involved. Vertebral bodies weakened by osteoporosis or tumor are especially prone to fracture from even minor trauma.

Compression fractures due to osteoporosis (Fig. 11.22) usually produce an anterior wedge deformity with preservation of the height and integrity of the posterior third of the vertebral body. Even in the presence of demineralization, neoplastic processes and, in particular, multiple myeloma still need to be considered since osteopenia is also a frequent component of these disorders. Children with spinal compression fractures (Fig. 11.23) may have tumor invasion by leukemia or histiocytosis X. Scheuermann's disease (Fig. 11.24) is a developmental disorder of adolescence that results in pressure retardation of the anterior growth plates of thoracic vertebra. This produces wedge-shaped vertebral bodies.

Traumatic compression fractures from motor vehi-

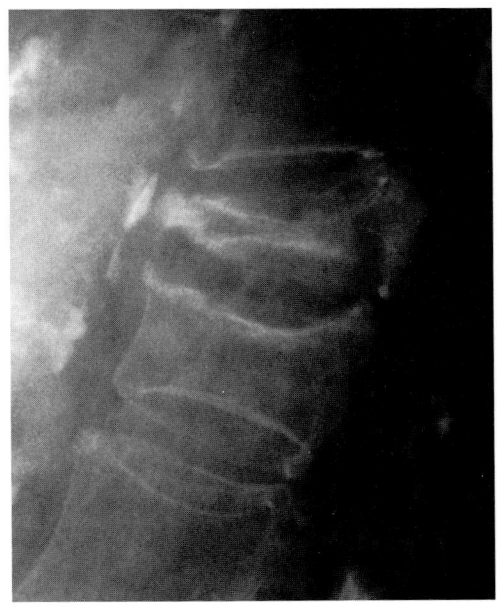

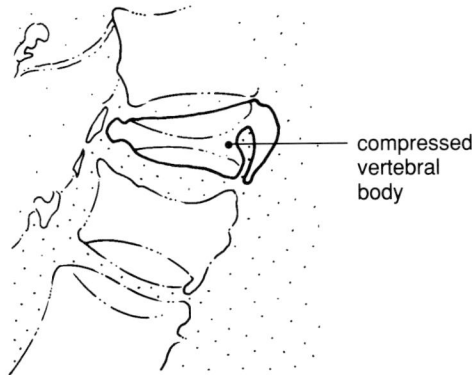

compressed vertebral body

Figure 11.22

Osteoporosis with compression fracture. Lateral view of the lower thoracic spine demonstrates a compression fracture of T11. There is marked loss of height and wedging of the anterior and mid-portion of the vertebral body with relative sparing of the posterior margin.

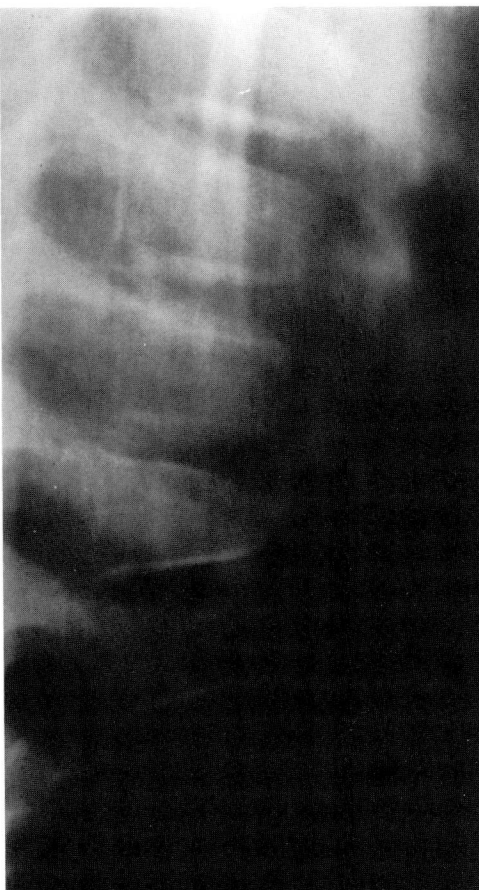

Figure 11.23

Compression fractures. Anterior, wedge-shaped compression fractures are demonstrated in this child. Although the etiology in this case was trauma, leukemia might also present with similar findings. Diffuse bony demineralization is present.

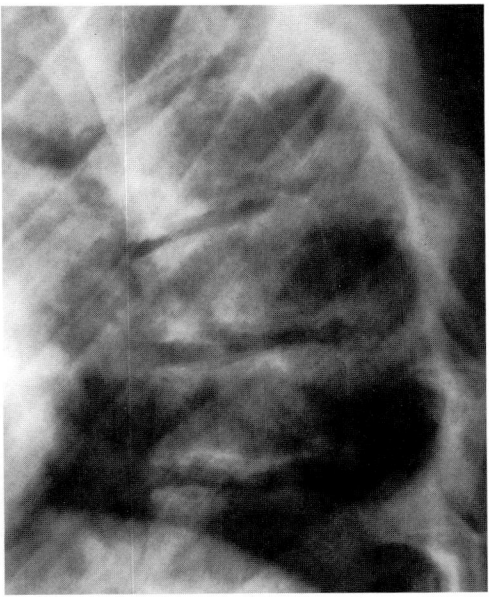

Figure 11.24

Scheuermann's disease. Lateral view of the thoracic spine shows anterior wedge deformity of multiple vertebral bodies.

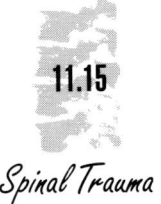

cle accidents often produce complex injuries (Fig. 11.25). Since fractures of the thoracic and lumbar spine are usually associated with a hyperflexion force, there is often posterior displacement of bony and soft tissue fragments into the spinal canal (Fig. 11.26) These may compress the spinal cord, conus medullaris, or nerve roots.

Slice fractures are transverse fractures through the vertebral bodies and posterior elements; there is resultant horizontal splitting of the vertebra into supe-

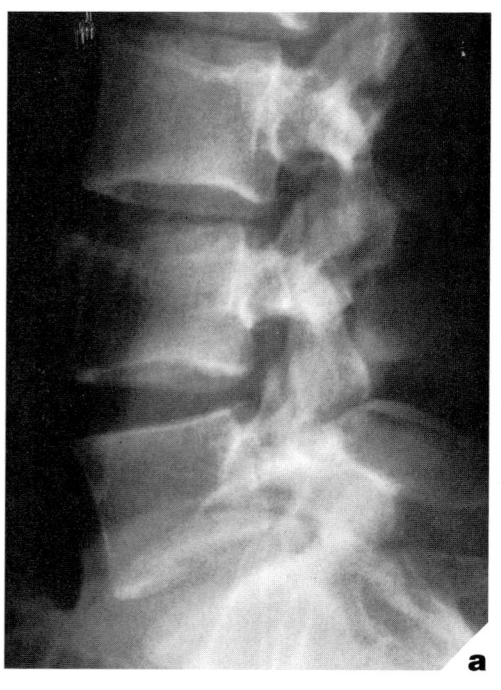
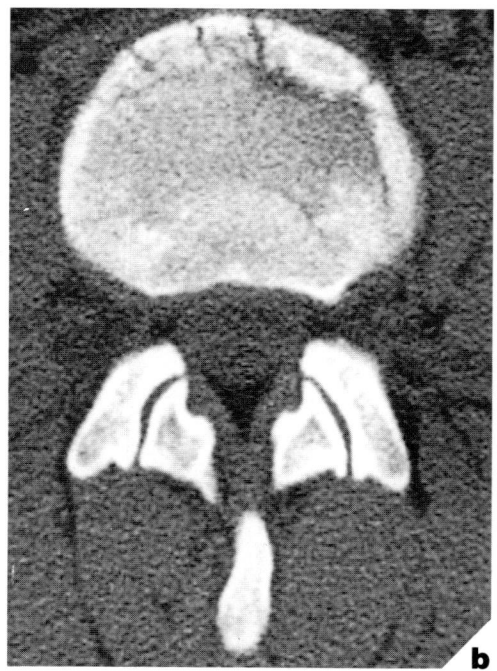
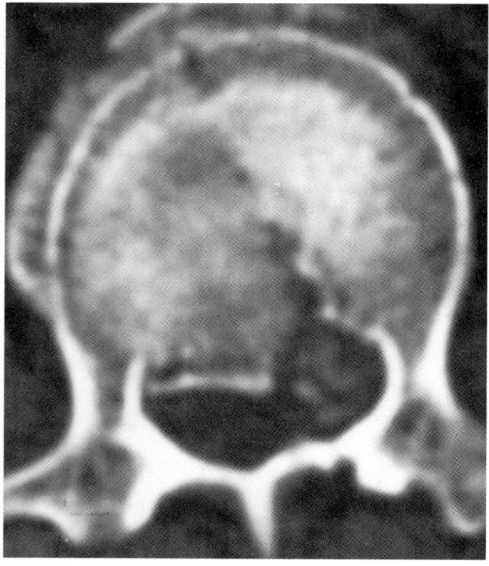

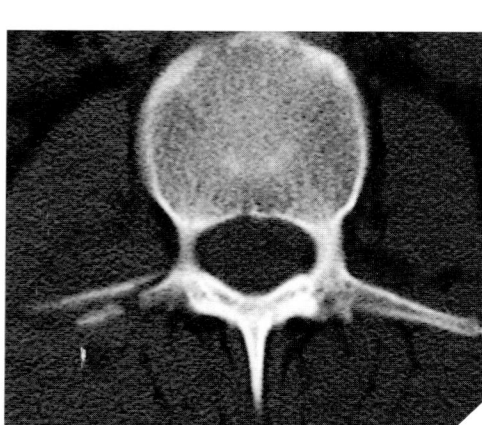
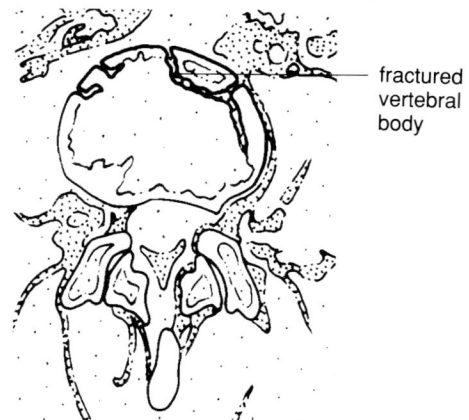
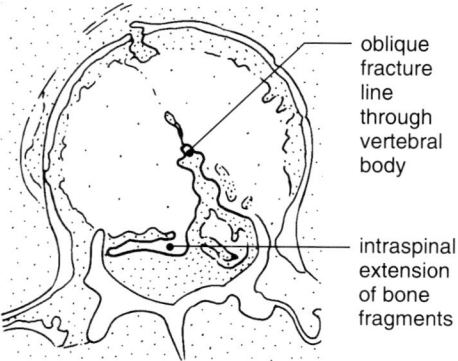

Figure 11.25

*L4 vertebral body and L3 transverse process fractures. **a,b** There is a fracture of the antero–superior aspect of the L4 vertebral body. **c** Right transverse process fractures, which were undetectable on plain films, are visualized on CT.*

Figure 11.26

Hyperflexion injury, L1. There is an obliquely oriented fracture through the L1 vertebral body. There is posterior extension of fracture fragments and soft tissue material into the spinal canal.

rior and inferior fragments ("Chance" fracture). These usually occur in motor vehicle accident victims who were wearing seatbelt restraints at the time of injury.

Burst fractures result from an axial compression force. Disc material is forced into the vertebral endplates and the vertebral body becomes crushed (Fig. 11.27). Fracture fragments extend radially in all directions. There may be associated fractures of the posterior elements.

CT is the most reliable method for detecting the presence of bone fragments and for evaluation of posterior element injuries. MR is superior for detecting intraspinal hemorrhage and soft tissue injuries.

Avulsion of cervical or lumbar (Fig. 11.28) nerve roots occur from injuries which result in pulling, twisting, or distraction of the extremities from the trunk. These are often seen in motorcycle accidents. A dural tear with pseudomeningocele formation results; this is optimally visualized by myelography.

SPONDYLOLYSIS AND SPONDYLOLISTHESIS

Spondylolysis (Fig. 11.29) represents a fracture of the pars interarticularis of one or more vertebra. This is best visualized on oblique plain films as a fracture of the "neck of the 'Scotty' dog." It is often associated with forward displacement of the vertebral body directly above it; this is termed *spondylolisthesis*. Spondylolisthesis may also be a result of severe facet joint hypertrophy which causes anterior slipping of one vertebra in relation to another. L5/S1 and L4/L5 are the most common levels for both types of spondylolisthesis. There is increase in the anteroposterior diameter of the spinal canal and kinking of the thecal sac and neural contents. These findings may be rather mild (Fig. 11.30) or may extend across the full length of a vertebral body. Various classifications of the severity of slippage have been proposed but the most informative description is based upon actual measurement of the distance of slippage. Occasionally, a superior vertebra becomes displaced posterior to the vertebra below it; this is termed *retrolisthesis*.

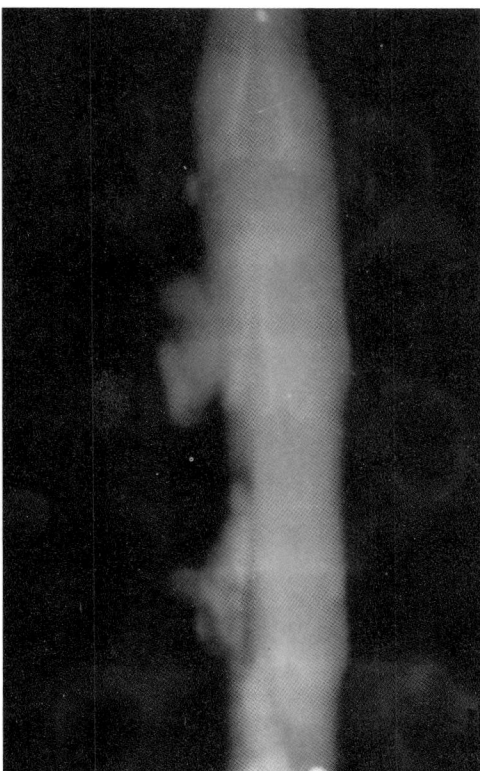

Figure 11.28
Avulsion of nerve roots. AP film from a myelogram shows extravasation of contrast material outside the spinal canal and pseudomeningocele formation.

Figure 11.27
Burst fracture L1. Postoperative plain film shows a burst fracture of the L1 vertebral body with diffuse increased transverse diameter of the vertebral body.

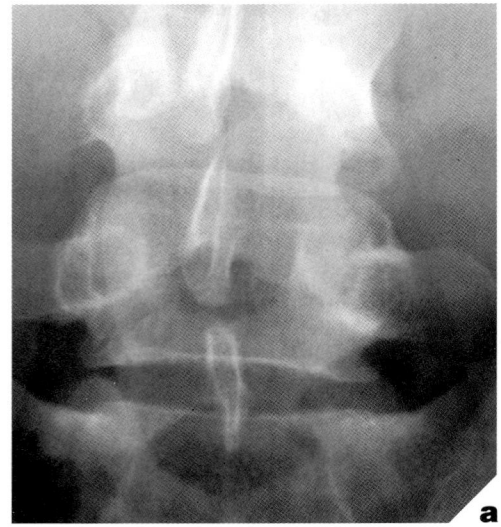

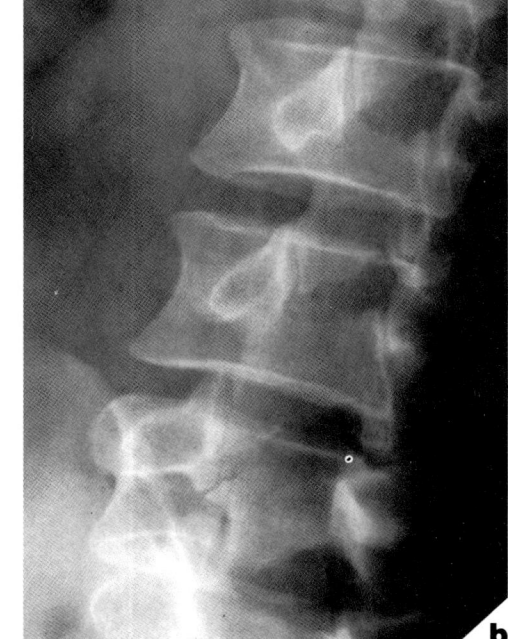

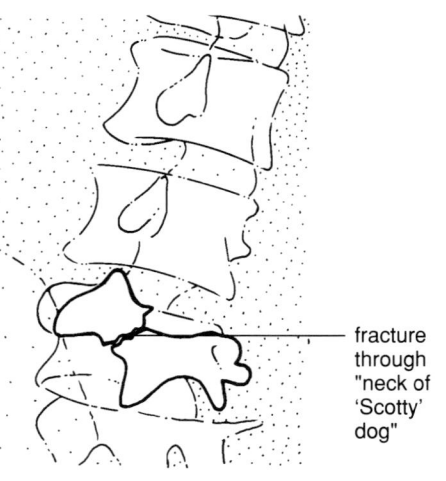

fracture
through
"neck of
'Scotty'
dog"

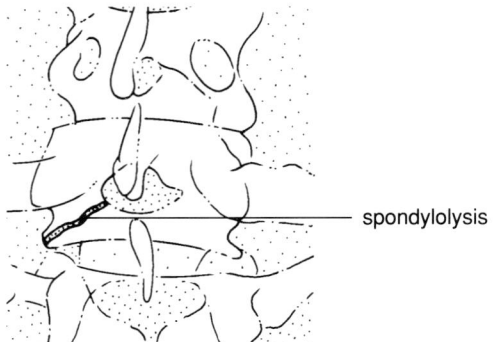

spondylolysis

Figure 11.29

*Spondylolysis L4/L5 on the right. **a** AP and **b** oblique plain films demonstrate a lucency through the pars interarticularis.*

This oblique view shows the fracture line extending through the "neck of the 'Scotty' dog."

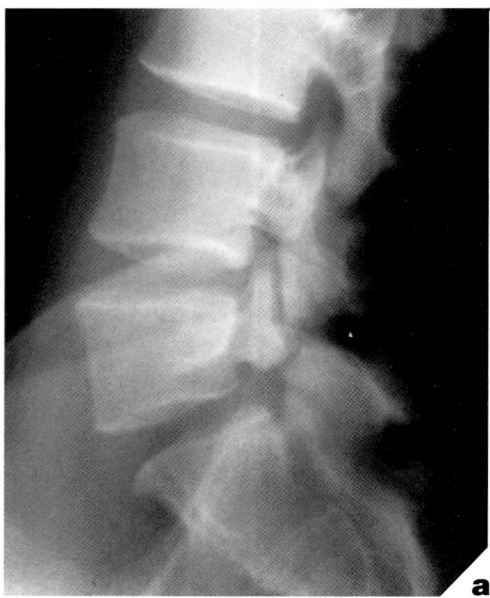

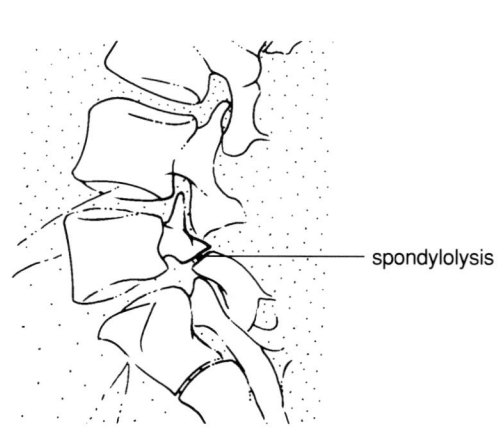

spondylolysis

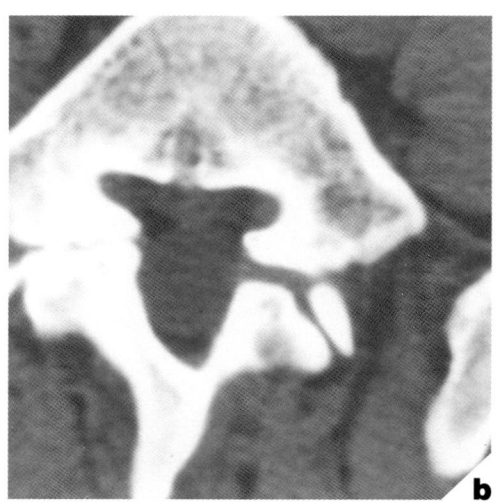

spondylolysis

widened
antero-
posterior
diameter

spondylolysis

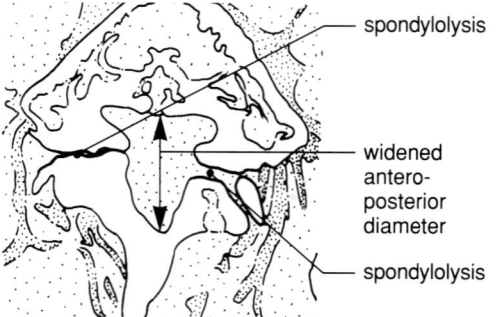

Figure 11.30

Spondylolisthesis and spondylolysis. There is an elongated AP diameter of the spinal canal associated with bilateral

*fractures of the pars interarticularis on the **a** plain lateral view and **b** CT images.*

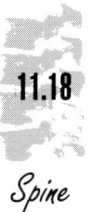

Degenerative Diseases of the Spine

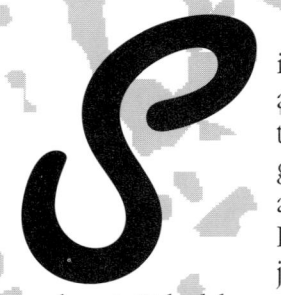

Since its original description by Mixter and Barr in the 1930s, herniation of the intervertebral disc has been regarded as a key cause of low back and cervical pain and radiculopathy. Low back pain continues to be a major cause of suffering and disability; it has probably existed since humans became bipedal creatures. The added pressure upon the spine by maintaining an upright posture may cause the soft, cartilaginous disc material to evenly bulge or focally protrude (herniate) from its normal location. If it extends posteriorly into the spinal canal, it may compress upon the thecal sac, nerve roots, or spinal cord.

HERNIATED NUCLEUS PULPOSUS

A disc herniation represents focal protrusion of the gelatinous nucleus pulposus through a tear in the an-ulus fibrosus. Most symptomatic disc herniations are posterolateral (Fig. 12.1). These may be identified on myelography as angled, sharply marginated extradural filling defects. CT scans show an extradural mass anterior and/or lateral to the thecal sac. On noncontrast CT scans, disc material is hyperdense to the mostly fluid-filled thecal sac. CT following myelography shows the denser, contrast-filled thecal sac compressed by the less dense herniated disc material. MRI also clearly shows the protruding disc material on most pulse sequences and offers the benefits of multiplanar imaging and the absence of ionizing radiation.

Disc herniations are most common in the lumbar and cervical spine; however, they occasionally occur in the thoracic spine (Fig. 12.2). In the lower thoracic spine they are often associated with bladder or bowel dysfunction; in the cervical spine they may be associated with long tract signs, spasticity, weakness, and/or radiculopathy.

In addition to the extradural mass effect upon the

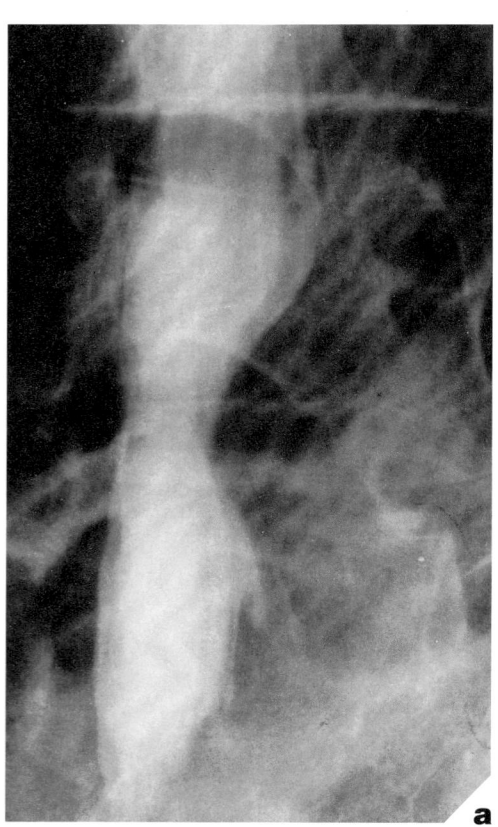

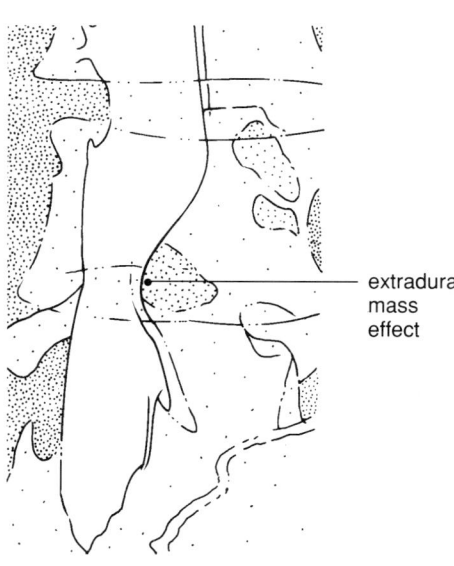

extradural mass effect

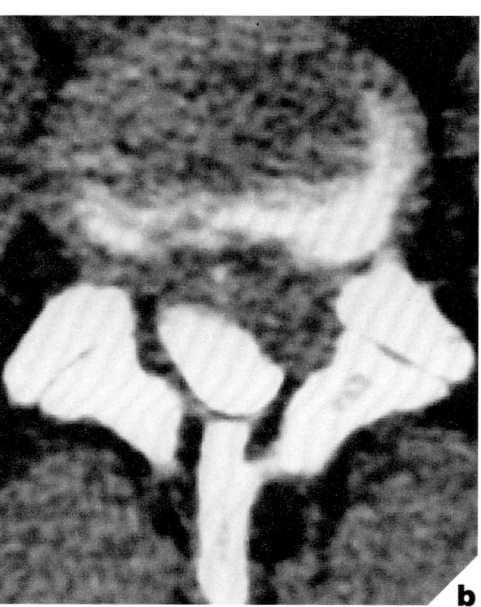

b

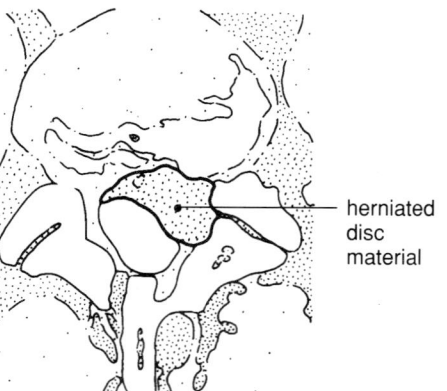

herniated disc material

Figure 12.1

*Herniated nucleus pulposus. **a** A lumbar myelogram demonstrates a large left-sided extradural defect at L4/L5 compressing the thecal sac and left L5 nerve root and displacing them medially. **b** The herniated disc material is well visualized on the postmyelographic CT scan which shows extension of disc material posteriorly and laterally and compression of the thecal sac. This finding was confirmed on **c** T2-weighted sagittal MRI and **d** T1-weighted axial MRI.*

thecal sac, disc herniations frequently cause compression of nerve roots; this results in swelling of the nerve root and myelographic foreshortening of the nerve root sleeve when compared to the opposite side.

A lateral disc herniation (Fig. 12.3) results from protrusion of disc material into a neural foramen, often resulting in compression of the nerve root exiting at that level. This type of disc herniation may be invisible on myelography since it usually does not compress the thecal sac or cause nerve root sleeve foreshortening.

INTERVERTEBRAL DISC BULGING AND SPINAL STENOSIS

Unlike disc herniation, diffuse bulging of the anulus fibrosus produces a smooth, extradural defect on myelography. Typically, disc bulges are central, al-though they may lateralize to either side. On CT or MRI, disc bulges do not result in the polypoid, angled extradural mass seen with disc herniations. Instead, there is a generalized increase in diameter of the disc, with preservation of its original contour.

Particularly in the elderly, disc bulges are often associated with thickening and hypertrophy of the ligaments and bony elements of the posterior arch of the spinal canal (Fig. 12.4). The facet joints become hypertrophic and sclerotic and the ligamenta flava thicken. This results in compression of the thecal sac laterally and posteriorly. Facet joint hypertrophy is usually bilateral although often it is asymmetric. When coupled with the ventral compression from a bulging disc, there is a focal, circumferential narrowing of the transverse diameter of the thecal sac. This is termed *spinal stenosis*. When severe, there may be a complete block to flow of contrast on myelography. More commonly, spinal stenosis produces an "hourglass" configuration of the contrast-filled thecal sac (Fig. 12.5).

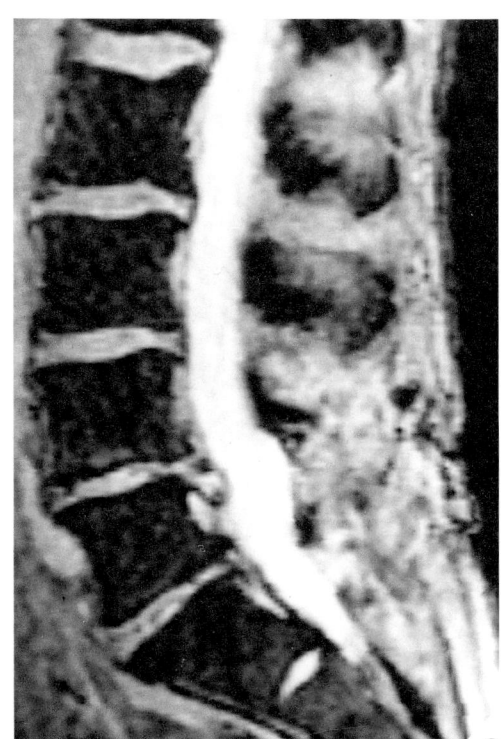

c

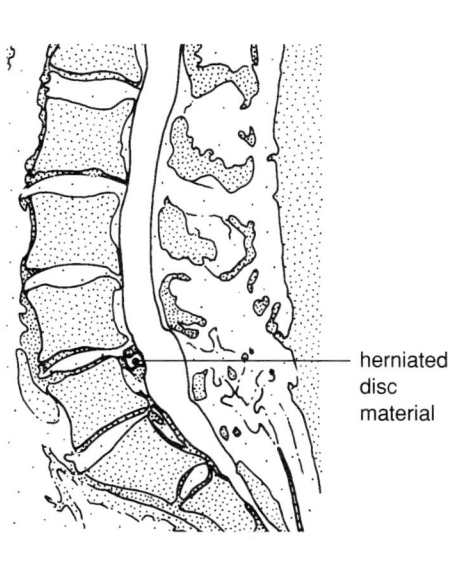

herniated
disc
material

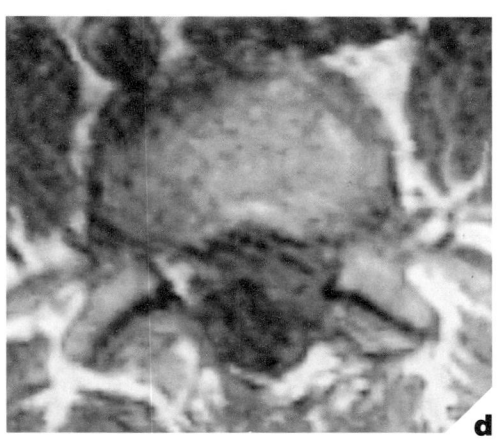

d

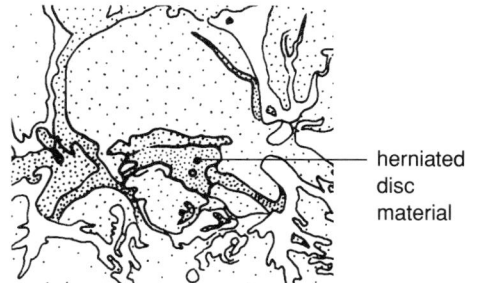

herniated
disc
material

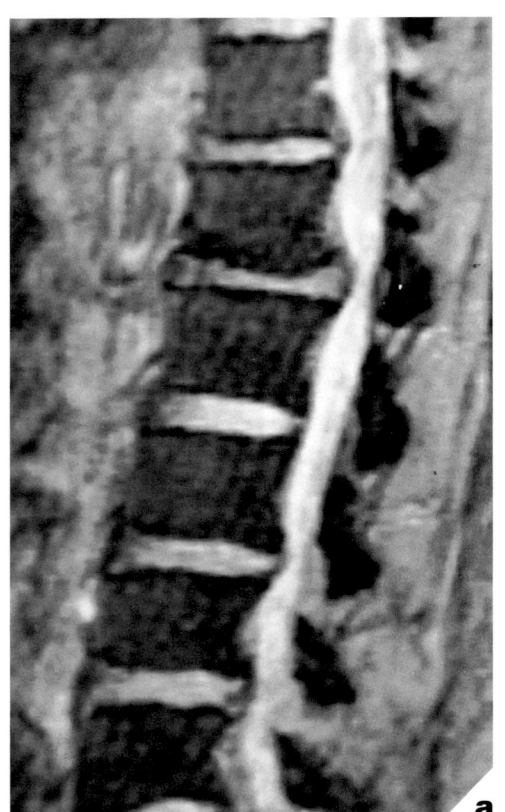

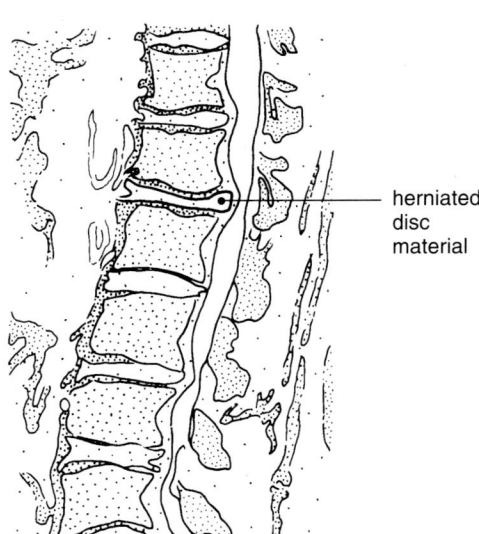

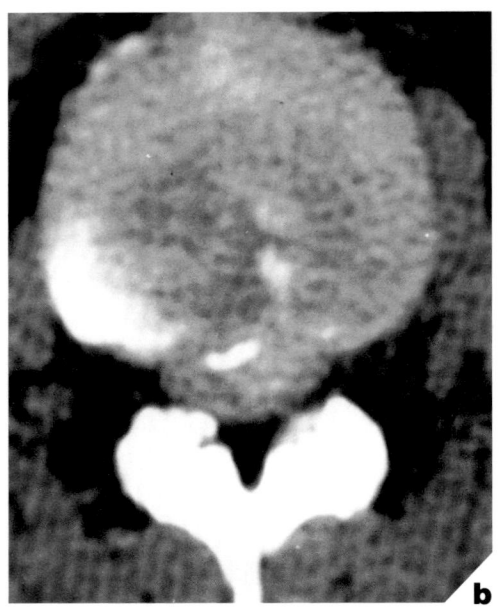

Figure 12.2

*L1/L2 disc herniation. There is herniation of disc material at L1/L2 on **a** T2–weighted sagittal MRI and **b** axial CT scan. There is associated facet joint hypertrophy demonstrated on the CT image.*

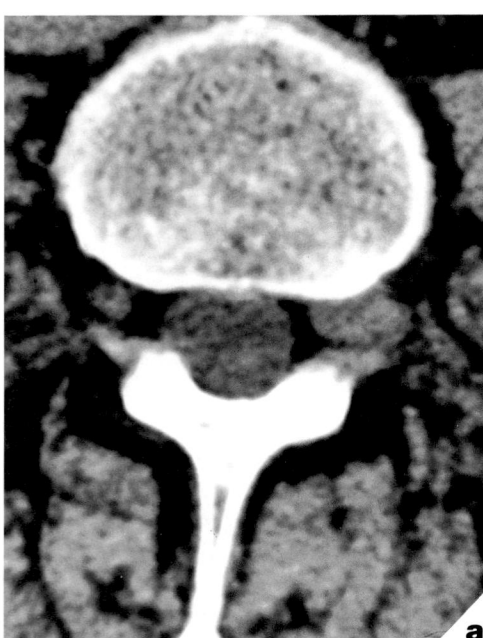

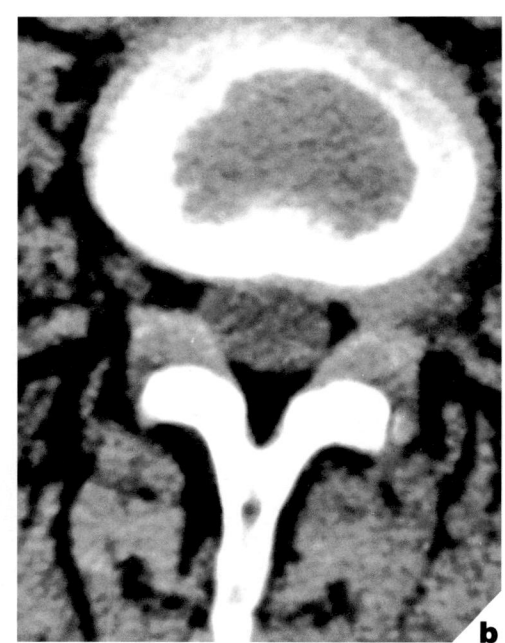

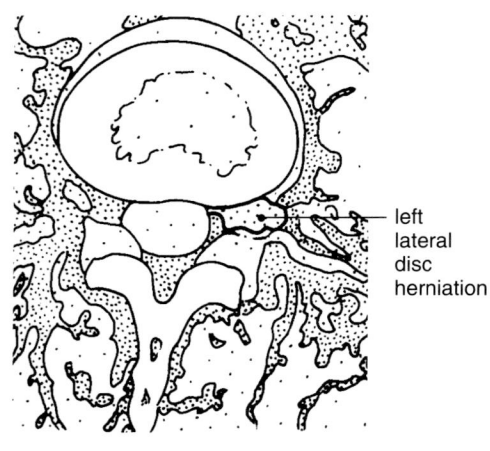

Figure 12.3

*Lateral disc herniation. **a,b** There is a herniation of disc material into the left L3/L4 neural foramen on these CT images. Such lateral herniations often result in no abnormalities on myelography.*

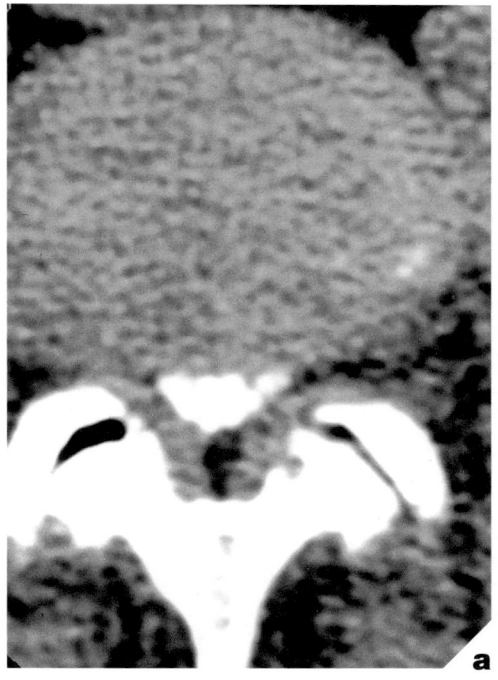
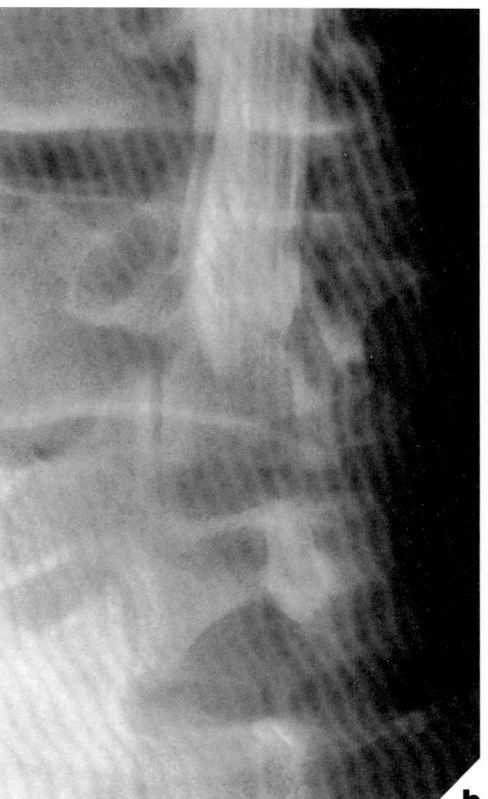
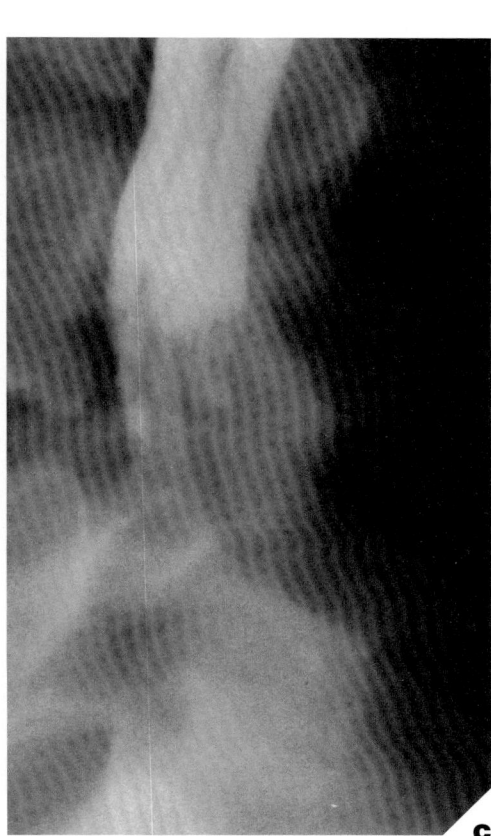

Figure 12.4

Spinal stenosis. **a** Postmyelographic CT scan at L4/L5 shows circumferential narrowing of the thecal sac by a moderate diffuse disc bulge, thickening of the ligamenta flava and hy-pertrophic facet joints. There is vacuum facet phenomenon. **b,c** At myelography there was a virtual complete block to flow of contrast medium at this level.

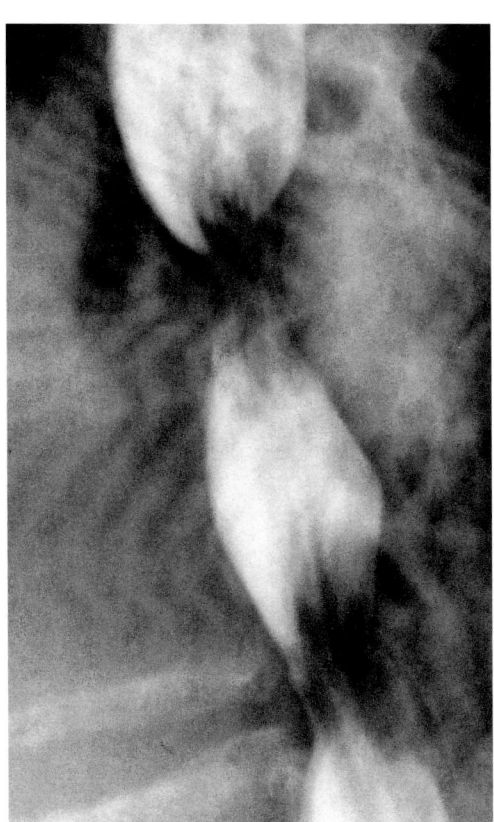
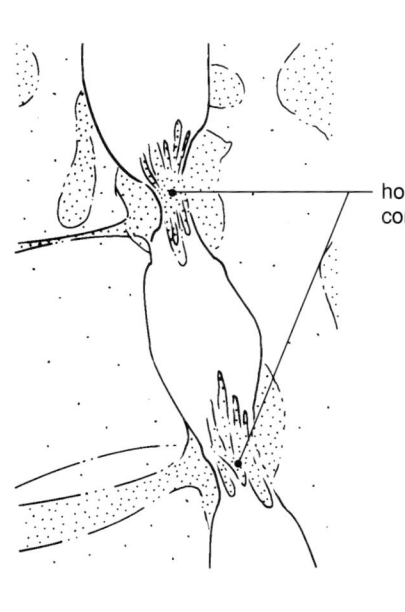

hourglass configuration

Figure 12.5

Spinal stenosis. This contrast–filled the-cal sac demonstrates an "hourglass" configuration at multiple levels due to multiple central disc bulges, facet joint hypertrophy, and thickening of the liga-menta flava.

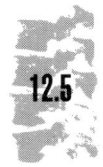

Lumbar spinal stenosis results in compression of the nerve roots of the cauda equina. These nerve roots may become redundant and swollen. Similarly, there may be compression and dilatation of epidural veins. These dilated, tortuous nerve roots and veins produce serpentine filling defects in the contrast-filled thecal sac (Fig. 12.6) which might be confused with an arteriovenous malformation.

Bony hypertrophy has a variety of typical patterns. In the lumbar spine, facet joint hypertrophy (Fig 12.7) and osteophyte formation occur. Osteophytes which form from vertebral endplates may be predominantly posterior, causing compression of neural elements. When osteophytes extend anteriorly, they produce no neurological signs or symptoms. These same alterations may occur in the cervical spine where, in addition, there may be prominent spurs arising posterolaterally from the uncovertebral joints (Fig. 12.8). This often causes neural foraminal stenosis.

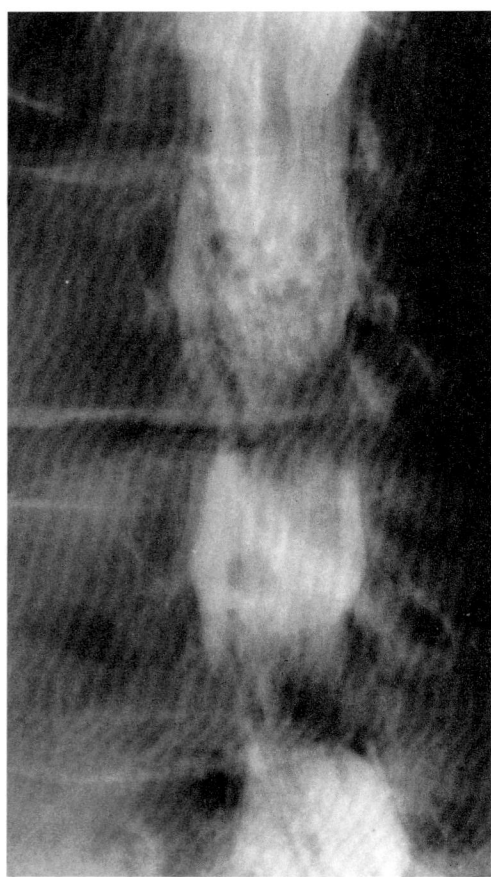

Figure 12.6

Spinal stenosis with tortuous epidural veins and nerve roots. Myelographic image shows multilevel circumferential narrowing of the thecal sac secondary to disc bulges, ligamentous thickening and facet joint hypertrophy. The epidural veins and nerve roots are compressed, dilated, and redundant.

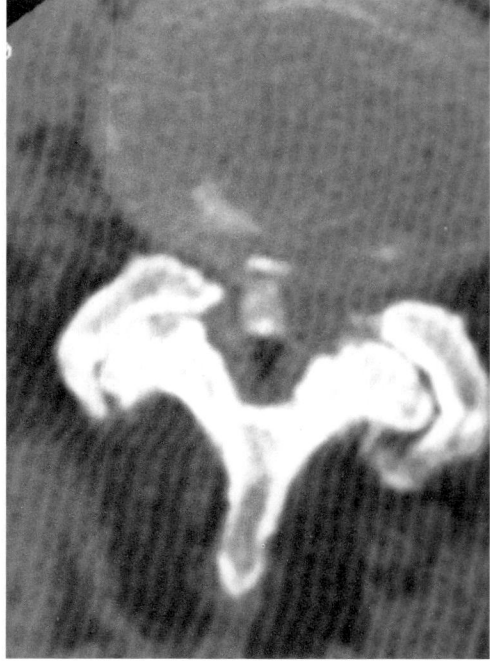

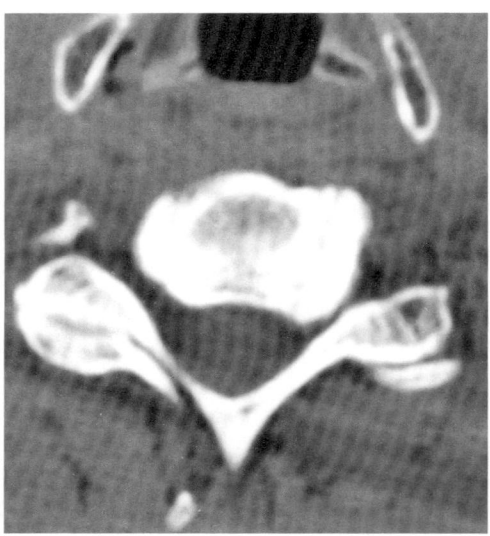

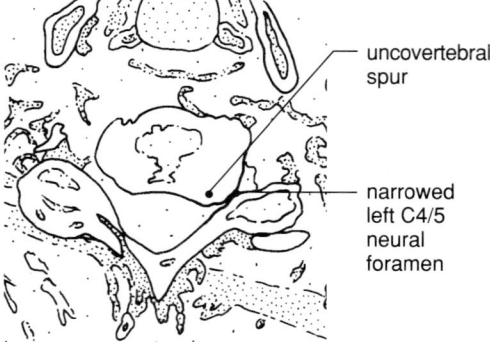

Figure 12.8

Uncovertebral spur. There is a prominent osteophyte extending from the left uncovertebral joint at C4/C5 with resultant narrowing of the adjacent neural foramen.

Figure 12.7

Facet joint hypertrophy. The facet joints bilaterally have become enlarged, irregular, and sclerotic. They impinge upon the neural foramina and central spinal canal. There is an associated, left-sided synovial cyst.

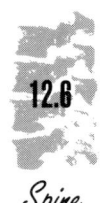

MISCELLANEOUS DEGENERATIVE CONDITIONS

Facet joint hypertrophy is sometimes associated with synovial cyst formation (Fig. 12.9). These cysts produce an extradural defect in the posterolateral thecal sac at myelography. On CT, the cysts are typically hypodense masses directly adjacent and medial to the hypertrophic facet joint. They may contain fluid or gas.

Disc material may herniate superiorly or inferiorly into the adjacent vertebral endplate (Fig. 12.10); this

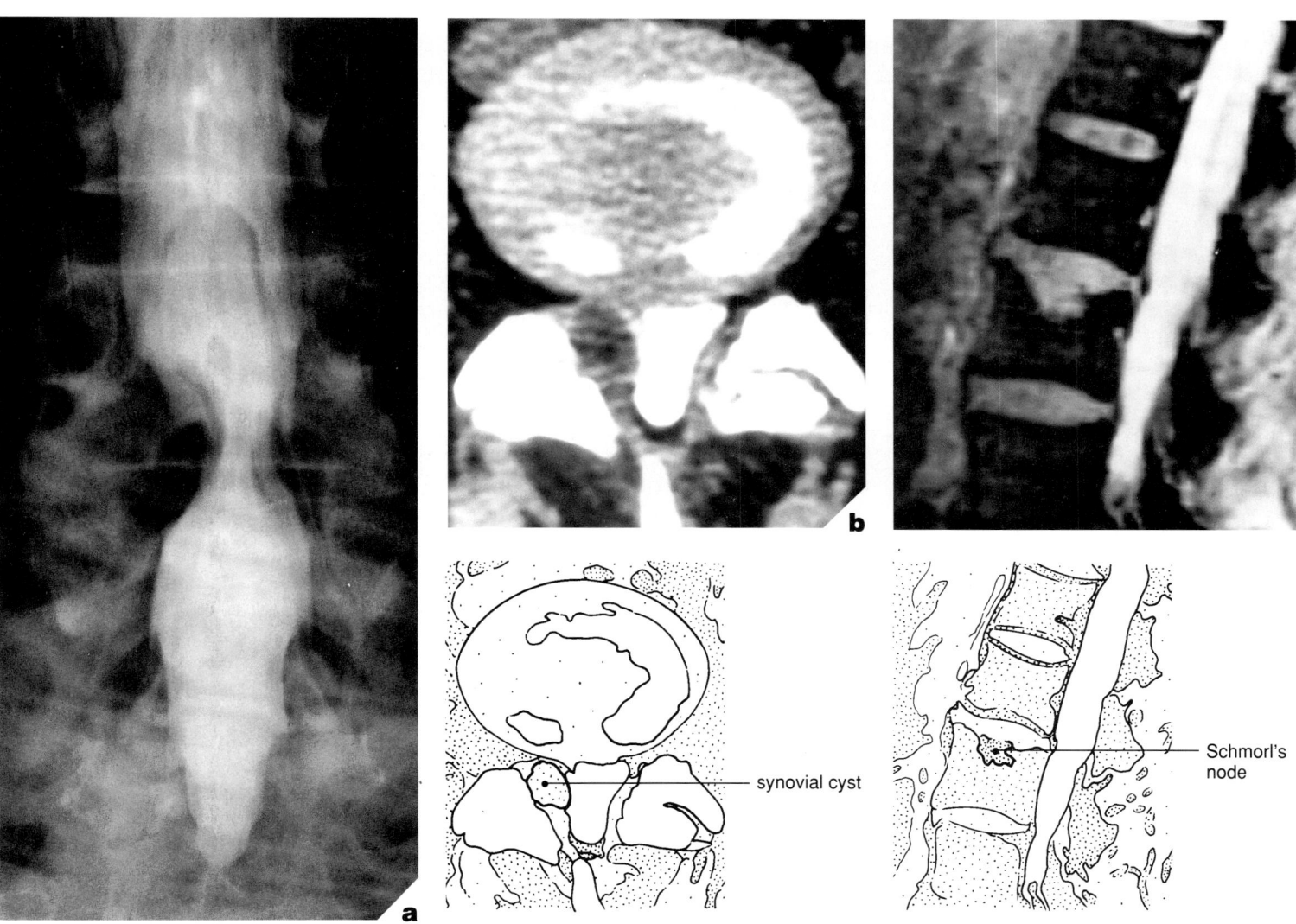

Figure 12.9

Synovial cysts. **a** There are bilateral extradural defects demonstrated on myelography at L4/L5 with compression and foreshortening of both L4 nerve root sleeves. **b** Postmyelographic CT scan shows a hypodense, fluid-filled synovial cyst adjacent to the facet joint on the right. A left-sided synovial cyst was present on other images (see Fig. 12.7).

Figure 12.10

Schmorl's node. T2–weighted sagittal MR image shows herniation of the L1/L2 intervertebral disc into the superior endplate of L2.

is called a *Schmorl's node*. Notch-like defects are seen in the affected endplate (Fig. 12.11).

Degenerated discs and facet joints may contain nitrogen gas which can be recognized on CT and plain films as the so-called "vacuum disc" or "vacuum facet" phenomenon. Although it is frequently associated with other significant degenerative processes, the vacuum itself is not clinically important. Similarly, loss of height of an intervertebral disc is only a sign of disc degeneration and, by itself, has no direct clinical implications.

In addition to synovial cysts, there are other extradural masses which may simulate disc herniation at myelography. These include extra-axial hematomas, abscesses, or neoplasms such as metastases or lymphoma.

Occasionally, two or more successive nerve roots from the same side of the spine exit together through

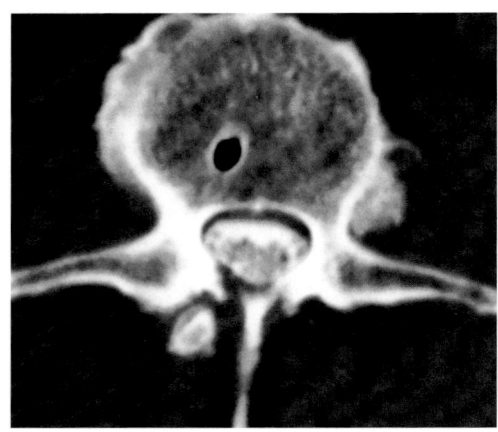

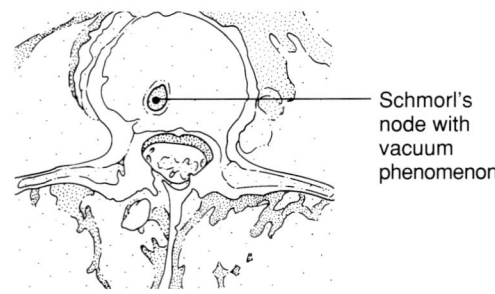

Schmorl's node with vacuum phenomenon

Figure 12.11

Schmorl's node. There is a defect within a vertebral body endplate on this post-myelographic CT scan. Due to degenerative disc disease, gas is present within this defect where there once had been herniated disc material.

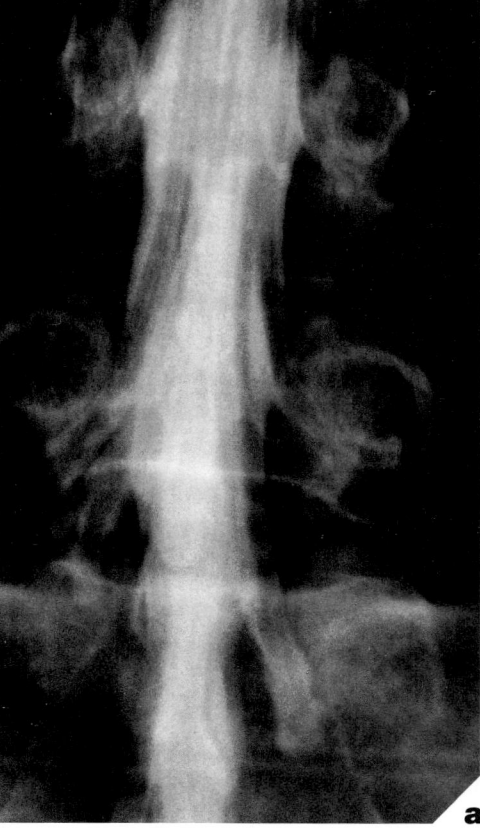

a

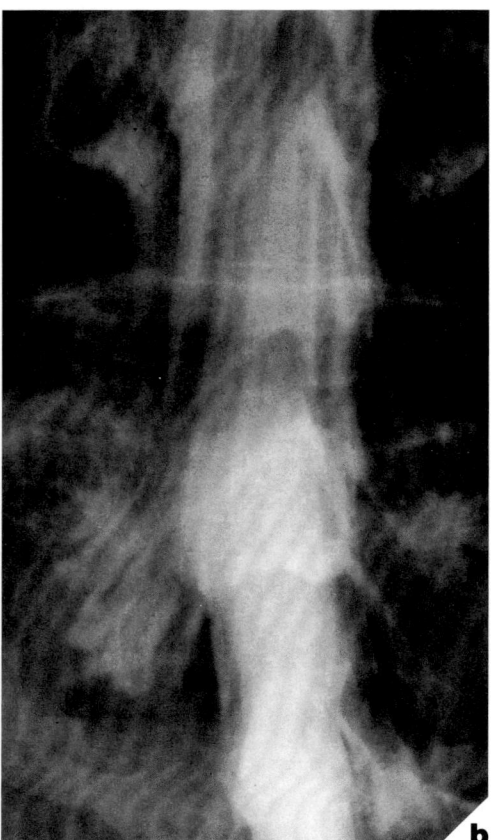

b

Figure 12.12

*Conjoined nerve roots. **a,b** There are multiple nerve roots exiting through the right L5/S1 neural foramen. The right S1 nerve root sleeve is absent.*

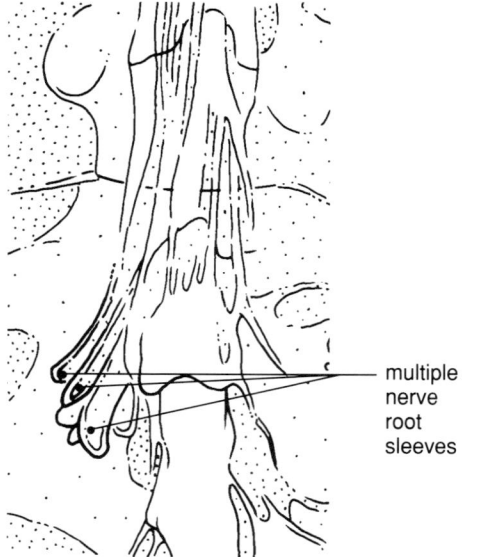

multiple nerve root sleeves

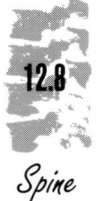

a common, enlarged dural sac. The combined sac and its contained nerve roots may mimic an extradural mass. Myelography (Fig. 12.12) shows atypical egress of nerve roots from the spinal canal.

Exuberant ossification of the posterior longitudinal ligament (OPLL) (Fig. 12.13) may produce compression of the thecal sac or spinal cord. This occurs especially in patients of Japanese ancestry. Ossification of the anterior longitudinal ligament does not cause neurologic symptoms although it may compress the esophagus and cause dysphagia.

Compression of the thecal sac or spinal nerve roots may occur in the postoperative spine due to epidural fibrosis (Fig. 12.14). This is best demonstrated on Gadolinium-enhanced MRI. Epidural fibrosis represents an important cause of "failed back surgery."

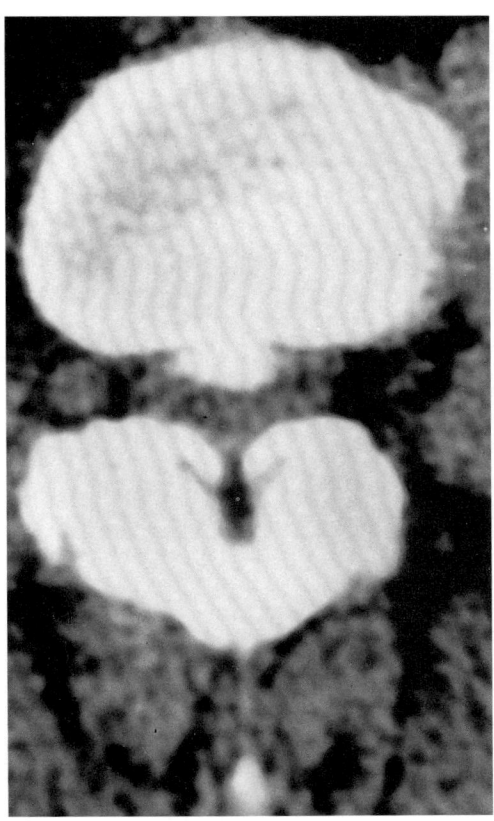

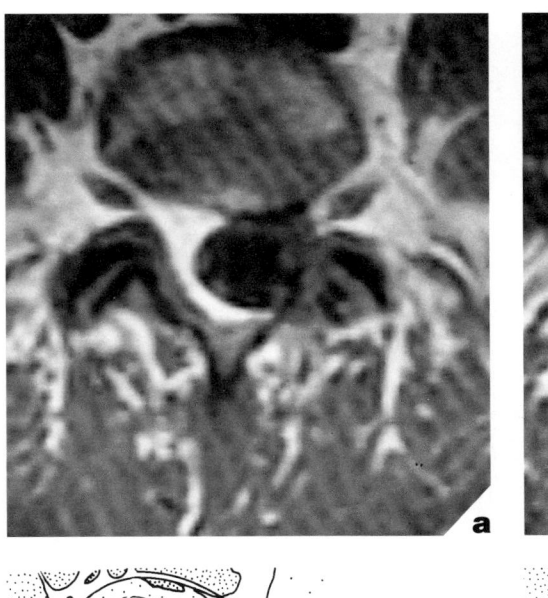

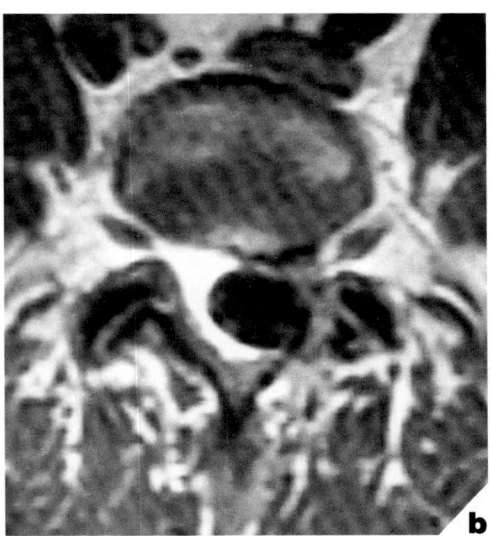

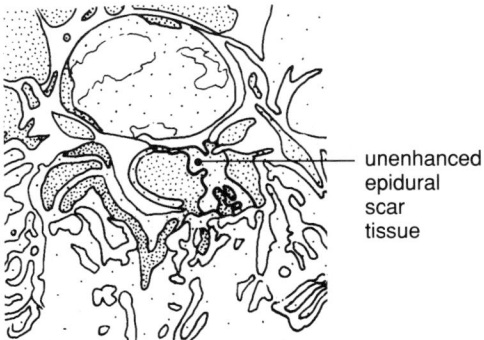

unenhanced epidural scar tissue

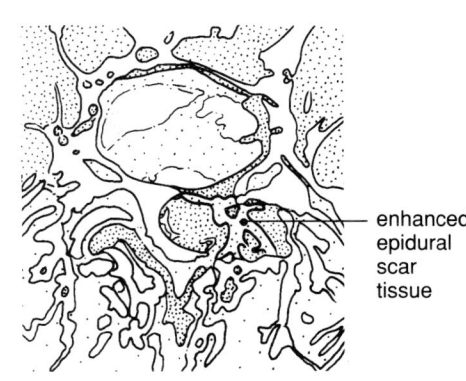

enhanced epidural scar tissue

Figure 12.13

Ossification of the posterior longitudinal ligament (OPLL). There is expansion and ossification of the posterior longitudinal ligament resulting in compression of the ventral thecal sac. The resultant spinal stenosis is further exacerbated by prominent facet joint hypertrophy at this level.

Figure 12.14

*Epidural scar tissue. **a** Unenhanced axial T1-weighted image shows prominent epidural soft tissue adherent to the anterior and left lateral margins of the thecal sac at the site of a prior laminec-tomy. **b** This soft tissue enhances moderately following Gadolinium-DTPA administration and represents postsurgical scar tissue formation.*

Arachnoiditis (Fig. 12.15) may produce an irregular, bizarre myelographic appearance of the thecal sac and nerve roots. Occasionally, a featureless thecal sac is demonstrated on myelography in patients with arachnoiditis.

An additional cause of thecal sac or spinal cord compression is proliferation of the epidural fat (Fig. 12.16). This is termed *epidural lipomatosis*. It is usually associated with Cushing's disease, steroid therapy, or alcoholism. Rarely, epidural lipomatosis develops in patients without an underlying metabolic or systemic disorder.

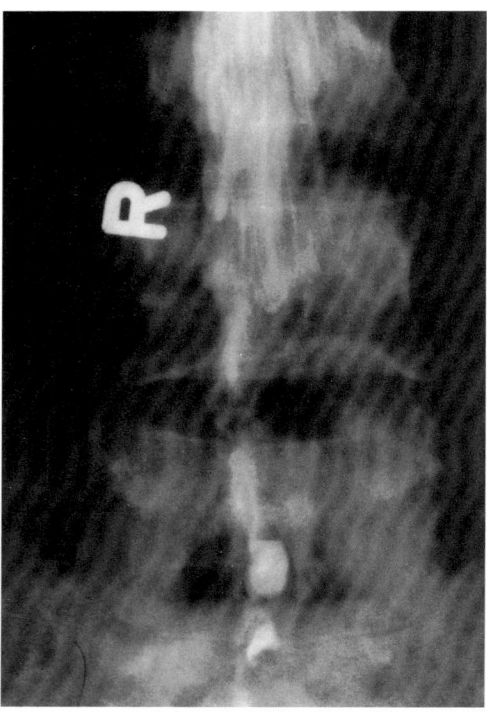

Figure 12.15
Adhesive arachnoiditis. Marked deformity and irregularity of the caudal thecal sac is demonstrated. This patient underwent an iophenyldate myelogram many years prior to this water-soluble contrast myelogram.

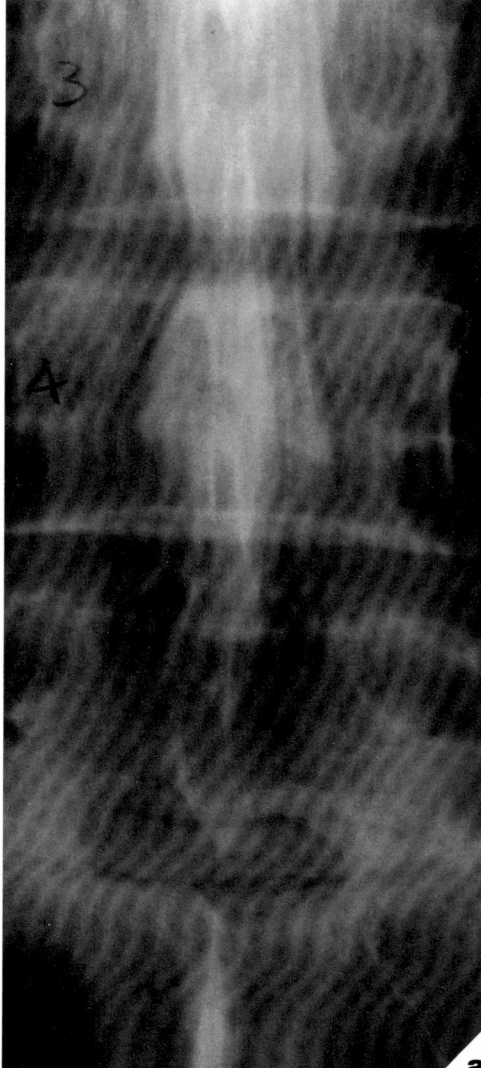

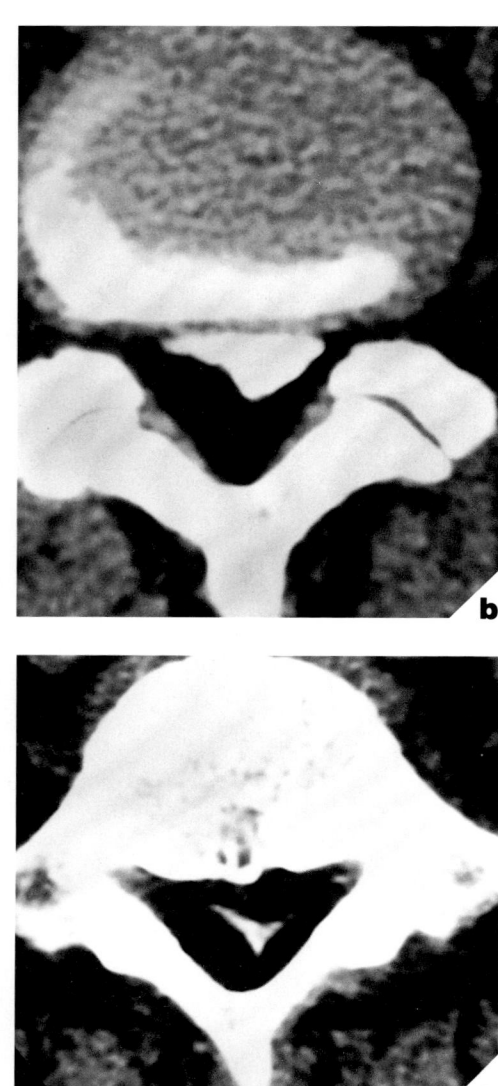

Figure 12.16
*Epidural lipomatosis. **a** Lumbar myelography demonstrates marked circumferential compression of the caudal thecal sac. **b,c** Postmyelographic CT images demonstrate marked proliferation of the epidural fat with severe compression of the caudal thecal sac.*

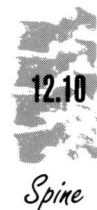

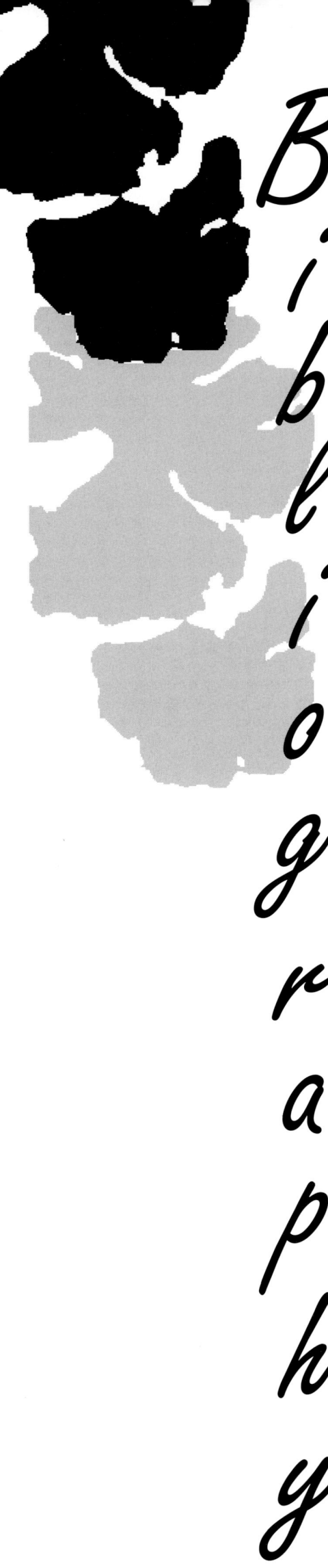

Bibliography

1

Aoki S, Barkovich AJ, Nishimura K, et al. Neurofibromatosis types 1 and 2: Cranial MR findings. Radiology 1989; 172:527

Byrd SE, Naidich T. Common congenital brain anomalies. Radiol Clin North Am 1988; 26:755

Kuhn MJ. Radiologic findings in Möbius syndrome. Mt Sinai J Med 1988; 55:167

Kuhn MJ, Clark HB, Morales A, et al. Group III Möbius syndrome: CT and MR findings. AJNR 1990; 11:903

Lee BCP, Engel M. MR of lissencephaly. AJNR 1988; 9:804

Nixon JR, Houser OW, Gomez MR, et al. Cerebral tuberous sclerosis: MR imaging. Radiology 1989; 170:869

Osborn RE, Byrd SE, Naidich TP, et al. MR imaging of neuronal migrational disorders. AJNR 1988; 9:1101

Van der Knapp MS, Valk J. Classification of congenital abnormalities of the CNS. AJNR 1988; 9:315

Wolpert SM, Anderson M, Scott RM, et al. Chiari II malformation: MR imaging evaluation. AJNR 1987; 8:783

2

Braffman BH, Zimmerman RA, Trojanowski JQ, et al. Brain MR: Pathologic correlation with gross and histopathology. 2. Hyperintense white matter foci in the elderly. AJNR 1988; 9:629

Grossman RI, Braffman BH, Brorson JR, et al. Multiple sclerosis: Serial study of gadolinium-enhanced MR imaging. Radiology 1988; 169:117

Horowitz AL, Kaplan RD, Grewe G, et al. Ovoid lesion: A new MR observation in patients with multiple sclerosis. AJNR 1989; 10:303

Jensen ME, Sawyer RW, Braun IF, et al. MR imaging appearance of childhood adrenoleukodystrophy with auditory, visual, and motor pathway involvement. Radiographics 1990; 10:53

Kuhn MJ, Johnson KA, Davis KR. Wallerian degeneration: Evaluation with MR imaging. Radiology 1988; 168:199

Kuhn MJ, Mikulis DJ, Ayoub DM, et al. Wallerian degeneration after cerebral infarction: Evaluation with sequential MR imaging. Radiology 1989; 172:179

Kuhn MJ, Taveras JM. Small bright foci (SBF) on T2 weighted MR images and associated disorders. In: Taveras JM, Ferrucci JT. Radiology: Diagnosis/Imaging/Intervention. Philadelphia, JB Lippincott, 1989

Mikulis DJ, Kuhn MJ. Multiple sclerosis. In: Taveras JM, Ferrucci JT. Radiology: Diagnosis/Imaging/Intervention. Philadelphia, JB Lippincott, 1990

Miller GM, Baker HL Jr, Okazaki H, et al. Central pontine myelinolysis and its imitators: MR findings. Radiology 1988; 168:795

Moriwaka F, Tashiro K, Maruo Y, et al. MR imaging of pontine and extrapontine myelinolysis. JCAT 1988; 12:446

Nowell MA, Grossman RI, Hackney DB. MR imaging of white matter disease in children. AJNR 1988; 9:503

Osborn AG, Harnsberger HR, Smoker WRK, et al. Multiple sclerosis in adolescents: CT and MR findings. AJNR 1990; 11:489

Runge VM, Wood ML, Kaufman DM, et al. MR imaging section profile optimization: Improved contrast and detection of lesions. Radiology 1988; 167:831

Uhlenbrock D, Seidel D, Gehlen W, et al. MR imaging in multiple sclerosis: Comparison with clinical, CSF, and visual evoked potential findings. AJNR 1988; 9:59

3

Barloon TJ, Yuh WTC, Knepper LE, et al. Cerebral ventriculitis: MR findings. JCAT 1990; 14:272

Chang KH, Han MH, Roh JK, et al. Gd-DTPA-enhanced MR imaging of the brain in patients with meningitis: Comparison with CT. AJNR 1990; 11:69

Chrysikopoulos HS, Press GA, Grafe MR, et al. Encephalitis caused by human immunodeficiency virus: CT and MR imaging manifestations with clinical and pathologic correlation. Radiology 1990; 175:185

Enzmann DR, Britt RR, Placone RC Jr. Staging of human brain abscess by computed tomography. Radiology 1983; 146:703

Haimes AB, Zimmerman RD, Morgello S. MR imaging of brain abscesses. AJNR 1989; 10:279

Mark AS, Atlas SW. Progressive multifocal leukoencephalo-pathy in patients with AIDS: Appearance on MR images. Radiology 1989; 173:517

Mathews VP, Kuharik MA, Edwards MK, et al. Gd-DTPA-enhanced MR imaging of experimental bacterial menin-gitis: Evaluation and comparison with CT. AJNR 1988; 9:1045

Post MJD, Tate LG, Quencer RM, et al. CT, MR, and pathology in HIV encephalitis and meningitis. AJNR 1988; 9:469

Riccio TJ, Hesselink J Jr. Gd-DTPA-enhanced MR of multiple cryptococcal brain abscesses. AJNR 1989; 10:565

Schoeman J, Hewlett R, Donald P. MR of childhood tuberculous meningitis. Neuroradiology 1988; 30:473

Sze G, Zimmerman RD. The magnetic resonance imaging of infectious and inflammatory disease. Radiol Clin North Am 1988; 26:839

Taccone A, Gambaro G, Ghiorzi M, et al. Computed tomography (CT) in children with herpes simplex encephalitis. Pediatr Radiol 1988; 19:9

Wehn SM, Heinz ER, Burger PC, et al. Dilated Virchow–Robin spaces in cryptococcal meningitis associated with AIDS: CT and MR findings. JCAT 1989; 13:756

Weingarten K, Zimmerman RD, Becker RD, et al. Subdural and epidural empyemas: MR imaging. AJNR 1989; 10:81

Weisberg LA, Greenberg J, Stazio A. Computed tomographic findings in acute viral encephalitis in adults with emphasis on herpes simplex encephalitis. Comput Med Imag Graph 1988; 12:385

Weisberg LA, Greenberg J, Stazio A. Computed tomographic findings in cerebral toxoplasmosis in adults. Comput Med Imag Graph 1988; 12:379

Zimmerman RD, Leeds NE, Danziger A. Subdural empyema: CT findings. Radiology 1984; 150:417

4

Atlas SW. Adult supratentorial tumors. Semin Roentgenol 1990; 25:130

Bilaniuk LT. Adult infratentorial tumors. Semin Roentgenol 1990; 25:155

Castillo M, Davis PC, Takei YD, et al. Intracranial ganglio-glioma: MR, CT, and clinical findings in 18 patients. AJR 1990; 154:607

Chakeres DW, Curtin A, Ford G. Magnetic resonance imaging of pituitary and parasellar abnormalities. Radiol Clin North Am 1989; 27:265

Chang T, Teng MMH, Guo W-Y, et al. CT of pineal tumors and intracranial germ-cell tumors. AJNR 1989; 10:1039

Dean BL, Drayer BP, Bird CR, et al. Gliomas: Classification with MR imaging. Radiology 1990; 174:411

Earnest F IV, Kelly PJ, Scheithauer BW, et al. Cerebral astrocytomas: Histopathologic correlation of MR and CT contrast enhancement with stereotactic biopsy. Radiology 1988; 166:823

Elster AD, Challa VR, Gilbert TH, et al. Meningiomas: MR and histopathologic features. Radiology 1989; 170:857

Jack CR Jr, O'Neill BP, Banks PM, et al. Central nervous system lymphoma: Histologic types and CT appearance. Radiology 1988; 167:211

Johnson PC, Hunt SJ, Drayer BP. Human cerebral gliomas: Correlation of postmortem MR imaging and neuro-pathologic findings. Radiology 1989; 170:211

Krol G, Sze G, Malkin M, et al. MR of cranial and spinal meningeal carcinomatosis: Comparison with CT and myelography. AJNR 1988; 9:709

Kulkanni MV, Lee KF, McArdle CB, et al. 1.5-T MR imaging of pituitary microadenomas: Technical considerations and CT correlation. AJNR 1988; 9:5

Kupfer MC, Zee C-S, Colletti PM, et al. MRI evaluation of AIDS-related encephalopathy: Toxoplasmosis vs lymphoma. Magn Reson Imaging 1990; 8:51

Lee SR, Sanches J, Mark AS, et al. Posterior fossa hemangioblastomas: MR imaging. Radiology 1989; 171:463

Lee Y-Y, Bruner JM, VanTassel P, et al. Primary central nervous system lymphoma: CT and pathologic correlation. AJNR 1986; 7:599

Lee Y-Y, VanTassel P. Intracranial oligodendrogliomas: Imaging findings in 35 untreated cases. AJNR 1989; 10:119

Lee Y-Y, VanTassel P, Bruner J. Juvenile pilocytic astro-cytomas: CT and MR characteristics. AJNR 1989; 10:363

Maeder PP, Holtas SL, Basibuyuk LN, et al. Colloid cysts of the third ventricle: Correlation of MR and CT findings with histology and chemical analysis. AJNR 1990; 11:575

Negendank WG, Al-Katib AM, Karanes C, et al. Lymphomas: MR imaging contrast characteristics with clinical–pathologic correlations. Radiology 1990; 177:209

Newton DR, Dillon WP, Norman D, et al. Gd-DTPA-enhanced MR imaging of pituitary adenomas. AJNR 1989; 10:949

Nov AA, Peirce KR, Mauney M, et al. Thalamic oligodendro-gliomas of childhood: CT and clinical course. J Neuroradiol 1988; 15:23

Orron DE, Kuhn MJ, Malhotra V, et al. Primary cerebral lymphoma in acquired immunodeficiency syndrome (AIDS)—CT manifestations. Comput Med Imag Graph 1989; 13(2):207

Pigeau I, Sigal R, Halimi P, et al. MRI features of cranio-pharyngiomas at 1.5 T: A series of 13 cases. J Neuroradiol 1988; 15:276

Press GA, Hesselink JR. MR imaging of cerebellopontine angle and internal auditory canal lesions at 1.5T. AJNR 1988; 9:241

Pusey E, Kortman KE, Flannigan BD. MR of craniopharyn-giomas. AJNR 1987; 8:439

Russell EJ, Geremia GK, Johnson CE, et al. Multiple cerebral metastasis: Detectability with Gd-DTPA-enhanced MR imaging. Radiology 1987; 165:609

Schwaighofer BW, Hesselink JR, Press GA, et al. Primary intracranial CNS lymphomas: MR manifestations. AJNR 1989; 10:725

Steiner E, Imhof H, Knosp E. Gd-DTPA-enhanced high resolution MR imaging of pituitary adenomas. Radiographics 1989; 9:587

Tampieri D, Melanson D, Ethier R. MR of epidermoid cysts. AJNR 1989; 10:351

Tien RD, Barkovich AJ, Edwards MSB. MR imaging of pineal tumors. AJNR 1990; 11:557

Wilms G, Marchal G, Van Hecke P, et al. Colloid cysts of the third ventricle: MR findings. JCAT 1990; 14:527

Yuh WTC, Wright DC, Barloon TJ, et al. MR imaging of primary tumors of trigeminal nerve and Meckel's cave. AJNR 1988; 9:655

Atlas SW. Intracranial vascular malformations and aneurysms. Radiol Clin North Am 1988; 26:821

Barkovich AJ, Atlas SW. Magnetic resonance imaging of intracranial hemorrhage. Radiol Clin North Am 1988; 26:801

Braffman BH, Zimmerman RA, Trojanowski JQ, et al. Brain MR: Pathologic correlation with gross and histopathology. 1. Lacunar infarction and Virchow–Robin spaces. AJNR 1988; 9:621

Brooks RA, DiChiro G, Patronas N. MR imaging of cerebral hematomas at different field strengths: Theory and applications. J Comput Assist Tomogr 1989; 13:194

Brown JJ, Hesselink JR, Rothrock JF. MR and CT of lacunar infarcts. AJNR 1988; 9:477

Davis KR, Kistler JP, Heros RC, et al. A neuroradiologic approach to the patient with a diagnosis of subarachnoid hemorrhage. Radiol Clin North Am 1982; 20:87

Gomori JM, Grossman RI, Hackney DB, et al. Variable appearances of subacute intracranial hematomas on high-field spin-echo MR. AJNR 1987; 8:1019

Kuhn MJ, Davis KR, Shoukimas GM, et al. Magnetic resonance imaging of migraine: Comparison with CT. AJNR 1987; 8:942

Kuhn MJ, Shekar PC. A comparative study of magnetic resonance imaging and computed tomography in the evaluation of migraine. Comput Med Imag Graph 1990; 14:149

Silver AJ, Pederson ME Jr, Ganti SR, et al. CT of subarachnoid hemorrhage due to ruptured aneurysm. AJNR 1981; 2:13

Edelman RR, Johnson K, Buxton R, et al. MR of hemorrhage: A new approach. AJNR 7:751

Fobben ES, Grossman RI, Atlas SW, et al. MR characteristics of subdural hematomas and hygromas at 1.5T. AJNR 1989; 10:687

Gomori JM, Grossman HI, Goldberg HI, et al. High field magnetic resonance imaging of intracranial hematomas. Radiology 1985; 157:87

Kelly AB, Zimmerman RD, et al. Head trauma: Comparison of MR and CT experience. AJNR 1988; 9:699

Zimmerman RA, Bilaniuk LT, Dolinskas C, et al. Computed tomography of acute intracerebral hemorrhagic contusion. J Comput Tomogr 1977 1:271

Zimmerman RA, Bilaniuk LT, Hackney DB, et al. Head injury: Early results of comparing CT and MR. AJNR 1986; 7:757

Braffman BH, Grossman RI, Goldberg HI, et al. MR imaging of Parkinson disease with spin echo and gradient echo sequences. AJNR 1988; 9:1093

Drayer BP. Imaging of the aging brain: Part I. Normal findings. Radiology 1988; 166:785

Drayer BP. Imaging of the aging brain: Part II. Pathologic conditions. Radiology 1988; 166:797

Gallucci M, Splendiani A, Bozzao A, et al. MR imaging of degenerative disorders of brainstem and cerebellum. Magn Reson Imaging 1990; 8:117

Gammal TE, Allen MB Jr, Brooks BS, et al. MR evaluation of hydrocephalus. AJNR 1987; 8:591

Jack CR Jr, Mokri B, Laws ER Jr. MR findings in normal-pressure hydrocephalus: Significance and comparison with other forms of dementia. J Comput Assist Tomogr 1987; 11:923

Maytal J, Alvarez LA, Elkin CM, et al. External hydrocephalus: Radiologic spectrum and differentiation from cerebral atrophy. AJNR 1987; 8:271

Savoiardo M, Strada L, Girotti F, et al. Olivopontocerebellar atrophy: MR diagnosis and relationship to multisystem atrophy. Radiology 1990; 174:693

Simmons JT, Pastakia B, Chase TN. Magnetic resonance imaging in Huntington disease. AJNR 1987; 7:25

Wikkelso C, Andersson H, Blomstrand C, et al. Computed tomography of the brain in the diagnosis of and prognosis in normal pressure hydrocephalus. Neuroradiology 1989; 31:160

Boisserie-Lacroix M, Bouin H, Joullie M, et al. Value of MRI in the study of spinal extradural arachnoid cysts. Comput Med Imag Graph 1990; 14:221

Brunberg JA, Latchaw RE, Kanai E, et al. Magnetic resonance imaging of spinal dysraphism. Radiol Clin North Am 1988; 26:181

Cecchini A, Locatelli D, Bonfanti N, et al. Lipomyelo-meningoceles: A neuroradiological approach. J Neuroradiol 1988; 15:49

Deeb ZL, Daffner RH, Rothfus WE, et al. Syringomyelia: Myelography, computed tomography and magnetic resonance imaging. CT 1988; 12:1

Gray L, Djang WT, Friedman AH. MR imaging of thoracic extradural arachnoid cysts. JCAT 1988; 12:646

Houang MTW, Stern M, Brew B, et al. Magnetic resonance imaging (MRI) appearances of syringohydromyelia. Australas Radiol 1988; 32:172

Kao SCS, Waziri MH, Smith WL, et al. MR imaging of the craniovertebral junction, cranium, and brain in children with achondroplasia. AJR 1989; 153:565

Merx JL, Bakker-Niezen SH, Thijssen HOM, et al. Tethered spinal cord syndrome: A correlation of radiological features and preoperative findings in 30 patients. Neuroradiology 1989; 31:63

Raghavan N, Barkovich AJ, Edwards M, et al. MR imaging in the tethered spinal cord syndrome. AJNR 1989; 10:27

Sklar E, Quencer RM, Green BA, et al. Acquired spinal subarachnoid cysts: Evaluation with MR, CT myelography and intraoperative sonography. AJR 1989; 153:1057

So CB, Li DKB. Anterolateral cervical meningocele in association with neurofibromatosis: MR and CT studies. JCAT 1989; 13:692

Barakos JA, Mark AS, Dillon WP, et al. MR imaging of acute transverse myelitis and AIDS myelopathy. JCAT 1990; 14:45

Kelly RP, Mahoney PD, Cawley KM. MR demonstration of spinal cord sarcoidosis: Report of a case. AJNR 1988; 9:197

Nesbit GM, Miller GM, Baker HL Jr, et al. Spinal cord sarcoidosis: A new finding at MR imaging with Gd-DTPA-enhancement. Radiology 1989; 173:839

Quencer RM, Montalvo BM, Katz BH, et al. Spinal infection: Evaluation with MR imaging and intraoperative US, Post MJD. Radiology 1988; 169:765

Van Lom KJ, Kellerhouse LE, Pathria MN, et al. Infection versus tumor in the spine: Criteria for distinction with CT. Radiology 1988; 166:851

Aoki S, Barkovich AJ, Nishimura K, et al. Neurofibromatosis type 1 and 2: Cranial MR findings. Radiology 1989; 172:527

Avrahami E, Tadmor R, Dally O, et al. Early MR demonstration of spinal metastases in patients with normal radiographs and CT and radionuclide bone scans. JCAT 1989; 13:598

Braffman BH, Bilaniuk LT, Zimmerman RA. Central nervous system manifestations of the phakomatoses on MR. Radiol Clin North Am 1988; 26:773

Carmody RF, Yang PJ, Seeley GW, et al. Spinal cord compression due to metastatic disease: Diagnosis with MR imaging versus myelography. Radiology 1989; 173:225

Colman LK, Porter BA, Redmond J III, et al. Early diagnosis of spinal metastases by CT and MR studies. JCAT 1988; 12:423

Forman HP, Leonidas JC, Berdon WE, et al. Congenital neuroblastoma: Evaluation with multimodality imaging. Radiology 1990; 175:365

Hurst RW, Newman SA, Cail WS. Multifocal intracranial MR abnormalities in neurofibromatosis. AJNR 1988; 9:293

Kroon HM, Schurmans J. Osteoblastoma: Clinical and radiologic findings in 98 new cases. Radiology 1990; 175:783

Kumar R, Guinto FC Jr, Madewell JE, et al. Expansile bone lesions of the vertebra. Radiographics 1988; 8:749

Parizel PM, Baleriaux D, Rodesch G, et al. Gd-DTPA-enhanced MR imaging of spinal tumors. AJNR 1989; 10:249

Rothwell CI, Jaspan T, Worthington BS, et al. Gadolinium-enhanced magnetic resonance imaging of spinal tumours. Br J Radiol 1989; 62:1067

Smoker WRK, Godersky JC, Knutzon RK, et al. The role of MR imaging in evaluating metastatic spinal disease. AJNR 1987; 8:901

Yuh WTC, Zachar CK, Barloon TJ, et al. Vertebral compression fractures: Distinction between benign and malignant causes with MR imaging. Radiology 1989; 172:215

Atlas SW, Regenbogen V, Rogers LF, et al. The radiographic characterization of burst fractures of the spine. AJNR 1986; 7:675

Goldberg AL, Daffner RH, Schapiro RL. Imaging of acute spinal trauma: An evolving multi-modality approach. Clin Imag 1990; 14:11

Goldberg AL, Rothfus WE, Deeb ZL, et al. Hyperextension injuries of the cervical spine: Magnetic resonance findings. Skeletal Radiol 1989; 18:283

Kim KS, Chen HH, Russell EJ, et al. Flexion teardrop fracture of the cervical spine: Radiographic characteristics. AJNR 1988; 9:1221

Kowalski HM, Cohen WA, Cooper P, et al. Pitfalls in the CT diagnosis of atlantoaxial rotatory subluxation. AJNR 1987; 8:697

Moss JG, Sellar RJ, Bradnock B. Atlanto-axial rotary fixation: Diagnosis by functional computed tomography. Br J Radiol 1989; 62:755

Murphey MO, Batnitzky S, Bramble JM. Diagnostic imaging of spinal trauma. Radiol Clin North Am 1989; 27:855

Roshkow JE, Haller JO, Hotson GC, et al. Imaging evaluation of children after falls from a height: Review of 45 cases. Radiology 1990; 175:359

Teng MMH, Shoung H-M, Chang C-Y, et al. CT and myelogram findings of os odontoideum. Comput Med Imag Graph 1989; 13:179

Teplick JG, Lassey PA, Berman A, et al. Diagnosis and evaluation of spondylolisthesis and/or spondylolysis on axial CT. AJNR 1986; 7:479

Vandemark RM. Radiology of the cervical spine in trauma patients: Practice pitfalls and recommendations for improving efficiency and communication. AJR 1990; 155:465

Bundschuk VC, Modic MT, Ross JS, et al. Epidural fibrosis and recurrent disk herniation in the lumbar spine. AJNR 1988; 9:169

Jackson DE Jr, Atlas SW, Mani JR, et al. Intraspinal synovial cysts: MR imaging. Radiology 1989; 170:527

Liu SS, Williams KD, Drayer BP, et al. Synovial cysts of the lumbosacral spine: Diagnosis by MR imaging. AJR 1990; 154:163

Mixter WJ, Barr JS. Rupture of intervertebral disc with involvement of spinal canal. NEJM 1934; 211:210

Ross JS, Masaryk TJ, Modic MT. MR imaging of lumbar arachnoiditis. AJNR 1987; 8:885

Silbergleit R, Gebarski SS, Brunberg JA, et al. Lumbar synovial cysts: Correlation of myelographic, CT, MR and pathologic findings. AJNR 1990; 11:777

Yamashita Y, Takahashi M, Matsuno Y, et al. Spinal cord compression due to ossification of ligaments: MR imaging. Radiology 1990; 175:843

Yu S, Haughton VM, Sether LA, et al. Anulus fibrosus in bulging intervertebral disks. Radiology 1988; 169:761

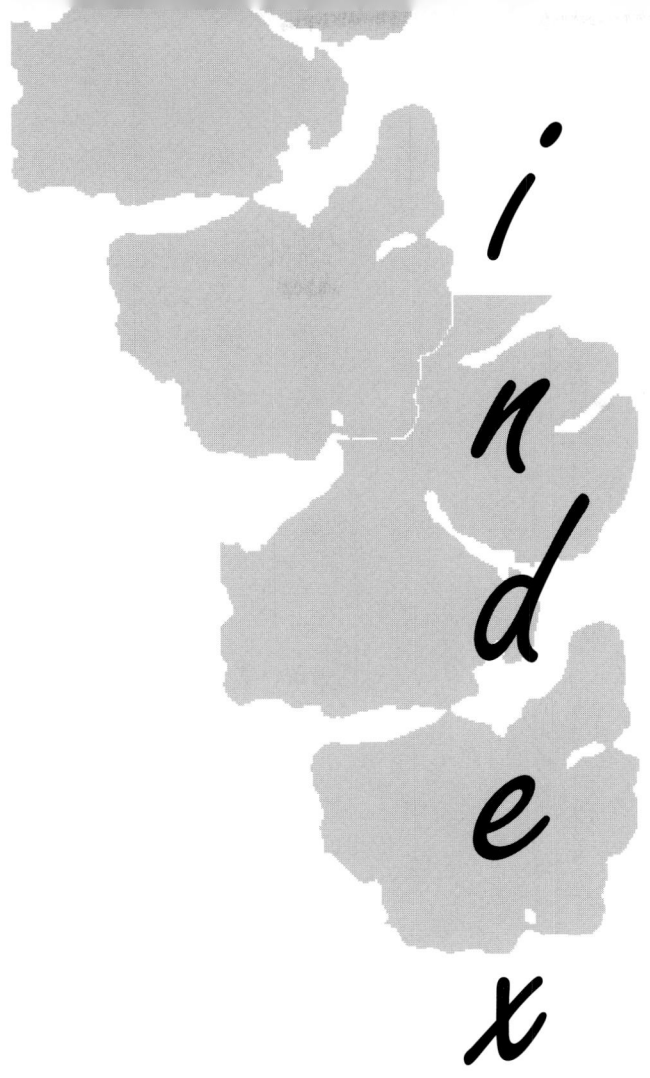

i n d e x